Praise for *Ultra-Processed People*

Longlisted for the Baillie Gifford Prize
Shortlisted for the Waterstones Book of the Year

"[*Ultra-Processed People*] is persuasive and scary. . . . [A]s [Chris van] Tulleken rightly insists, there is simply something creepy about eating things whose composition we can't comprehend."
—Adam Gopnik, *The New Yorker*

"*Ultra-Processed People* makes the case that corporate interests have given rise to highly addictive ultra-processed foods. . . . A brisk and engaging read, though it might piss you off. That's kind of the point."
—Ashwin Rodrigues, *GQ*

"In *Ultra-Processed People*, a persuasive mix of analysis and commentary, [Chris van Tulleken] shows how [ultra-processed] foods affect our bodies and how their popularity stems in part from shady marketing and slanted science."
—Matthew Rees, *Wall Street Journal*

"Van Tulleken is at his best when using his own scientific expertise to help readers through otherwise unnavigable science, data and history, explaining with precision what we are actually eating."
—Jacob E. Gersen, *New York Times Book Review*

"Before reading van Tulleken's work, I felt pretty confident that junk food was bad. That didn't stop me from eating it, however. Learning about UPF is a different experience—you begin to realize that some of this stuff is barely food at all."
—Helen Lewis, *Atlantic*

"There is much to cheer about calories being cheap and abundant. . . . But as Chris van Tulleken's new book, *Ultra-Processed People*, explains, that cheapness and abundance come at a cost."
—*Economist*

"An unsettling examination of the food we eat [and] a fascinating, but frankly horrifying, investigation into our industrialised food system."
—Ben Spencer, *Sunday Times*

"More than just a great science book: [*Ultra-Processed People*] breaks down a complex issue of cultural, social, economic and political importance with clarity and sensitivity but without moralising; it competently evaluates the scientific literature; and it roams the globe in search of answers." —Anjana Ahuja, *Financial Times*

"Deeply researched and persuasive."
—Sophie McBain, *New Statesman*

"[*Ultra-Processed People*] is highly readable and van Tulleken . . . writes with the confidence of a doctor who has a reassuring bedside manner." —Dave Hage, *Minneapolis Star Tribune*

"Eye-opening. . . . *Ultra-Processed People* is a tremendously important book that will help readers choose less processed, better food."
—Vincent Lam, *Toronto Star*

"Chris van Tulleken . . . would simply like people to know what they are eating and be equipped to make a conscious choice."
—Rachel Dixon, *Guardian*

"[A] slice of packaged supermarket loaf is more than likely a dietary devil than a time-saving treat. And thanks to Dr. Chris van Tulleken, author of the bestselling book *Ultra-Processed People*, it's a term now popping up everywhere."
—Sue Quinn, *Telegraph*

"Additives, preservatives and artificial colorings in food are America's gateway drugs to overconsumption. . . . [Van Tulleken] explores the effects of ultra-processed food in a world where profit is the goal and purposeful addiction is part of the recipe." —Evan Kleiman, KCRW

"Ultra-processed foods are not only limited to things you eat occasionally. . . . Dr. van Tulleken explain[s] the impact this type of diet has on your body and just how bad it can be."

—Diana Buntajova, *Express*

"Witty, pacy and (despite a lot of academic stuff) approachable."

—Adam Leyland, *Grocer*

"[A] scathing takedown. . . . This impassioned polemic will make readers think twice about what they eat."　　—*Publishers Weekly*

"A painfully eye-opening study of food and health."

—*Kirkus Reviews*

"Astonishingly well-researched. . . . Read it and fight back!"

—Rob Delaney, comedian, actor,
and author of *A Heart That Works*

"If you only read one diet or nutrition book in your life, make it this one."

—Bee Wilson, author of *Consider the Fork* and *The Secret of Cooking*

"A devastating, witty, and scholarly destruction of the food we eat and why."

—Adam Rutherford, author of *Control* and coauthor of *The Complete Guide to Absolutely Everything* (*Abridged)

"*Ultra-Processed People*. . . . changed forever how I think about what I eat."

—Hannah Fry, author of *Hello World* and coauthor of *The Complete Guide to Absolutely Everything* (*Abridged)

"Wonderful and fascinating."

—Dr. Michael Mosley, BBC presenter
and best-selling author of *The Fast Diet*

"Everyone needs to know this stuff."
                        —Tim Spector, author of *Spoon Fed* and *Food for Life*

"Incendiary and infuriating, this book is a diet grenade."
                        —Chris Packham, television presenter, naturalist,
                                    and author of *Amazing Animal Journeys*

"Urgent and captivating."
                        —Giles Yeo, author of *Gene Eating*
                                    and *Why Calories Don't Count*

"Mindblowing. You'll never see food—or your body—the same way again."   —Alice Roberts, author of *Anatomical Oddities*

"Read it; your diet will never be the same again!"
                        —Mariella Frostrup, coauthor of *Cracking the Menopause*

Ultra-Processed People

Chris van Tulleken
is an infectious diseases doctor at the
Hospital for Tropical Diseases in London.
He trained at Oxford and has a PhD in
molecular virology from University College
London, where he is an Associate Professor.
His research focuses on how corporations
affect human health, especially in the context of
child nutrition, and he works with UNICEF and the
World Health Organization. As one of the BBC's
leading broadcasters for children and adults,
his work has won two BAFTAs. He lives in
London with his wife and two children.

On Twitter and Instagram @DoctorChrisVT

Ultra-Processed People

Why We Can't Stop Eating
Food That Isn't Food

CHRIS VAN TULLEKEN

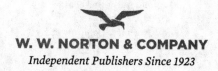

W. W. NORTON & COMPANY
Independent Publishers Since 1923

For Dinah, Lyra and Sasha

For information about permission to reproduce selections from this book,
write to Permissions, W. W. Norton & Company, Inc.,
500 Fifth Avenue, New York, NY 10110

For information about special discounts for bulk purchases, please contact
W. W. Norton Special Sales at specialsales@wwnorton.com or 800-233-4830

Manufacturing by Lakeside Book Company

Library of Congress Control Number: 2023951869

ISBN 978-1-324-07626-1 pbk.

W. W. Norton & Company, Inc.
500 Fifth Avenue, New York, N.Y. 10110
www.wwnorton.com

W. W. Norton & Company Ltd.
15 Carlisle Street, London W1D 3BS

10 9 8 7 6 5 4 3 2 1

Contents

Introduction

Every Wednesday afternoon in the laboratory where I used to work, we had an event called journal club. The word 'club' makes it sound more fun than it was. The ritual, practised in labs around the world, worked like this: one member of the lab would present a recent publication from the scientific literature that they felt was relevant to our work, and the rest of us would tear it to pieces. If the paper wasn't of sufficient quality, then the unhappy person who had selected it would also be torn to pieces.

The lab, which is run by Greg Towers, is still based at University College London (UCL), in a converted Victorian hospital built by the same architect who designed the Natural History Museum. It is a beautiful old building, full of mice and leaks. It seemed like an improbable venue for the world-class molecular virology research it produced, when I arrived in 2011 to do a PhD.

At these journal clubs, Greg and the other senior lab members taught me that science is not a list of rules or facts, but a living argument. Greg was more up for the argument about any data point in any paper than anyone I have met before or since. Nothing went unexamined. It was the best scientific training I could have hoped for.

The lab specialty was the ongoing competition between viruses like HIV and the cells they need to infect in order to reproduce. This competition is like a military arms race. All cells have defences against viral attack, and all viruses carry weapons to overcome those defences. As the cells evolve ever more sophisticated defences, so too are the viruses constantly evolving better weapons, which in turn drives the evolution of more cellular defences, and so on.

Most of us studied HIV and its viral cousins for exciting reasons, like the development of new drugs and vaccines, but there was a splinter group within the lab that studied a different type of virus, one that barely seemed like a virus at all. Almost half of the DNA in every cell of your body is made of ancient dead virus genes. Known for a long time as 'junk' DNA, this topic seemed to be a scientific backwater until, in October 2014, one of the members of the splinter group presented a paper at journal club from the publication *Nature*, its title dense with jargon: 'An evolutionary arms race between KRAB zinc-finger genes *ZNF91/93* and *SVA/L1* retrotransposons'.[1]

I gave the paper a quick skim before the meeting and found it incomprehensible. Out of every ten papers presented at journal club, roughly seven would be demolished, two would stand up and provide useful new information, and one would betray evidence of naked fraud. It wasn't clear to me which category this paper would fall into.

As we talked through the data, I noticed a shift in the atmosphere. Everyone sat forward as the data made the case that these old, dead viruses found throughout the human genome aren't dead at all. They have functioning genes, ready to make more viruses. Every cell in the human body is a potential virus factory, but something keeps these viral genes quiet. It turned out that they're suppressed by other genes in the cell.

The paper was saying that one part of our genome is constantly at war with another part.

The implications of this were immediately obvious to everyone in a lab familiar with the nature of arms races. Whether they involve competition between viruses, neighbourhood disputes, sports teams, political campaigns or global superpowers, all arms races must generate complexity. As insurgency develops, so must counterinsurgency. Intelligence begets counterintelligence, with double and triple agents. It's the development of ever more sophisticated weapons that drives the evolution of ever more sophisticated defences.

Because the human genome is in an internal arms race, with one piece of DNA at war with another, this means that it must inexorably be driven towards ever greater complexity. Over thousands of generations, as those old 'dead' viruses evolve, so the rest of the genome must evolve to keep them quiet.

This arms race within our genes has been going on since the dawn of life, and it may very well be the engine of the evolution of complexity itself. The major difference between the human genome and that of chimpanzees is not in the parts that code for proteins (which are around 96 per cent similar) but in the parts that seem to come from the old, dead viruses.[2]

The paper transformed my understanding of myself, even if it took me a while to get my head around the idea that, at least in part, I'm an assembly of old viruses at war with my other genes. It may change the way *you* see yourself, too. You aren't simply living alongside this arms race between different genes – you're the product of it, an uneasy coalition of competing genetic elements.

These coalitions and competitions extend beyond our genes. Where 'you' end and 'not you' begins is far from clear. You're covered in microbes that keep you alive – they're a part of you as much as your liver is – but those same microbes can kill you if they get into the wrong area of the body. Our bodies are much more like societies than like mechanical entities, comprising billions of bacteria, viruses and other microbial life forms, but just one primate. They're full of odd, negotiated compromises and imperfections. Arms races blur boundaries.

I worked in Greg's lab for six years before going back to being a doctor, but the idea of arms races, the complex systems they create and the boundaries they blur became a key part of the way I think about the world. I continued to do research, but my focus shifted from studying viruses, towards investigating scientific research that was biased or fraudulent. Now I mainly study the food industry and how it affects human health. My laboratory grounding has proved crucial for this: arms races and their effects will come up a lot throughout this book.

For a start, to eat is to compete in an arms race that has lasted billions of years. The world around us has a relatively fixed amount of available energy, and all life is engaged in a competition against other forms of life for that energy. Life has, after all, only two projects: reproduction and extracting energy to fuel that reproduction.

Predators are locked in competition not only with each other to obtain prey, but also of course with the prey itself, which generally wants to hang onto the energy contained in its meat. The 'prey' animals also compete for vegetation both with each other and with the plants themselves, which produce toxins, thorns and other defences against being eaten. Plants compete with each other for sun, water and soil. Microbes, bacteria, viruses and fungi constantly assault all the organisms in the ecosystem to extract what energy they can. And no one gets ahead for long in an arms race: wolves may be well adapted for eating deer, but deer are superbly adapted to avoid being eaten by wolves and do, on occasion, kill them.*

We eat, then, as part of a set of interlinking, entangled arms races, competing for energy flowing between life forms. Like all arms races, this competition has generated complexity, and so everything about eating is complex.

Our senses of taste and smell, our immune system, our manual dexterity, our tooth and jaw anatomy, our eyesight: it's hard to think of any aspect of human biology, physiology or culture that isn't primarily shaped by our historic need for energy. Over billions of years our bodies have superbly adapted to using a wide range of food.

But over the past 150 years food has become … not food.

We've started eating substances constructed from novel molecules and using processes never previously encountered in our evolutionary history, substances that can't really even be called 'food'. Our calories increasingly come from modified starches, from invert

---

* There is a significant scientific literature on wolves being killed by their prey. In one analysis, 40% of wolf skulls had evidence of prey injuries, and wolves are well documented to have been killed by moose, musk oxen and deer.[3, 4]

sugars, hydrolysed protein isolates and seed oils that have been refined, bleached, deodorised, hydrogenated – and interesterified. And these calories have been assembled into concoctions using other molecules that our senses have never been exposed to either: synthetic emulsifiers, low-calorie sweeteners, stabilising gums, humectants, flavour compounds, dyes, colour stabilisers, carbonating agents, firming agents and bulking – and anti-bulking – agents.

These substances entered the diet gradually at first, beginning in the last part of the nineteenth century, but the incursion gained pace from the 1950s onwards, to the point that they now constitute the majority of what people eat in the UK and the USA, and form a significant part of the diet of nearly every society on earth.

And, at the same time as we've entered this unfamiliar food environment, we've also moved into a new, parallel ecosystem, one with its own arms races that are powered not by the flow of energy, but by the flow of money. This is the new system of industrial food production. In this system we are the prey, the source of the money that powers the system. The competition for that money, which drives increasing complexity and innovation, occurs between an entire ecosystem of constantly evolving corporations, from giant transnational groups to thousands of smaller national companies. And their bait for extracting the money is called ultra-processed food, or UPF. These foods have been put through an evolutionary selection process over many decades, whereby the products that are purchased and eaten in the greatest quantities are the ones that survive best in the market. To achieve this, they have evolved to subvert the systems in the body that regulate weight and many other functions.*

UPF now makes up as much as 60 per cent of the average diet in the UK and the USA.[5–7] Many children, including my own, get most of their calories from these substances. UPF is our food culture, the

---

* A strange inversion of a standard ecosystem, in which the things that get eaten the least are the fittest.

stuff from which we construct our bodies. If you are reading this in Australia, Canada, the UK or the USA, this *is* your national diet.

UPF has a long, formal scientific definition, but it can be boiled down to this: if it's wrapped in plastic and has at least one ingredient that you wouldn't usually find in a standard home kitchen, it's UPF. Much of it will be familiar to you as 'junk food', but there's plenty of organic, free-range, 'ethical' UPF too, which might be sold as healthy, nutritious, environmentally friendly or useful for weight loss (it's another rule of thumb that almost every food that comes with a health claim on the packet is a UPF).

When we think about food processing, most of us think about the physical things done to food – like frying, extruding, macerating, mechanically recovering and so on. But ultra-processing also includes other, more indirect processes – deceptive marketing, bogus court cases, secret lobbying, fraudulent research – all of which are vital for corporations to extract that money.

The formal UPF definition was first drawn up by a Brazilian team back in 2010, but since then a vast body of data has emerged in support of the hypothesis that UPF damages the human body and increases rates of cancer, metabolic disease and mental illness, that it damages human societies by displacing food cultures and driving inequality, poverty and early death, and that it damages the planet. The food system necessary for its production, and of which it is the necessary product, is the leading cause of declining biodiversity and the second largest contributor to global emissions. UPF is thus causing a synergistic pandemic of climate change, malnutrition and obesity. This last effect is the most studied, and the hardest to talk about, because discussions of food and weight, however well intentioned, make a lot of people feel very bad.*

Much of this book will be about weight because much of the evidence around UPF is related to its effect on weight, but UPF causes

---

* Many of the health outcomes associated with obesity are a direct result of stigma: research shows that anti-fat bias is more ingrained among doctors and other healthcare professionals than prejudice against almost any other form of bodily difference. This is a huge barrier to care.

suffering in many ways that are independent of effects on weight. UPF doesn't cause heart disease and strokes and early death simply because it causes obesity. The risks increase with the quantity of UPF consumed irrespective of weight gain. Additionally, people who eat UPF and don't gain weight have increased risks of dementia and inflammatory bowel disease, but we don't tend to blame patients for having these problems. So, obesity gets a special mention because it is unique among diet-related diseases – in fact unique among almost all diseases – because doctors blame patients for having it.

In fact, let me back up a moment on obesity. We're still figuring out the language for this discussion. The word is rightly offensive to many people and calling obesity a disease is stigmatising. Many people don't live with obesity as a disease but as an identity. For others it's just a way of being, and an increasingly normal way of being at that. Weight gain is not inevitably associated with increased risk of health problems and the risk of death is in fact lower for many people who live with overweight than for those who live at a 'healthy' weight. Nonetheless, I will sometimes use the word obesity, and I will sometimes frame it as a disease, because diseases get funding for research and treatment, and sometimes the disease label reduces stigma: a disease is not a lifestyle or a choice, and the word can help to shift the burden of responsibility away from the affected person.

This is important because every discussion of weight gain, whether in the press or in our own heads, is suppurating with blame, which is always directed at the people who live with it. The idea that they are to blame has survived scientific and moral scrutiny because it is simplistic to the point of transparency. It's based on there being some failure of willpower – a failure to move more or to eat less. This idea doesn't stand up to scrutiny, as I will show repeatedly. For example, since 1960, the US National Health surveys have recorded an accurate picture of the nation's weight. They show that – in white, Black *and* Hispanic men *and* women of *all* ages – there was a dramatic increase in obesity, beginning in the 1970s.[8] The idea that there has been a simultaneous collapse in personal responsibility in both men and women across age and ethnic groups is not plausible. If you're living with obesity, it isn't due to a lack of willpower; it isn't your fault.

In fact, we're a lot less responsible for our weight than a skier is for breaking their leg, a footballer for injuring their knee, or a bat scientist for getting a fungal lung infection from working in caves. Diet-related diseases come from the collision of some ancient genes with a new food ecosystem that is engineered to drive excess consumption and that we currently seem unable, or perhaps unwilling, to improve.

For the past thirty years, under the close scrutiny of policy-makers, scientists, doctors and parents, obesity has grown at a staggering rate. During this period, fourteen government strategies containing 689 wide-ranging policies have been published in England,[9] but among children leaving primary school rates of obesity have increased by more than 700 per cent, and rates of severe obesity by 1600 per cent.[10]

Children in the UK and the USA, countries with the highest rates of UPF consumption, aren't just heavier than their peers in nearly all other high-income western countries, they're shorter too.[11, 12] This stunting goes hand in hand with obesity around the world, suggesting that it is a form of malnutrition rather than a disorder of excess.

By the time those children reach adulthood they will have been joined by so many of their peers that the proportion of the population that lives with obesity will rise to one in three. The chances of an adult living with severe obesity being able to achieve and maintain a healthy body weight without specialist help are less than one in a thousand. Severe obesity is thus, for the majority of those affected, an incurable condition without drugs or surgery. Overweight now affects more than a quarter of children and half the adult population.[13]

Policies in the UK and almost every other country have failed to solve obesity because they don't frame it as a commerciogenic disease – that is, a disease caused by the marketing and consumption of addictive substances. Comparisons to drugs and cigarettes risk yet more stigma, but I will make them with due care in the pages that follow. Like all diet-related disease, obesity has deeper causes than UPF, including genetic vulnerability, poverty, injustice, inequality, trauma, fatigue and stress. Just as smoking is the number one cause of lung cancer, poverty is the main cause of smoking. Smoking rates in the UK are four times higher among the most disadvantaged than among the wealthiest, and half the difference in death rates between rich and poor in the UK is explained by smoking.[14]

Like cigarettes, UPF is a collection of substances through which these deeper societal problems harm the body. It is a tangible way in which these injustices are manifested, mediating trauma and poverty and allowing the expression of genes that might otherwise remain hidden. Fix poverty and you prevent a lot of both lung cancer and obesity. That's another book though.

This is a book about the systems that provide our food and tell us what we should eat. I want to prompt you to imagine a world structured in a different way, a world that would offer everyone more opportunity and choice. So, there are no proposals to tax things or ban them – only a demand to improve information about UPF, and access to real food.

This is not a weight-loss book because first, no one has yet devised a method that helps people safely and sustainably lose weight, and second, I don't accept that you *should* lose weight. I don't have a 'correct' body and I don't have an opinion about what one would look like. I don't have an opinion on the food you *should* eat; that's up to you. I make choices that are not 'healthy' the whole time, whether it's dangerous sports or eating junk. But I feel strongly that to make choices we all need accurate information about the possible risks of our food, and that we should be less exposed to aggressive, often misleading marketing.

So, you'll find almost no advice in these pages about how to live your life or how to feed your children. Partly it's none of my business, but mainly I think advice is a bit pointless. What we eat is determined by the food around us, its price and how it's marketed – this is what needs to change.

But I do have one suggestion about how you read this book. If you feel like you might want to quit UPF – don't. Eat along.

Let me explain. You're a participant in an experiment you didn't volunteer for. New substances are being tested on all of us all the time to see which of them are best at extracting money. Can a synthetic emulsifier be used instead of an egg? Can a seed oil replace a dairy fat? Can a bit of ethyl methylphenylglycidate be chucked in instead of a strawberry? By buying UPF, we're continuously driving its evolution. We take the risk in this experiment while the benefits are handed to the owners of the companies producing UPF and the results are largely concealed from us – apart from the effects on our health.

My proposal is that, for the duration of reading this book, you continue the experiment of eating UPF, but that you do it for you, not for the corporations that make it. I can tell you about UPF, but the stuff itself will be your greatest teacher. Only by eating it will you understand its true nature. I know this because I did the experiment myself.

In the course of researching the impact of UPF, I partnered with colleagues at University College London Hospital (UCLH). I was the first patient in this study. The idea was to get data from me that would help us get funding for a much larger study (one we're now undertaking). The idea was simple: I would quit UPF for a month, then be weighed and measured in every possible way. Then, the next month I would eat a diet where 80 per cent of my calories came from UPF – the same diet that around one in five people in the UK and the USA eat.

I didn't deliberately overeat during that second month, I just ate as I normally do, which is whenever I feel like it and whatever food is available. As I ate, I spoke to the world's leading experts on food, nutrition, eating and ultra-processing from academia, agriculture and, most importantly, the food industry itself.

This diet of UPF should have been enjoyable, as I was eating food that I typically deny myself. But something odd happened. The more I spoke to experts, the more disgusted by the food I became. I was reminded of Allen Carr's best-selling book, *The Easy Way to Stop Smoking*. The book is unusual in the self-help genre in that it has actually been studied and the intervention it recommends is pretty good. The idea is that you keep smoking while you read about how bad smoking is. Eventually, the cigarettes begin to seem disgusting.

So, give in – allow yourself to experience UPF's full horror. I'm not urging you to binge or to overeat, but simply to stop resisting UPF. I did it for four weeks – if you feel like trying this then do it for as long as it takes to finish the book. There is an ethical question about encouraging you to do this, but I'm comfortable with it. First of all, you're already being encouraged to eat UPF all day long. Second, if you are typical, you're already eating around 60 per cent of your calories from UPF, so increasing that to 80 per cent for a month probably won't make a big difference.

As you read this book, I hope you'll also read the lists of ingredients on the back of the packets of food that you eat. You'll find many more substances than I am able to unpack individually in these pages, but by the end I hope you'll have begun to understand how everything from the marketing campaign to the strange lack of satisfaction you feel after eating is driving ill health. And you may see that many of the problems in your life that you've been putting down to getting older, or having children or work stress, are caused by the food you eat.

I can't promise that the UPF will become bizarre and disgusting as you read, but you may find that it does, and if you are able to give it up, the evidence suggests that this will be good for your body, your brain and the planet. It's happened to a number of people involved in the process of making this book, and the podcast that came before it, and I'd love to know if it happens to you.

PART ONE

Wait, I'm eating what?

Why is there bacterial slime in my ice cream? The invention of UPF

The first weekend of my 80 per cent UPF diet was one of those freakish autumn days when summer briefly returns. We headed to the park, and I bought myself and the rest of the family ice cream. Dinah, my wife, had a Freeze Pop, a tube of frozen bright-blue liquid made by a brand called Swizzels, and I had a Wall's Twister. Our three-year-old, Lyra, had a giant scoop of pistachio ice cream from a brand called 'Hackney Gelato'. Her one-year-old sister, Sasha, managed to scrounge licks off the rest of us.

Lyra met two friends and sat around in the blazing sunshine with her ice cream, talking about whatever three-year-olds talk about, before going to play on the swings. She handed me her tub of ice cream as she ran off. It was more or less untouched, a perfect glistening green ball of pistachio. It took me a moment to realise that this was peculiar. How was it still a ball? The outside of the tub was actually warm to the touch. Why hadn't the ice cream melted?

I tried a spoonful. It was a tepid gelatinous foam. Something had stopped the ice cream from melting.

I took a look at the ingredients online: 'fresh milk, sugar, pistachio paste (Bronte pistachios 4%, almonds 2%, sugar, soy protein, soy lecithin, coconut oil, sunflower oil, chlorophyll, natural flavours including lemon), dextrose, fresh double cream, glucose, skim milk powder, stabilisers (locust bean gum, guar gum, carrageenan), emulsifier (mono and diglycerides of fatty acids), Maldon sea salt'.

Stabilisers, emulsifiers, gums, lecithin, glucose, a number of different oils … these are the hallmarks of UPF. The definition (which is long, and which I'll explore properly in the next chapter) encompasses far more than the addition of additives, but remember the presence of those ingredients you don't have in your kitchen is one indicator that a food *is* UPF. As we'll see further on, other aspects of processing are equally, if not more, important than additives when it comes to effects on the human body.

And Hackney Gelato are not alone in using these types of ingredients – they are nearly universal in ice cream you buy in shops but are not found in typical kitchens. I didn't get exactly why they were all necessary from the manufacturer's perspective. Surely it would be simpler and cheaper to use fewer ingredients?

To try to understand why UPF is made the way it is, and why it's so ubiquitous, I arranged a meeting with a man named Paul Hart. Paul's a food-industry insider. He went straight from school into an apprenticeship at Unilever and stayed for over twenty years, first training as a biochemist and then designing food-production systems. There is almost nothing he doesn't know about UPF or the industry that makes it. And he's an original: 'I worked in the Big Food Industry, man and boy. Too old to die young now!'

Paul's speech is peppered with little phrases like this – quotes, aphorisms – that seem to be shortcuts to deeper thoughts. It's as if his brain works faster than his mouth can speak, so he has to reduce everything to the minimum number of words (although there's still a lot of words). Asking Paul questions feels like uncorking a bottle under pressure. When I asked if we could have a chat, he sent me a five-page briefing.

I met Paul with his wife Sharon in the McDonald's on Pentonville Road in London. He had just returned from the vast Food Ingredients Europe trade show in Frankfurt, and he pulled out bundles of literature from ingredients companies I'd never heard of, spreading them all over the sticky plastic table: 'Exhibit A. Dearie me. This is dreadful. Blimey! Look at this yoghurt shot.'

Paul showed me a label with extravagant claims about prebiotics, probiotics and omega 3, and explained that the yoghurt is nothing more than a vehicle to make claims about these other ingredients: 'You lure the consumer in on the basis that some defect in their diet is going to be fixed by swallowing a yoghurt full of additives.'

Conversations with Paul can become enjoyably, if incomprehensibly, obscure. But yoghurt felt like a good segue for me to ask about why Lyra's ice cream hadn't melted. 'Chris, we can use ice cream as an example to explain nearly everything about UPF,' he told me.

This sounded ideal. We left McDonald's for a walk down the Regent's Canal to the station where Sharon and Paul needed to catch their train home. They've been married for forty years, and they're fun to spend time with, still interested in each other's ideas. Sharon is a retired nurse, and she helpfully explained things that I seemed confused by. It was the perfect setting to get really into the topic of ice cream ... so Paul started talking about a tortilla conference he'd been to. 'One company was boasting, in jest, that their products were essentially embalmed, with a shelf life extending for years,' he said. I must have looked horrified, because he quickly clarified that 'Everyone was delighted!'

We ambled along the canal, going under and over little bridges and dodging cyclists. The blazing sunshine gave me a chance to get back onto ice cream. As I guided Sharon and Paul through London, pointing out local landmarks, Paul guided me through ice cream. I had looked at the ice creams at my local Tesco and almost all of them had xanthan gum, guar gum, emulsifiers and glycerine. Could Paul explain why? 'It's all about price and costs. Those ingredients save money.'

This is important to British consumers who in 2017, even before the current cost-of-living crisis, spent just 8 per cent of their household budget on food, lower than almost anywhere else other than the USA (where people spend 6 per cent). Our European neighbours – Germany, Norway, France, Italy – all spend 11–14 per cent of their budget on food, and households in low-income countries spend 60 per cent or more.[1, 2]

In the UK (and many other countries), housing, fuel and transport are fantastically expensive, squeezing that food budget. For rich people this isn't a problem. But an analysis by the Food

Foundation[3] shows that the poorest 50 per cent of households would need to spend almost 30 per cent of their disposable income on food if they wanted to eat a diet that adheres to our national healthy-eating guidelines. The poorest 10 per cent of households by income would need to spend almost 75 per cent. UPF is almost universally cheaper, quicker and supposedly just as nutritious – if not more so – than foods and meals that need home preparation. The combination of low wages, loss of time and the promise of something delicious all probably contribute to the high levels of UPF in our diets – perhaps it's no surprise that UPF is eaten in greater quantities in countries like the UK and USA that are more economically unequal than similar high-income countries.

In any event, Paul explained how ingredients like emulsifiers and gums help in the making of UPF – and in cutting costs. First, they make the ice cream tolerant of warmth, which makes the process of moving the ice cream around easier. From factory to truck, truck to supermarket, supermarket to your freezer at home, ice cream will go from –18°C to –5°C and back down again many times. The gums, glycerine and emulsifiers all stop ice crystals forming by holding water close to them. This means that ice cream can be made in bulk in one factory and then transported around the country. It allows the supply chain to be a little less rushed at each stage and reduces the need to maintain very low temperatures. 'Customers like creaminess,' Paul said, 'not shards of ice!' Centralised manufacturing also allows the companies to negotiate a price with a retailer for shops around the whole country, which further cuts their costs.

One of Paul's first jobs at Unilever was in an ice-cream development lab. He described the scale of the ambition there. The aim was to make blocks of foam that were stable at room temperature which could be distributed worldwide and then frozen onsite. If this could be achieved, the savings would be immense. In fact, many ice creams aren't far off this goal now, as I had discovered in the park. 'The only remaining problem,' Paul told me, 'is the bugs – bugs love ice cream. So, it does all still need to be frozen.'

Paul gave an example of an artisanal brand, Cream o' Galloway, whose vanilla ice cream appears to be made from more or less the same ingredients that you might use at home: milk, cream, sugar, skimmed milk powder, egg yolk, vanilla essence. This is great, but the result is that the product isn't sold nationwide, because their ice cream is just a little less tolerant of all the transporting around. This choice of ingredients is also reflected in the price: Cream o' Galloway vanilla ice cream costs £3.60 for 500ml. That's about fourteen times more expensive than, for example, Ms Molly's Vanilla, exclusive to Tesco, which is £1 for two whole litres. Unsurprisingly, Ms Molly uses very different ingredients in her recipe: reconstituted skimmed milk concentrate, partially reconstituted whey powder (milk), glucose syrup, sugar, dextrose, palm stearin, palm oil, palm kernel oil, emulsifier (mono- and di-glycerides of fatty acids), stabilisers (guar gum, sodium alginate), flavouring, colours (carotenes).

According to Paul, another reason these ingredients save money is that many of them – palm stearin, palm kernel oil, the reconstituted milks, the emulsifiers – are simply mimicking real and expensive ingredients like milk, cream and eggs.* This kind of molecular replacement is the key to all UPF. Traditional food (or, as we might more properly call it, 'food') is made from three broad categories of molecules that give it its taste, texture and calories: fats, proteins and carbohydrates.

Traditional ice cream gets its texture from a complex arrangement of ice crystals, liquid water (which stays liquid because it contains dissolved sugar), milk protein and milk fat globules, all wrapped around cells of air. It's a foam – typically around 50 per cent air – which is why it's not too hard even when it's cold, and

---

* When it comes to food, manufacturers can't reduce personnel, factory overheads or energy costs – competition with other companies means that all those factors have been stripped back as far as they can already. 'The one thing the accountants can play Whac-A-Mole with is the ingredients,' Paul told me. This highlights the complexity of pushing back against UPF: these lower costs of production and distribution are, sometimes, passed onto us.

why it's not easy to make at home since you have to continuously whip while you freeze it.*

The secret to those ultra-processed ice creams, like all UPF, is that they are constructed from the cheapest possible versions of those three essential molecules: fats, proteins and carbs.

Sometimes entirely novel products and textures are created – things like gummy sweets or lentil-foam crisps – but usually the aim of UPF is to replace the ingredients of a traditional and much-loved food with cheaper alternatives and additives that extend shelf life, facilitate centralised distribution and, it turns out, drive excess consumption.

Pies, fried chicken, pizza, butter, pancake mix, pastries, gravies, mayonnaise – all these began as real food. But the non-UPF versions are expensive, so their traditional ingredients are often replaced with cheap, sometimes entirely synthetic, alternatives. These alternatives are generally molecules that are extracted from crops grown for animal food, which in some countries are significantly subsidised. The molecules are refined and modified until, as Paul told me, they can be used to make practically anything.

'We can replace almost any ingredient with a cheap modified alternative,' he said. 'I'll talk you through starch and butter. It's simple enough.' It was not simple. As we paused at the entrance to the long Islington Canal Tunnel and a pair of mating damsel flies settled on some rushes, Paul began a compelling but dense explanation of the chemistry of synthetic carbohydrates.

He started by talking about starches. Starches are how plants store energy – either as fuel in a seed for the growing seedling, or

---

* Manufacturing of factory-processed ice cream accelerated in the USA from the 1850s as a use for waste milk that would otherwise be thrown away. People, after all, can only drink so much fresh milk, and it goes off quite quickly. Turning waste milk into ice cream not only extends the shelf life, it also shows how processing adds value. As we will repeatedly see, repurposing waste is a crucial part of UPF, and is another reason, alongside cheapness, why the advent of UPF has in part been seen as a positive development rather than a problem.

in their roots to fuel the resprouting of a tuber. When you bury a seed or a potato, it essentially eats itself to produce roots and leaves.

Starch is made up of microscopic granules made from chains of glucose sugar molecules. How these chains are organised and tangled affects the properties of the starch when it comes to things like heating, cooling and how they feel in our mouths. It's complex chemistry. Yet even without understanding the exact nature of the molecules, humans have perfected a lot of starch science over the past 10,000 years, through cooking and domestication of crops.

Take the potato, for example. Waxy potatoes like Jersey Royals have sturdy granules of starch, meaning they stay firm when you boil them, and can hold their structure in a potato salad. Floury potatoes like russets, on the other hand, contain sugar-molecule chains that aren't stuck together so well. That's why, though they roast brilliantly, they have a mealy quality that makes them disintegrate in a potato salad, turning it into a mayonnaise mash. Then you have potatoes like Maris Pipers, whose starch hits a sweet spot between the other two, meaning they can be used for pretty much anything – it's the UK's most popular potato for a reason.

If you extract the different starches made by different plants, you find that they have contrasting properties. You can mix them with water to make all kinds of different gels and pastes with different textures at different temperatures. Chemists realised in the nineteenth century that by chemically modifying starch they could create the exact properties they required. Modified starches, which you will start to notice in so many UPF ingredients lists, can replace fats and dairy, hold water during freezing and bulk out any sauce. With the taming of starch, came the possibility of turning very cheap crops into unimaginable amounts of money.

By the 1930s, Kraft had started to use a paste of corn and arrowroot starches in the production of mayonnaise, ingredients that were much cheaper than eggs or oil, but still gave the same creamy mouth-feel. By the 1950s, thanks to scientists with extraordinary industrial names like Carlyle 'Corky' Caldwell, Moses Konigsberg and Otto Wurzburg, the use of modified starches really began to take hold.[4]

Once you can modify a starch precisely, there's very little you can't do.* Thin your starch with acid, and it's useful for textiles and laundry. Treat it with propylene oxide, and you get that gloopy feel for salad dressings. Mix it with phosphoric acid and you can improve stability through multiple cycles of freezing and thawing – perfect for pie fillings. And maltodextrins (short glucose polymers – a form of modified starch) can do things like giving a surface sheen and creaminess to what people think is a 'milkshake'. No more need for expensive dairy fats: these starches come from crops that can be grown at vast scales and at a fraction of the cost.

Paul then moved seamlessly on to the gums that I had noticed listed in the ingredients of Lyra's ice cream.

You might recognise the names of some of these: guar gum, locust bean gum, alginate, carrageenan and the near-ubiquitous xanthan gum. The last of these is, revoltingly, a bacterial exudate: slime that bacteria produce to allow them to cling to surfaces. Think of xanthan gum when you next scrape the accumulated gunk from the filter on your dishwasher.

Like the modified starches, these gums can be used to replace more expensive molecules and to give food a longer shelf life. Paul has particular experience with gums. In the 1980s, he joined a world-class team at Unilever whose work on these gums led to massive advances in the texture of low-fat – and even zero-fat – products, including dressings and spreads. You will probably have eaten the molecules that he worked on many times.

These low-fat products were very much in line with the 1970s guidelines advising people to eat less fat. Today, even though carbs may have replaced fats as the problem molecule in the minds of many people, low-fat dressings are still big business.

---

* Modified starches became nearly universal in the early UPF of the 1950s, but they were also useful in mining and oil drilling, in which starches are used to adjust the viscosity of drilling muds so they aren't too thick or too thin to be pumped or screwed to the surface.

The Centre for Industrial Rheology – that's the science of how materials deform, which is the property that gives them texture in our mouths – compared the fat-replacement strategies in the low-fat offerings of two big mayonnaise manufacturers: Hellmann's and Heinz.[5] Removing the fat from a product like mayonnaise, which is almost all fat, is not a trivial task. The fat affects the taste and the very particular texture of traditional mayonnaise, which behaves like a solid when you don't bother it, and then like a 'structured' liquid when you do.

The two manufacturers went for different solutions: Hellmann's uses gums and starch for thickening, while Heinz uses modified starch only. These differences were apparent in the texture. The low-fat Heinz behaved very much like the full-fat version in terms of the way it flows, whereas the low-fat Hellmann's is a whole lot thicker than its full-fat counterpart. Those gums bring a risk of stringiness like mucus, and snotty mayonnaise isn't appealing. But, used properly, the gums give more lubrication, which is very desirable because it feels like oil in the mouth. In both cases, the starches and the gums give the manufacturers the opportunity to reduce their costs while claiming that they're improving consumer health.

I'm not saying that everyone should make their own mayonnaise, but I am saying that the low-fat versions probably provide no health benefit. In fact, the jury is pretty much in on these low-fat substitutes. Just as artificial sweeteners don't seem to reduce overall calorie intake or protect against disease (something I'll come back to), using novel synthetic molecules to make these low-fat versions of mayonnaise, and many other products, doesn't seem to work. The best independent evidence shows that UPF products like these are strongly associated with weight gain and other diet-related diseases (as we'll see in the next chapter). Additionally, since the introduction and widespread use of such low-fat products, rates of obesity have continued to rise. This may be because we eat more of these products (since we're not quite getting the fat that we're actually after), or it may be because some of the molecules that replace the fat seem to have a range of directly harmful effects (which I'll also come back to later … a lot).

The mayonnaise talk brought to an end Paul's explanation of starches and gums. But he wanted to continue talking about fat. As we stood in the early evening sun, the light reflecting off the canal onto a pretty bank of flowers, Paul started to tell me about melting-point profiles and carbon-chain saturation.

Almost all the aromatic molecules that give food flavour in the mouth, the ones that evaporate off the tongue and go up the back of the nose, are fat soluble. That makes fat pretty important. Because butter makes bread delicious, and oily dressings make salad edible. In fact, it's hard to think of a food that *isn't* improved by some creamy dip or a fatty spread. And there are precise mixtures of fat and sugar that seem to be especially intrinsically palatable.

But fats aren't just tasty and a source of calories – they also bring structure to food. Solid fat is especially useful for this second purpose, as every baker knows. Butter in particular has a perfect melting profile for so many dishes. It's made by churning milk, which causes the fat to separate out into clumps, preserving all the fat-soluble vitamins while getting rid of the sugar and protein.

Paul explained the value of butter compared with milk, which is a liquid emulsion (meaning that the fats, sugars and proteins are all dispersed in water): 'A bug can easily drift through [milk], eating and replicating. It's a nearly perfect bacterial culture medium. But butter …' – he paused to ensure my absolute attention – 'butter is an *inverted* emulsion.'

This means that butter is mainly fat with a little water dispersed. Since butter is not a liquid, bacteria can't move through it, so it keeps for a long time without refrigeration and it's full of those fat-soluble vitamins and essential fatty acids. 'It's a fantastic food,' Paul said. 'It would have transformed early human societies.' Paul was right: it did.

***

Some of the earliest evidence of butter production is found in an unlikely place: an immense sandstone escarpment where the borders of Libya, Algeria and Niger meet in the middle of the Sahara Desert. Search online for Messak Mellet. You'll see the dark yellow rock of the Tadrart Acacus mountains surrounded by the great yellow sand seas on every side. From the satellite images, you might not expect this to be a place where you'd find caves with paintings and carvings of crocodiles, elephants and giraffes.[6] Yet there they are. And there are other even more surprising images, including scenes of cattle, with a few being milked.* The pictures are hard to date, but nearby bones show that cattle, sheep and goats were present in the area from 8,000 years ago and had become very common by 7,000 years ago. The unequivocal evidence of dairying came in 2012, when a team from Bristol University found milk residues on shards of pottery in the Takarkori rock shelter dated to 5000 BC.[8] Analyses indicated that the milk was being processed into cheese or a butter-like product.

Back then, adult humans, like all other mammals, had never drunk milk past weaning, and so didn't produce lactase, the enzyme that enables many of us to digest lactose (the major carbohydrate in milk). But recent research shows that inability to produce lactase made remarkably little difference to our ability to enjoy milk.[9] The major motivation for early processing would probably have been preservation: yoghurt (made when the lactose sugar is consumed by *Lactobacillus* bacteria to produce the natural preservative lactic acid) and butter keep much longer than milk. Over the next few millennia butter became central to food cultures around the world.

The problem with butter is that it's always been expensive. After all, you have to raise and then milk an animal to get it. Plant fat is far cheaper but most of it is liquid oil – harder to store and less useful in giving food texture. It just isn't butter. So, it's not surprising that

---

* 12,000 years ago, the Sahara was lush and green after the end of the last ice age. There was a sedentary hunter, fisher and gatherer population who started to change their way of life around 10,000 years ago, becoming semi-nomadic cattle, sheep and goat herders.[7]

the quest to make a cheap, artificial, solid-fat butter substitute began as long ago as 1869.

That year, Napoleon III – nephew of the most famous Napoleon[*] – offered a prize to anyone who could pull off this fatty alchemy. The winner was a French chemist and pharmacist named Hippolyte Mège-Mouriès, who had already won the Legion of Honour for improvements in baking technology. His description of his production method for his butter substitute may be the first of an *ultra*-process.[10–13]

Mège-Mouriès took cheap solid fat from a cow (suet), rendered it (heated it up with some water), digested it with some enzymes from a sheep stomach to break down the cellular tissue holding the fat together, then it was sieved, allowed to set, extruded from between two plates, bleached with acid, washed with water, warmed, and finally mixed with bicarb, milk protein, cow-udder tissue and annatto (a yellow food colouring derived from seeds of the achiote tree).[14] The result was a spreadable, plausible butter substitute.

Mège-Mouriès branded his creation Oleomargarine, but the slight hitch, as you might have spotted, was that the original margarine recipe still called for animal fats.[†] Breakthroughs in industrial chemistry in the nineteenth and early twentieth centuries opened the door to making margarine from plant oils instead.

The key was to find a way of making the plant oils solid, which was achieved at the turn of the twentieth century via a process called hydrogenation. It was discovered that, if you heat oil in the presence of hydrogen gas at high pressure, you can modify its

---

[*] Napoleon III was the nephew of Napoleon I (the one with the arm tucked in who was exiled to Elba, escaped and then lost the Battle of Waterloo). He was generally popular, and throughout his reign he promoted projects which aimed at improving life for the working class, including giving French workers the right to strike and organise, and gave women the right to be admitted to university. He didn't do any hand tucking, but he did follow in his uncle's footsteps in at least two ways: by losing a battle (Sedan) and by dying in exile (England not Elba).

[†] By 1930, it was possible to produce a solid margarine from liquid *whale oil*. The spread melted at 30°C and would therefore melt in the mouth. By 1960, whale oil made up 17 per cent of the total fats used in margarine production.[15]

chemical structure and change its melting properties. If you hydrogenate the oil fully, you get fat that's hard like ice. But if you only
partially hydrogenate, you can make any melting profile you like,
which makes it possible to produce a fat that's solid at room temperature but still easy to spread out of the fridge.*

The next step was to find the cheapest possible oil. Cottonseeds
were a worthless byproduct of the cotton industry, and were
regarded as garbage up to 1860. Cotton gins were set up on the
banks of rivers so that the seeds would just be washed away. But by
1907, the early Procter & Gamble company (who would go on to
make Pringles) had worked out how to turn cottonseed oil into solid
edible fat.† One difficulty was that the oil contained a toxin called
gossypol, which protects the plant from insects but also leads to
reduced fertility in men, as well as a number of other impurities
that made it taste foul.[16]

---

* There *is* one unfortunate side-effect, in that the process creates trans fats,
which have been linked to heart disease and other health problems. These days,
partial hydrogenation is often replaced by blending different oils, using heat to
separate different molecule sizes (fractionation) and using enzymes to swap
around chains of hydrocarbons between different fats (enzymatic interesterifi-
cation). However, despite widespread concerns that trans fats are harmful,
some food manufacturers still continue to use hydrogenation. In the UK, in
2010, then Health Secretary Andrew Lansley rejected an outright ban of trans
fats. Both Lansley and his special adviser had previously worked for firms that
advised many of the companies that the ban would have affected, such as Pizza
Hut, Kraft and Tesco. Some might feel that this is a conflict of interest.

† In *Life on the Mississippi*, published in 1883, Mark Twain gives a lovely description of the emerging science: 'You see, there's just one little wee speck, essence,
or whatever it is, in a gallon of cotton-seed oil, that gives it a smell, or a flavor,
or something – get that out, and you're all right – perfectly easy then to turn the
oil into any kind of oil you want to, and there ain't anybody that can detect the
true from the false. Well, we know how to get that one little particle out – and
we're the only firm that does. And we turn out an olive-oil that is just simply
perfect – undetectable! We are doing a ripping trade, too – as I could easily show
you by my order-book for this trip. Maybe you'll butter everybody's bread
pretty soon, but we'll cotton-seed his salad for him from the Gulf to Canada,
and that's a dead-certain thing.'

The solution to these problems was a process now known as RBD, whereby oils are refined, bleached and deodorised.

Take palm oil, for example. When freshly pressed, it's an almost luminous crimson, highly aromatic, spicy and flavourful, and full of antioxidants like palm tocotrienol. But, for UPF manufacturers, all that flavour and colour is a problem rather than an advantage. You can't make Nutella with spicy red oil. Oil for UPF needs to be bland, plain and flavourless, so that it can be used to make any edible product – thus the use of RBD. So, manufacturers refine the oil by heating, use phosphoric acid to remove any gums and waxes, neutralise it with caustic soda, bleach it with a bentonite clay, and finally deodorise it using high-pressure steam.* This is the process used to make soybean oil, palm oil, canola (rapeseed) oil and sunflower oil – four oils that make up 90 per cent of the global market – and any other non 'virgin' or 'cold-pressed' oils.

Having solved the problems of cottonseed oil, P&G began a large campaign marketing de-toxified oil as Crisco, an acronym for crystallised cottonseed oil. (They considered but rejected the name 'Cryst' because of its potential religious connotations.) By 1920, use of the product was widespread. Crisco shortening, essentially a fake lard, was possibly the first mass-produced UPF.†

---

* Although the antioxidant palm tocotrienol is removed during the RBD process, it is then added back in to prevent rancidity. As Paul said: 'You couldn't make it up!'

† Initially people hated margarine and the new fake butters. As imports and manufacturing began in the USA, the margarine wars started. Maine, Michigan, Minnesota and some other states not beginning with 'M' banned margarine. Other states put huge tariffs on it. Lucius Hubbard, the governor of Minnesota, a dairy state, declared that 'the ingenuity of depraved human genius has culminated in the production of oleomargarine and its kindred abominations'. Senator Joseph Quarles (of Wisconsin, another dairy-heavy state) said, 'I want butter that has the natural aroma of life and health. I decline to accept as a substitute caul fat, matured under the chill of death, blended with vegetable oils, and flavored by chemical tricks.' *Harper's Weekly* commented: 'Affrighted epicures are informed that they are eating their old candle-ends and tallow-dip remnants in the guise of butter.'

The long lists of fats (many of which have never previously been in a human diet) that you'll start noticing on everything from biscuits to ice cream are the legacy of this technology for processing fat: shea fat, palm fat, mango kernel fat, palm stearate, coconut fat. Once they've been given the RBD treatment, they are essentially interchangeable. Standing in dappled sunlight, as Sharon looked at her watch, Paul explained the advantage of this to all manufacturers of UPF – not just those that make ice cream: 'They can simply use whichever happens to have the cheapest market price. And to avoid the cost of re-writing packaging, they can stick on these Uncle Tom Cobley labels* with all the different fats listed.'

If you see any of these fats on a label, ones that you wouldn't use at home (like any modified palm fat for example), then the product is UPF. The fluctuating market prices may end up resulting in even more unusual ingredients in our food. The war in Ukraine caused sunflower oil prices to spike, and Indonesia temporarily placed a ban on exports of palm oil at the same time in an effort to reduce soaring domestic food prices. This may have the effect that the cost of some of these vegetable fats starts to approach the cost of butter. 'They're already at about the same level as tallow dripping and schmaltz, which is chicken fat,' Paul said. 'So, we may start to see chicken fat in ice cream before long. Just imagine!'

And with that final disgusting thought, Paul and Sharon went to catch their train.

---

* I hadn't heard this expression, and at first thought that Uncle Tom Cobley was an ingredients company. The phrase comes from a folk song, in which the chorus ends with a long list of people, including 'Old Uncle Tom Cobley and all'. I have started to use this expression a lot.

2

I'd rather have five bowls of Coco Pops: the discovery of UPF

Exactly seven days before Lyra's ice cream didn't melt, I had begun my UPF diet with a breakfast of Coco Pops.

'Is it for me?' asked Lyra. No, I told her. She was having porridge.

'I want the Mickey Mouse cereal!' Lyra said, pointing at Coco Monkey.*

I had assumed that, having never tried Coco Pops, she wouldn't have any interest in them. But Kellogg's had got her hooked before she'd had a mouthful. She *knew* that here was a product designed with a three-year-old in mind. Again, I told her no, so she collapsed on the floor crying and screaming with rage, bringing Sasha into the room (carried by Dinah).

I had made Lyra porridge because my instincts told me that Coco Pops weren't a healthy breakfast for a three-year-old, although everything on the package seemed to indicate otherwise. The box was covered in reassuring nutritional information: '50% of your daily vitamin D', '30% less sugar'.† In the UK we have 'traffic lights' to

---

* This mascot has been enthusiastically selling Coco Pops in the UK since before I was born, and (according to YouTube cereal mascot history afficionado Gabe Fonseca) in countries where the cereal is known as Coco/Choco Pops or Choco Krispies. In the USA, where it's sold as Cocoa Krispies, there have been monkeys and elephants, but the current mascots are Snap, Crackle and Pop, who also represent Cocoa Krispies in Canada.

† There's a little asterisk by that 30 per cent less sugar claim: it turns out that Coco Pops have on average 30 per cent less sugar than other chocolate-flavoured toasted-rice cereals – essentially meaningless.

indicate whether a food is healthy. The Coco Pops nutritional information showed two green values (for fat and saturates) and two
ambers (for salt and sugar). And there was that cartoon monkey on
the box, suggesting that the cereal was not merely safe for kids, but
deliberately intended for them. Maybe it was fine.

My lingering doubts were irrelevant anyway. As I was considering all this, Lyra had crawled out from under the table, filled her
bowl and started to eat great fistfuls of dry Coco Pops, wide-eyed
and ecstatic. Defeated, I poured out the milk, and read the ingredients: rice, glucose syrup, sugar, fat reduced cocoa powder, cocoa
mass, salt, barley malt extract, flavourings.

Coco Pops meet the definition of UPF because of the glucose
syrup, the cocoa mass and the flavourings. They are a spectacular
triumph of engineering.

If you eat puffed rice cereal every day, you may no longer notice
the snapping, crackling and popping, but that morning I was transported to the breakfasts of my childhood. Lyra put her ear to the
bowl and shut her eyes, entranced. She then began to eat again.

And eat. And eat. As I watched her, it seemed she wasn't fully in
control. The pack said that a recommended serving for an adult is
30g (roughly a handful). But 30g in, Lyra had hardly taken a breath.
I normally have to do a little cajoling at mealtimes, but the first
bowl of Coco Pops had simply disappeared. When I tried to suggest
that one bowl was enough, the idea was immediately dismissed. It
felt like advising a smoker to stick to one cigarette. Her eating
wasn't just mindless: it was trancelike.

***

If Coco Pops don't seem like a typical diet food, that's because I had
started the month-long dietary experiment that I was conducting
with help from colleagues at UCLH, where I work. The idea came
from two papers that a colleague, the television producer Lizzie
Bolton, had urged me to read. They'd been sitting in a pile on my
desk for several weeks by the time I got round to them. At first

glance they didn't seem particularly appealing, but they would turn out to be two of the most important papers I've ever read.

The first was published in Portuguese, more than a decade ago, in a relatively obscure Brazilian public health journal. It had a modest, rather specific title: 'A new classification of foods based on the extent and purpose of their processing'. The lead author was Carlos Monteiro, a professor of nutrition in São Paulo.

The second paper sounded even less enticing. It was a dietary experiment about weight gain, perhaps promoting another fad: 'Ultra-processed diets cause excess calorie intake and weight gain: an inpatient randomized controlled trial of ad libitum food intake' (lead author: Kevin Hall).

In the first paper, Monteiro advanced a theory; in the second, Hall described an experiment that tested that theory and, at least at first glance, seemed to confirm it. Here's the theory: the main reason for the rapid increase in overweight and obesity throughout the world, especially since the 1980s, is the correspondingly rapid increase in production and consumption of ultra-processed food and drink products.

I had never heard of UPF and was sceptical of a single overarching explanation of the obesity pandemic, which is widely known to be complex and multifactorial. But there was something about Monteiro's proposed classification system that felt fresh and interesting.

The classification system is now called the NOVA system, and it divides food into four groups.[1] The first is 'unprocessed or minimally processed foods' – foods found in nature like meat, fruit and vegetables, but also things like flour and pasta. Group 2 is 'processed culinary ingredients', including oils,[*] lard, butter, sugar, salt,

---

[*] Paul Hart suggests that most modern oils, having been refined, bleached and deodorised, should be in group 4. It's a reasonable point, but the classification comes from Monteiro's Brazilian data suggesting that use of these oils is associated with people making their own food, meaning that, like sugar on the table, they are a sign of health. There is persuasive emerging evidence that these seed oils are harmful in lots of ways at the doses we consume them, but there is a world of difference between cooking with sunflower oil and eating an industrially produced product in which sunflower oil is one of many ingredients. This discussion of what should and shouldn't be in each NOVA group is one we'll return to many times.

vinegar, honey, starches – traditional foods that might well be prepared using industrial technologies. They're not things we can survive on, because they tend to be nutrient-poor and energy-dense. But mix them with stuff from the first group, and you've got the basis of some delicious food. Group 3 is 'processed food', ready-made mixtures of groups 1 and 2, processed mainly for preservation: think tins of beans, salted nuts, smoked meat, canned fish, chunks of fruit in syrup and proper freshly made bread.

And then we come to Group 4, 'ultra-processed foods'. It's long, perhaps the longest definition I'd ever read of a scientific category: 'Formulations of ingredients, mostly of exclusive industrial use, made by a series of industrial processes, many requiring sophisticated equipment and technology.'

That's just the first bit. It continues: 'Processes used to make ultra-processed foods include the fractioning of whole foods into substances, chemical modifications of these substances …'

Exactly as Paul described, crops like corn and soy are turned into oil, protein and starch, which are then further modified. The oils are refined, bleached, deodorised, hydrogenated and interesterified, the protein may be hydrolysed, the starch modified. These modified food fractions are then combined with additives and assembled using industrial techniques like moulding, extrusion and pressure changes. This is a pattern I would encounter throughout my diet. Ingredient lists, from pizza to chew bars, started to look the same.

The definition of UPF continues for a long time before concluding in a way that suddenly resonated:

'Processes and ingredients used to manufacture ultra-processed foods are designed to create highly profitable (low-cost ingredients, long shelf life, emphatic branding) convenient (ready-to-consume) hyperpalatable products liable to displace freshly prepared dishes and meals made from all other NOVA food groups.'

The idea that the purpose of a food could be important barely registered the first time I encountered Monteiro's work, and yet it began to crystalise a cloud of ideas that had been floating around in my head for many years. I could understand that at least in theory physical and chemical processes might affect how the food interacts with the body. But to include, as part of the definition the *purpose* for the processing – 'to create highly profitable products' – was completely new.

Considerations about whether traditional food might have a different *purpose* from substances made by transnational corporations with hundreds of billions in revenue had been almost entirely absent from scientific and policy discussions of food and nutrition. It wasn't a big mental leap to imagine that products that subvert the body's evolved mechanisms that signal when to stop eating might survive better in the marketplace.

Having read Monteiro's work, I found that the NOVA system and UPF had some initial appeal as ideas, but it was just a hypothesis. So, then I read Hall's experiment, which put the idea to the test.

It was published in *Cell Metabolism*, a respectable – if specialist – journal. The experiment was simple enough. Volunteers were fed either an ultra-processed diet or a diet that was identical in terms of fat, salt, sugar and fibre but without any UPF. After two weeks, both groups then switched to receive the other diet. During both phases, participants could eat as much as they liked. On the ultra-processed diet, participants ate more and gained weight, whereas on the unprocessed diet they actually lost weight, despite having access to as much food as they wanted. At the time, I had no great expertise in these sorts of experiments, so the details were hard to critique. But the report had real heft and the data seemed sound.

Yet I still wasn't convinced. Even the most prestigious journals – perhaps *especially* the most prestigious journals – are full of appealing ideas, presented well and seemingly backed up with promising data, which in the end turn out to be utterly wrong. In fact, there are credible estimates that *most* scientific papers might be wrong.[2] Two papers aren't sufficient to turn an entire field around. And I found it odd that none of the dozens of UK-based nutrition experts I'd interviewed while researching other articles and documentaries had ever mentioned Carlos Monteiro, Kevin Hall or UPF. Processing is not mentioned in the UK or US national nutrition guidelines. There's no labelling on packets about whether food is ultra-processed.

Nonetheless, I remember my feeling of cautious excitement reading these papers after I'd put Lyra and Sasha to bed that night. The way we'd been thinking about food previously had shown no signs of solving the growing problem of diet-related disease.

The next day, I went to see a friend and colleague at UCLH, Rachel Batterham. She's a professor of obesity, diabetes and endocrinology and is internationally renowned for her obesity research, having published some of the most important science around appetite regulation and eating behaviours, including a ground-breaking paper in *Nature*. She's smart and funny, and she's transformed the way I think about obesity and the people who live with it.*

I showed Rachel the papers. She, too, had barely heard of UPF, but she knew Kevin Hall's work more generally and she was immediately able to make connections between how physical processing of ingredients might affect the quantity of a food that would be eaten before the body said 'stop'. And, always keen to tackle big questions with absolute scientific rigour, she immediately started to draw up an approach to testing these hypotheses.

We decided to do an experiment: I'd go on a month-long diet of UPF and Rachel's team would monitor every aspect of my brain and body. If there were any interesting results, then we would use them as pilot data to get funding for a larger study.† At the time, the only paper looking at the body's responses to a UPF diet was Hall's, and that had been conducted in a lab setting. We'd take the experiment out into the real world.

---

* One of the main effects is that I no longer use obese as a descriptor. People 'have' overweight and obesity just like they have cancer or diabetes. It's not their identity. There is a helpful trend in this direction in medicine generally. People live with stuff, they don't need it to define them.

† Small, well-conducted studies can be very informative, although their conclusions have to be carefully tested in larger groups. Historically, many, many discoveries – from the effects of sildenafil (Viagra) to the efficacy of vaccines – have been initially discovered in studies of a tiny number of patients.

The terms of my diet were simple. I would eat like a child. In the UK, one in five people gets at least 80 per cent of their calories from UPF, and this figure is typical for children and adolescents too.[3] In the population as a whole, the average figure is 60 per cent.[4-7]

So, I would eat 80 per cent UPF but I wasn't going to force the food in – this wasn't *Super Size Me*. I'd just eat when I felt like it. Frankly, neither Rachel nor I expected anything much to happen in only a month, but we thought we might find something that would justify further investigation.

The first step was to stop eating UPF for four weeks as preparation. I was still in the mindset of thinking that UPF was synonymous with 'junk food', so I was surprised to find from keeping a food diary over a typical week that I was generally getting around 30 per cent of my calories from UPF.

After years of writing and broadcasting about food – and slow but steady weight gain – my usual diet looked something like this: black coffee for breakfast, a sandwich and crisps for lunch, and a fairly healthy home-cooked dinner (chicken, rice and broccoli is a staple), followed by a supermarket dessert. Every few nights, rather than cooking the main course, we'd have a UPF microwave lasagne or a UPF oven pizza. I'd have a takeaway about once per week, usually UPF thanks to liberal use of modified starches and flavour enhancers.

Quitting this UPF intake was surprisingly hard. I craved those microwave meals, snack bars and takeaways. But, as I started to look at labels and ingredients lists, I also found that most food from the sandwich shops and the hospital canteen was ruled out. I couldn't buy a sandwich for lunch because of the emulsifiers in the bread and the maltodextrin and preservatives in the spreads. So, I had to make my own sandwiches – mainly cheese, butter and proper sourdough bread from a local bakery. I couldn't even add my favourite Hellmann's mayonnaise.*

---

* Hellmann's: rapeseed oil (78%), water, pasteurised egg & egg yolk, spirit vinegar, salt, sugar, flavourings, lemon juice concentrate, antioxidant (calcium disodium EDTA), paprika extract.

My belt got a little looser, sure, but I started really looking forward to my UPF diet. The foods that were forbidden became hugely desirable. I started to obsess over stuff that I didn't typically think about as my mind focused more than usual on all the tempting options around me – especially the McDonald's and KFC across the road from the hospital.

The day before the diet was due to begin, I visited the lab at UCL to spend half a day being weighed and measured. I got on the body-composition scales. Weight: 82kg. Height: 185 centimetres. BMI: 24.2. Body fat: 17 per cent. All in all, I was in depressingly average shape for a man of my age. Rachel's team took some blood to measure my inflammation levels and to check how my body responded to food. I had fasted overnight. They fed me a delicious banana milkshake with precise quantities of fat, protein and sugar and then looked at the increase in fullness hormones and my insulin response. I also did psychometric tests, and filled in mood and appetite questionnaires.

Last, I went for an MRI scan to build up a map of how different parts of my brain were connected to each other. I remember thinking, as I lay in the scanner, that this test seemed absurd. We weren't going to find noticeable changes on an MRI scan in just four weeks of eating a diet that is totally normal for millions of people around the country.

As I watched Lyra finish her first bowl of Coco Pops and clumsily pour herself another, I started to wonder when she would stop. I thought more about the comparison with smoking while we ate. The first spoonful was ecstatic for both of us. The cereal is rich, complex and intensely chocolatey, far more so than I remembered. The texture of the first mouthful is extraordinary, some of the 'pops' becoming chewy almost instantly while others remain crisp, crackling on the tongue.

But three spoons in, the joy was gone: what remained was a brown sludge, consumed only to relieve a craving. Lyra and I were drawn to our next mouthfuls just like smokers to the next drag. The experience of the first pull couldn't be replicated, yet something about the cereal made us keep trying.

Lyra wasn't up for any chat, so I looked at the box, which seemed to illustrate very clearly the way that we think about food in the UK and the USA – in terms of its 'nutritional profile'. Food contains 'good' and 'bad' nutrients, and the nutritional profile details the quantities of these. To work out if a food is healthy, most of us ask how much saturated fat, salt, sugar, fibre, vitamins and minerals it contains. How many calories are in a portion? Does it have vitamin C? It's so ingrained that it's hard to think about food in any other way.

This approach to food was termed, somewhat scornfully, 'nutritionism' by Gorgy Scrinis, an associate professor of food politics and policy at the University of Melbourne (and one of the first people to put forward the idea that perhaps food is more than the sum of its component parts). But nutritionism does solve an important problem. Whenever you decide to study something, you need to 'operationalise' it. This is at the core of most modern science: we often need to define things we can't measure in terms of things that we can. Wealth and health are good examples. Wealth is easy: you can directly measure it and give it a number. But health is more slippery: it exists, but there's no specific unit to quantify it, so, we instead define it in terms of a frailty index, BMI, blood pressure, the presence of chronic medical conditions, iron levels, and so on.

Food is like health, in that it lacks a specific measurable dimension. To study it scientifically, you need to break it down into measurables like nutritional components, which *do* have dimensions – calories, grams of vitamin C and so on. We exhaustively documented the effects of these nutrients on almost every aspect of our physiology as diet-related disease exploded around the world. But before Carlos Monteiro no one involved in health and nutrition had spent much time worrying about how to describe diet in any other way.

As Lyra lifted her second bowl to carelessly slurp the brown dregs of milk, I started to think that nutritionism wasn't very helpful for trying to work out how much or what she should eat. Had she eaten too much sugar for a child her age for instance? I was almost certain she had, but there was no question of intervening. The pack had a little data table with the amount of sugar and salt per gram, but I didn't know how many grams she'd eaten. And the pack didn't say how many grams of Coco Pops were OK for a three-year-old, which seemed odd given that so much space on the box is devoted to a cartoon monkey that markets the product directly to children.

I then started to look at the salt content. Coco Pops is 0.65 per cent salt, but I had no idea what this meant. So, for context, I looked up the salt content of other foods. I think a more useful way of explaining the salt in Coco Pops might be: this cereal contains 20 per cent more salt per gram than a typical microwave lasagne. This incredible saltiness is true of most breakfast cereals – it helps to make them taste amazing. So, why isn't there a salt warning?

I think it's because the recommended serving size for an adult is 30g, which is four large spoonfuls. If you're a grown-up and you eat that amount then you won't eat too much salt, but I was pretty sure that Lyra had consumed more than 30g of cereal while I was looking up lasagne nutrition tables.

Those nutritional 'traffic lights' (two green, two amber) started to seem more and more absurd as I watched her. In the UK, this system of highlighting the levels of fat, saturated fat, salt and sugar is entirely voluntary (many other countries have similar systems). But imagine driving a car with a three-year-old in the back seat and being faced with four lights, two of which are green and two of which are amber. Do you drive or not?

As well as the traffic light system, in the UK there *is* another way of thinking about food, and it crops up fairly often in the UK press: the designation High in (saturated) fat, salt and sugar, or HFSS. For marketing purposes in the UK, packaged food is formally categorised as HFSS (or not) by something opaquely called the Nutrient

Profile Model (or NPM 2004/5), which was developed as a tool to regulate food advertisements targeted at children.*

If you struggle to make sense of the nutrient data table on the pack to guide healthy eating for your child, then the NPM 2004/5 is going to blow your mind. You can't look up the NPM score of a food easily – you have to calculate it using the following three steps, which I write out only to illustrate their complexity.

First, you award a score for the bad stuff: calories, saturated fat, sugars and sodium. These are called 'A' points. Second, you add up the points for the good stuff: fruit, vegetables, nuts, fibre and protein. These are called 'C' points. (By the way, you may need to pay for access to something like the NielsenIQ Brandbank nutritional database to gather all this information.) After you've calculated the A and C points, there are other rules to be factored in, like: 'If a food or drink scores 11 or more A points then it cannot score points for protein unless it also scores 5 points for fruit, vegetables and nuts.'

Clear so far? Well, *then* you subtract the C points from the A points to calculate a score out of thirty. Any food that scores more than four is classified as HFSS. But, even if you do all that, it isn't clear whether children should eat these HFSS foods, or in what amounts. The designation determines only whether a food can be *marketed* to children at particular times and in particular ways.

According to a 2018 review of the NPM 2004/5 calculator, 'There is no single, simple measurement that defines these foods as "healthier" or "less healthy".'[8] But as Lyra dabbed a spillage of chocolate milk from her pyjamas, it seemed like Carlos Monteiro's UPF

---

* The NPM 2004/5 was developed by the Food Standards Agency to provide Ofcom, the broadcast regulator, with a tool to differentiate foods on the basis of their nutritional composition, in the context of television advertising of foods to children. HFSS is one of the categories in the NPM 2004/5. Currently, if a food is categorised as HFSS, then advertising of that particular product to a child is restricted online and on TV. However, children can still see an ad for the brand (McDonalds or Coca-Cola, for example) and they can have that brand marketed to them with a toy and a cartoon character in a shop.

definition might be a little simpler – provided, of course, that the evidence supported his definition and the links to health.

Certainly, the traffic lights, the nutrition data tables, the HFSS designation all seem to represent a delusion about the way people choose and eat food. It's not just that no normal person can understand the information mixed in among the manufacturers' claims. The delusion is the idea that we can eat according to numbers rather than appetite.

Humans, like all animals, have evolved systems that control nutritional intake. As I read more, I started to wonder whether it's the normal regulation of appetite that UPF disrupts, so that we keep eating, no matter what's written on the box.

The original paper, outlining Monteiro's hypothesis, seemed to be as potentially important as some of those papers in journal club in the lab, the ones that forever changed my understanding of the world. But how had he come up with this idea of categorising food according to its level of processing?

I started looking back through Monteiro's published papers. It's a journey through the history of nutrition and obesity.

He was born in 1948 to a family that sat in a very particular position in the Brazilian social hierarchy, at the upper edge of poverty and the lower edge of wealth. Carlos could see in both directions. Perhaps his interest in social justice came from the idea that falling into the desperate poverty so visible around him would be very easy, perhaps a matter of luck more than anything else.

He was the first person from his family to go university and was accepted to medical school in 1966, just after the US-backed military coup. His medical career started against a backdrop of successive military regimes and increasing state violence, and his interest in the health of the most marginalised communities grew.

His research career began in one of the most impoverished regions near São Paolo, the Ribeira Valley. He was studying how social class – as opposed to education or income – affected nutritional status in the plantation workers. It was a project with a number of fuzzy boundaries: defining 'social class' and 'nutritional status' isn't easy. Monteiro combined skills in mathematics, medicine, anthropology and economics to organise and analyse diverse sets of data. He was starting to learn the skills he'd later apply to creating the category of UPF.

His early papers, starting in 1977, focused on malnutrition, a huge problem in Brazil at that time. There's work on breastfeeding, on stunted growth, and on iron supplementation in children. A crisis of overweight was all but unimaginable.

This is how nutrition science began around the world: studying diseases of deficiency. Scurvy in sailors looking for the Northwest Passage. The 'Lancashire neck' of iodine deficiency. Beriberi, pellagra, rickets: familiar names for diseases of vitamin deficiency. Nutritional science was forged in a world where the most pressing question was the minimum requirements for a healthy body and where terrible suffering could be relieved with the addition of a single nutrient. This probably has a lot to do with the emergence of the idea that a healthy diet can be broken down into individual chemicals, each with its own exact dose.

Our understanding of how the body responds to excess lags far behind. And excess is what Monteiro started to observe from the mid-nineties. The once-impossible crisis of overweight had suddenly become not just plausible, but evident everywhere he looked. He saw what he called a 'nutritional transformation', a confusing rise in obesity among the poorest communities as obesity rates in more affluent areas were beginning to fall.

While his papers are full of complex equations, the content feels routine. It doesn't feel like curing cancer or sequencing the genome – it's looking at shopping bills, albeit using multiple linear regression models to do so. Even with my scientific training, glancing superficially at Monteiro's work, I felt that it was being obscured by the same issue that hinders so many important ideas – being complicated and dull. But when I stepped back from the statistical methods section of any one of his papers and looked at the body of work, I could see that he was meticulously documenting something extraordinary: Brazil's nutritional transformation from a country where obesity was of merely academic interest into a country where it is arguably the dominant public health problem.

The reason this was so exciting is that, in countries like the UK and the USA, we really missed the moment when our diets changed from largely unprocessed foods to UPF. We have almost no directly collected individual dietary data about what people were eating in the fifties, sixties or seventies beyond national household consumption data. But Monteiro knew what had happened in the USA and the UK, and he was watching it unfold at an accelerated pace in Brazil.

From around 2003, he began to produce more papers on how much fat and sugar people were eating, which looked at the data in an unusual way. Indeed, his papers about overweight, obesity, sugar and fat revealed a peculiar paradox.

Traditional advice recommends a diet based on carbohydrates, like cereals, bread, rice, pasta, potatoes as well as fruit and vegetables. Oils, fats, salt and refined sugar, conversely, should be consumed only sparingly. Yet Carlos found that, between the mid-eighties and the 2010s, the period in which Brazilian obesity rates had exploded, purchases of the supposedly healthy stuff – cereals, pasta, bread – had been increasing, while there had been an enormous decline in apparently unhealthy purchases of oil and sugar as ingredients.[9] Judged conventionally, the shift was towards better diet, not worse.

In an effort to solve this apparent paradox, Carlos decided that, rather than focusing on single nutrients or food items, he would look at the overall dietary *pattern*. He and his team would approach the task of drawing a boundary around 'bad food' in a different way. Rather than starting at the beginning, down at the microscopic level, they'd start at the end. They'd identify what foods were causing the problems, and then work backwards to see what they all had in common.

This required statistical methods that hadn't been used in nutrition before. What emerged from the mathematics were two separate patterns of eating in Brazil: one that comprised mainly traditional foods, such as rice and beans, and another that consisted mainly of foods like soft drinks, cookies, prepared desserts, instant noodles and cereals. The latter was taking over, pushing out the traditional foods. Biscuit consumption in Brazil had grown by 400 per cent between 1974 and 2003, and soft-drink consumption was also up 400 per cent. The link between the popular products causing the problem was clear: they were all made from deconstructed, modified ingredients that were mixed with additives and frequently aggressively marketed.

When analysing the food purchases that were associated with health, Monteiro and his team found that they included sugar and oil. It wasn't that sugar or oil were healthy, but rather they indicated a household that still cooked rice and beans.

This brought Monteiro and his team up against a long-standing issue. When it comes to obesity, the problem *is* food. The difficulty since 1980 – in fact, since 1890 – has been the question of which food, exactly.

Clearly, there's bad food, but how do you define it?

You might be feeling like you've heard all this before. Lots of smart people have long expressed concern about 'processed food', but have found that it's not an easy idea to nail down – my mother, for example.

Back around the time Monteiro was studying the plantation workers in the Ribeira Valley, my mother was an editor at Time Life. She worked on lots of different books, but her passion project was a series called 'The Good Cook', written by a food purist called Richard Olney. He was the kind of cook who would grow wheat to make his own flour. People like him, and my mother, talked about 'junk food'.

As my brothers and I became scientifically literate, we'd argue with Mum that she was being snobby. We'd remind her that her own (delicious) cooking was laden with just as much salt and fat as the McDonald's we were hardly ever allowed. The way of thinking about food that we learned at medical school doesn't distinguish between the salty fatty foods that mum cooked and their industrial equivalents. But Carlos Monteiro's data did make a distinction, and this distinction has become clearer ever since.

Take a pizza for example. In terms of nutrition, a pizza is a pizza. Flour, tomato, cheese. You can buy one from Sweet Thursday, the pizza restaurant at the end of my road, for around £10. It's made with about six ingredients and is not UPF. But it has approximately the same nutritional profile as a £1 UPF pizza from the supermarket next door that contains preservatives, stabilisers and antioxidants. Both pizzas have roughly the same number of calories, fat, salt and sugar. But one is a traditional food not associated with obesity or diet-related disease, while the other isn't.

Any discussion of food descends quickly into a quagmire of snobbery because, typically, people with more money to spend on food eat different types of food and a wider variety of foods from people with less disposable income. And this, as we will see, contributes to the fact that, overall, people with less money have higher rates of obesity. It is also a mainstay of the argument that obesity and other diet-related diseases are not a choice.

My mum's generation was far from the first to worry about 'junk' or 'processed' food, either. Even before processed food was associated with poverty, there were concerns. Hugh MacDonald Sinclair, the father of much of our understanding of fat and its metabolism in the body, was already worrying about processing years before my mother was editing cookery books or Monteiro came on the scene. A charismatic and eccentric Oxford biochemist, Sinclair wrote a letter to *The Lancet* in 1956, described (by Sinclair himself) as 'the longest and rudest letter *The Lancet* ever published'.

In the letter, he linked chronic deficiency of essential fatty acids to lung cancer, coronary thrombosis and leukaemia. The deficiency, he asserted, was due to the high processing levels of wheat and to the manufacture of margarine: 'With no sympathy for long-haired naturalism, I humbly plead that we should give more thought and perform more research before extracting and "improving" wheat, and manufacturing margarine, before foisting upon the public sophisticated fodder which it unsuspectingly accepts.'

Still earlier than Sinclair, there was a Chicago paediatrician named Clara Davis. A towering – if mysterious – figure in human nutrition, whom we'll meet properly later, she was worrying about white flour and baked goods and sugar back in the 1920s. Before Davis, the 1820s saw the publication of the first major piece of academic writing on the harms of food adulteration and processing: *Death in the Pot: A Treatise on Adulterations of Food, and Culinary Poisons, and Methods Of Detecting Them* by Frederick Accum.

And I think it's safe to assume that when, about 6,000 years ago, a North African pastoralist decided to store milk in an animal stomach and ended up accidentally inventing cheese, not everyone would have welcomed the new form of processing, despite the increase in shelf life.

Dividing food into processed and unprocessed is an impossible task. Try to think of a single food that's truly unprocessed, which you can eat whole and raw and that was never selectively bred. A few wild berries, oysters, raw milk, some mushrooms and not much else. Processing started barely a million years after we diverged from chimpanzees. Hacking a chunk of meat off a mammoth carcass? That's food processing. Cooking with fire? Also processing. Genetically modifying crops and animals by breeding them selectively, a method that predates writing? Processing.

The fact that almost all our food is processed to some extent probably has a lot to do with why nutritional guidelines have simply never worried about processing when it comes to health. 'Junk food' had been considered harmful simply because it contained too much of the 'bad' things – salt, saturated fat and sugar – and too little of the good stuff.

In 2007, while Monteiro was grappling with this problem, a couple of articles were published that greatly influenced him and his team. The first, by Michael Pollan, was published in the *New York Times* and began with the well-known lines: 'Eat food. Not too much. Mostly plants.'[10] Pollan underlined the point that almost any kind of traditional diet seemed to be associated with health, regardless of what they contained – including in the case of the French, for example, large quantities of alcohol and saturated fat, or in the case of the Italians, lots of pizza and pasta.

The second article, written by David Jacobs, an epidemiologist from the University of Minnesota, and Linda Tapsell, from the University of Wollongong in Australia, was published in the rather less mainstream *Nutrition Reviews*. Its title was 'Food, not nutrients, is the fundamental unit in nutrition', and it pointed out an as-yet unexplained phenomenon: that a number of good studies had iden-tified foods, such as whole grains, nuts, olives and oily fish, that seemed to reduce chronic disease risk, but that the benefit of the relevant nutrient – beta-carotene, fish oil, vitamin B, etc – vanished as soon as they were extracted from the food and taken instead as a supplement.

In short, there aren't any supplements that work for healthy people. Beneficial nutrients only seem to help us when we consume them in context. Fish oil doesn't benefit us, but oily fish do. It seems unbelievable, I know. There's no supplement, vitamin or antioxi-dant that decreases risk of death, or even of disease of any kind in healthy people. Almost all the large-scale independent studies of multivitamin and antioxidant supplements have shown that, if any-thing, they increase the risk of death. This is especially true for vitamin E, beta-carotene and high-dose vitamin C.[11-13] If you can understand that outside the context of possible deficiency vitamins supplements don't work, then you have begun to understand that food and food extracts are not the same. Remember the effect of arms races: food is complex.

These two articles laid the intellectual foundation for Monteiro's next step: to describe the bad food formally so that it could be stud-ied. It was a task for which his time on the plantations had prepared him. He and his team looked at the foods associated with poor health outcomes in their data and started to try to describe them. By 2010, they had come up with the NOVA classification. Monteiro himself denies it was his idea, insisting it was a collective piece of work. And he denies that there was any kind of 'Eureka!' moment either. Instead, he says the definition came from many years of studiously analysing data. No one on Monteiro's team could even tell me exactly how or even when they arrived at the definition, only that Jean-Claude Moubarac came up with the name 'NOVA' one day in the university canteen.

***

At breakfast, I found myself humming the jingle from the old TV ad: 'I'd rather have a bowl of Coco Pops!' It turned out that Lyra would rather have a bowl of Coco Pops than almost anything else. She ate until her belly was drum taut. By the time she stopped, she had consumed two adult servings covered in whole milk: most of her day's worth of calories. After we had finished, I got out my digital scales and refilled her bowl and checked all the weights of what we had eaten. I have a digital scales because many of my best recipes come from lab colleagues who write them out like experimental protocols with weights to the nearest gram. One colleague got into measuring spices on a microbalance, such that her recipes would say things like '100mg of ground cloves'. I have not bought a microbalance.

At the same time, I had eaten five portions, an appropriate first meal of my UPF diet. Invented in the late 1950s, Coco Pops were a staple of breakfasts for my parents' generation and were by far the most popular cereal of my own childhood. Far from feeling like something to be concerned about, they've almost begun to feel like a 'traditional' food.

Since the first publication of Monteiro's NOVA classification system there has been significant backlash. How, critics asked, could a group of processes that don't add calories or change the chemical composition of a food* cause weight gain or ill health? It's an understandable objection. You may have had an uneasy feeling about something else, too: that the definition of UPF feels just a little bit ... arbitrary?

---

* Cooking does change chemical composition, but many of the other processes don't.

The contrarian journalist Christopher Snowdon made this point exactly when, in January 2022, he wrote a blogpost titled 'What is "ultra-processed food"?'.[14] The piece had been inspired, Snowdon said, by a 'deranged' op-ed about UPF in the *British Medical Journal*. His summary of this 'arbitrariness' of the definition is neat: '"Junk food" is too narrow since most people interpret it to mean "fast food" from a handful of restaurant chains. And so, in the absence of an obvious dietary culprit, the "public health" lobby is shifting towards a crusade against "ultra-processed food".'

Snowdon had particular beef with one of the op-ed's rules of thumb for identifying UPF: that UPF is likely to contain more than five ingredients. 'What kind of ludicrous, arbitrary threshold is that??' he wrote. 'None of this has any scientific standing whatsoever!'

It *is* easy to see what he means. Why not six ingredients? Why not four? But arbitrariness simply doesn't matter if you're a scientist.

Let's imagine Monteiro's team had started with something explicitly arbitrary, like star signs. Instead of UPF, they might have suggested that being a Leo is the cause of obesity – in scientific terms, it just doesn't matter, *so long as you can back it up with evidence*.

Let's imagine someone had observed that Leos *did* have more obesity. Well, then the researchers would have to build an intellectual model to explain why that might be: seasons, weather at conception, maternal diet, circulating viruses at birth and so on. They could have done animal experiments, breeding mice to be born between 23 July and 22 August, and then comparing them to mice born on other dates. Then imagine that, having tested their model to destruction, they found that being born when the sun is transiting the 120th to 150th degree of celestial longitude, the constellation of Leo, made all the difference and nothing else mattered. Well, we'd have to live with it. It would be weird, but it would still be true, even though the starting point had been completely and utterly arbitrary.

Philosophers of science aren't in total agreement about where knowledge comes from, but most accept that science starts with an observation, followed by building a model and then testing that observation. Sometimes the observational data feel very science-y: measurements of the movement of celestial objects, or numbers read out from a fancy machine like a linear collider. But other times a dog walker finds a dead goose in a park and it's the first data point in a bird flu pandemic.

Of course, in reality, the arbitrary astrological proposition would be supported by none of the data and the model would collapse. The researchers would need to go and look for another cause, like a food system that compels people to eat lots of industrially produced food, or being a Sagittarius. The power of good science is that it can handle a bad, wrong or arbitrary hypothesis. That, really, is the defining characteristic of science.

Real-life science *often* starts with something arbitrary. Sticking things in boxes. Grouping things together. Naming them. We have to draw a line somewhere and describe the object of interest. In the physical sciences, the boundaries are often clearer. In physics, particles are grouped and described according to how they behave in gravitational or electromagnetic fields. In chemistry, elements are ordered in the periodic table according to their subatomic composition and chemical behaviour. The systems are objective and discrete.

Sometimes, in the biosciences, we also have well defined categories. HIV is, now, a binary diagnosis: you have it or you don't. But many of the most pressing problems are much fuzzier. Obesity in adults is defined, arbitrarily, as having a BMI of 30 or above. It wouldn't matter if the threshold was 29 or 31 instead.* There's no sudden change in health that happens at 30 exactly – the risks are

---

* There are too many problems with the limitations of using BMI to go into here. For now, it remains the best tool we've got for thinking about populations. For a dissection of the problems with BMI, I recommend 'The bizarre and racist history of the BMI' by Aubrey Gordon.[15]

just gradually increasing. Almost all biological measurements – blood pressure, haemoglobin, lung capacity – fall along a continuum. At some point we draw a line, somewhat arbitrarily, and say the people on one side of the line have high blood pressure or anaemia or obesity and those on the other side don't.

That was Monteiro's team's genius: they drew a line. Or perhaps their genius was to decide that a line could be drawn at all – that there *is* harmful food and that it can be defined. And while the exact place to draw the line is arbitrary, the idea that there are dietary patterns that cause disease and others that don't is not arbitrary. That idea comes from a huge volume of carefully collected and analysed data. And it's also not arbitrary to propose that food produced for profit might be designed, deliberately or inadvertently, to make us consume it to excess.

The NOVA classification was a hypothesis, a model that sorted foods into categories for rigorous testing by Kevin Hall and many others. And it sidesteps, at least partially, the social minefield of studying food. Whether a particular pizza will drive excess consumption has nothing to do with how much it costs or who's eating it. The only question is whether it's UPF.

Having created a definition in 2010, UPF was operationalised for study. But would the hypothesis stand up to scrutiny?

3.

Sure, 'ultra-processed food' sounds bad, but is it really a problem?

The second weekend of my diet I went on a camping trip with my brother Xand and my two brothers-in-law, Chid (Richard) and Ryan. We drove west from London toward Wales, stopping at Leigh Delamere services, a festival of UPF. I bought Cool Original Doritos, two cans of Red Bull and packets of Skittles and Haribo Supermix for the rest of the journey.

We slept in a beautiful spot near a waterfall in the Brecon Beacons National Park, spoiled only by my waking dreams about food and my body. I imagined my blood had become thick and sticky, as if it had become too concentrated from the salt and sugar. I woke up early, feeling sad and unwell.

I diluted myself with some water and cheered up over breakfast looking at the ridge of mountains. We had Kellogg's Crunchy Nut Clusters (with wholegrain and no artificial colours or flavours and a promotion for adults to go free at Legoland) and Alpen Original Recipe 'naturally wholesome muesli'.

Ryan, an internationally renowned psychology professor from Australia, was astounded to see I was eating Alpen on my UPF diet: 'What's wrong with Alpen? It's natural and wholesome.' I told him that it technically qualified as UPF because it has milk whey powder in it, an ingredient that isn't typically used in home cooking.

He looked genuinely baffled. 'But the mountains on the pack look pristine!' I responded that it was still UPF. Chid and Xand agreed. 'Well, it tastes good,' he insisted. If the packaging can persuade Ryan, it can persuade anyone.

As we drove home, I got a phone call from a producer at BBC Radio. They wanted me to make a short radio documentary introducing people to the idea of UPF. It seemed like this documentary could maybe help us get funding for our study should we discover anything interesting from my 80 per cent UPF diet (funders love to know that the research they've sponsored will be communicated widely). It would also be an opportunity to build relationships with potential research collaborators. So, I got in touch with Kevin Hall, the author of the paper that tested Monteiro's hypothesis to see if UPF did in fact cause weight gain.

I called Hall from a soundproof radio booth in Broadcasting House and asked him about his experiment. 'When I first came across this idea – that we should not be concerned about the nutrients in our food, but about the extent and purpose of the processing – I thought it was absolute nonsense,' he told me. It was a surprising start.

Hall was in his office in Bethesda, Maryland, where he is a senior investigator at the US National Institute of Diabetes and Digestive and Kidney Diseases. His somewhat bureaucratic job title – 'section chief: integrative physiology section, Laboratory of Biological Modeling' – belies the fact he's one of the major figures of twenty-first century nutrition science, despite not being a trained nutritionist. He's a physicist with a PhD in mathematical modelling – something called non-linear dynamics.

Born in Canada to blue-collar British parents – his father was a skilful machinist who built turbines for some of the first nuclear power stations, while his mother was an administrative assistant at a physiotherapist office – Hall was, like Carlos Monteiro, the first in his family to go to university. Hall excelled during his undergraduate physics degree at McMaster University, ranking near the top of his class in high-energy particle physics. He is characteristically modest discussing his achievements there: 'The guy at the very top found it all so effortless, I realised I'd need to find something I was better at.'

He got a summer job in an electrophysiology lab, studying how dog guts organise their contractions. It was there that he started building mathematical models of biological processes, which diverted him into the field of nutritional research, which he subsequently transformed.

'Depending on who you run into, I'm known for one of three things,' Hall told me. He laid these out neatly.

First, there is his mathematical model of adult human metabolism.[1] Using models like this Hall predicted several years ago that a low-carb diet would not have a significant effect on weight.

His next achievement was to test this model against the idea that had been growing since the turn of the millennium, that sugar was the main problem when it came to obesity. He did some of the defining work on how sugar affects our metabolism, which we'll look at later.

Then there was his '*Biggest Loser* study'.[2] For this, Hall followed the participants in the smash-hit American TV series, *The Biggest Loser*, for six years. They all started the programme with a BMI of greater than 40 – class 3 obesity (or, as it used to appallingly be known, 'morbid' obesity) – and were then isolated for several months on a ranch where they were subjected to a programme of extreme calorie restriction and exercise. At the end of the competition, mean weight loss was around 60kg. Six years later, mean weight regain was 41kg, despite participants maintaining high levels of exercise. Hall's study underlined the enormous difficulty in maintaining weight loss.

'And, finally, my work on ultra-processed foods ... I guess it's four things, in fact,' Hall said. This last study was why I was speaking with him. I certainly hadn't been expecting him to start by saying he'd originally thought that Monteiro's UPF theory was nonsense. He told me that he was at a conference, sitting next to a Pepsi executive, when he first heard about UPF. This was back in 2017, when a few papers on UPF were starting to appear: '[The Pepsi executive] said there was this new way of thinking about foods that they were concerned about, and they wanted to get my opinion on it. My initial response was: how could anyone take it seriously?'

From Hall's perspective, there had been decades of important progress in discovering which nutrients in our food supply are good (and bad) for us and how to cure diseases of deficiency. 'Nutrition science,' he continued, 'is called nutrition science because it's about the nutrients, right? And here comes this Monteiro group saying, "No, no, no, you've got it all wrong."'

He particularly didn't like the way Monteiro described UPF as 'formulations of mostly cheap industrial sources of dietary energy and nutrients, plus additives, using a series of processes and containing minimal whole foods'. He thought it was a fuzzy, unsatisfying definition that didn't say anything about what the problem with these foods actually was.

Hall had a few questions that he thought needed asking:

1. Isn't this 'UPF' bad for you because it's made of salt, fat and sugar and doesn't have much fibre? If that's the case, isn't UPF simply another way of saying 'high fat salt sugar'?
2. Or were these people saying it's bad because it displaces good food from people's diet?
3. Or was it a proxy for other things, like smoking and poverty?
4. Or was it some combination of these?
5. *Or* were Monteiro and his colleagues claiming that it was something else that was the problem? Something about the actual processing itself – the chemicals, the physical processes, the additives, the marketing and so on?

He asked the people who first told him about UPF (who were not part of Monteiro's team) for answers. They replied that the issue was the high salt, sugar and fat content, combined with a lack of fibre. At this point in our conversation, Hall became quite excited: 'I said, "Wait a second guys – you can't have it both ways! You can't say it's not about the nutrients and then, when I ask you for a mechanism, tell me it *is* about the nutrients: salt, sugar, fat, and fibre!"'

It seemed to Hall that the very idea of UPF was confused, so he decided to run an experiment to disprove the UPF hypothesis. He wanted to demonstrate that anything to do with processing made no difference at all – that the only thing that matters is a food's chemical, nutritional composition.

The experiment he devised was appealingly simple: he'd put two different diets head-to-head.[3] One would comprise 80 per cent NOVA group 1 food (stuff like milk, fruit, vegetables and so on), with some foods from NOVA groups 2 (kitchen ingredients like oil and vinegar) and 3 (processed foods including tinned goods, butter and cheese) but no UPF (NOVA group 4). The other diet would consist of at least 80 per cent NOVA group 4 foods – i.e. 80 per cent UPF.

Crucially, the diets would be matched with each other exactly in terms of salt, sugar, fat and fibre content, and the participants would be able to eat as much of the food as they wanted. All participants wore baggy clothes so they couldn't easily tell if they were putting on weight.

Twenty men and women of varying shapes and sizes with relatively stable weight were included in the study. The average age of participants was around thirty years old. These volunteers spent four weeks living continuously – twenty-four hours a day, seven days a week – in the National Institutes of Health's Clinical Center. Half started on the UPF diet, and half on what Hall called 'the unprocessed diet'.* After two weeks, they'd swap over, so that everyone would eat each diet for a fortnight. The UPF was bought from shops, a typical American diet. The other would be made using only whole ingredients by the research centre's talented pool of dieticians and in-house chefs.

'They looked at me like I was crazy when I said I wanted them to match the ingredients in the ultra-processed diet,' Hall recalled. In the supplemental information to the paper about the experiment, there's a detailed list of the meals, along with photographs of each of them. From the photos, the unprocessed diet looks appetising while the ultra-processed one looks to me, frankly, repellent.†

---

* This diet did actually contain some 'processed food' like cheese, pasta and so on, but no UPF.
† I asked Hall about this, and he said that lots of people preferred the look of the UPF diet.

Take day 5 lunch on the UPF diet for example: lunch was a spam sandwich accompanied by diet lemonade. The sandwich had been cut into triangles and mangled bits of spam were falling out onto the plate. Even the lemonade looks grey and sad, like dishwater. And the dinners were no better: two of the saddest, most withered-looking burgers, tinned grey-green beans, tinned sweetcorn, mac-and-cheese that looks like some sort of wound exudate – a relentless parade of dry beige and brown, exaggerated by the floral placemat on which the dishes are photographed. It made me feel constipated just looking at it. Because of the low fibre content of UPF, most meals had extra NutriSource fibre added to them.

By comparison, the unprocessed food looks like it might be the advertisement for a fabulous new restaurant. Lunch on day 1 was a spinach salad with chicken breast, apple slices, bulgur wheat, sunflower seeds and grapes. There's a vinaigrette dressing made with olive oil, fresh squeezed lemon juice, apple cider vinegar, ground mustard seed, black pepper and salt. Dinner was roast beef with basmati rice, steamed broccoli, a tomato side salad, balsamic vinaigrette, some orange slices and a scattering of pecans. Everything is presented like the cooking team's talents hadn't quite been exhausted by the food prep, so sliced meats are fanned out on the plate with little garnishes.

Whatever the photographs show, the participants rated the meals almost identically in terms of familiarity and pleasantness. No one ever managed to finish all their food. This is important. The test was very much like 'normal life' in the USA, where most people have access to as many calories as they like.

When the results came in, Hall was shocked. He had proved himself wrong and Monteiro right. On the grey, tinned, ultra-processed diet, people ate an average of 500 calories more per day than those on the unprocessed diet, and they gained weight in line with that. Perhaps even more surprisingly, participants actually *lost* weight when they were on the unprocessed diet, even though they could eat as much of it as they liked. As already mentioned, it wasn't that the UPF was more delicious, either. There was some other quality beyond 'deliciousness' that was driving the UPF group to overeat.

If anything, the study probably underestimates the effect of UPF. The UPF foods weren't marketed to the participants during the study, after all. There were no posters or health claims, and the food had been removed from its packaging covered in attractive photographs. In the real world, part of the processing is that packaging and the adverts, which are nearly universally for UPF. You almost never see an ad for beef or mushrooms or milk, and there are no health claims on their packaging. But you do see cartoon characters and vitamin-enriched claims printed all over UPF. I'll talk through the strong evidence that marketing, in all its forms, drives excess consumption later on.

Moreover, the study's participants didn't have to pay for or prepare their food. It cost Hall's team about $100 a week to provide 2,000 calories per day of UPF; for the unprocessed diet, the equivalent cost was more like $150. That's a massive cost saving with UPF. There is also a time saving, too. Hall underlined the skills of the centre's chefs. They can make any food, any way, but lots of people don't have the time to make fresh granola and chop four different fruits and vegetables for every meal, or to prepare little bowls of dressing and nuts. A fairer test would probably have been UPF set against the sort of unprocessed meal that most of us are able to make at home in a hurry. My attempts at home-made pizza usually end up involving microwaving cheese and tomatoes on toast (little surprise that Lyra prefers a frozen ultra-processed option).

The fact that Kevin proved himself wrong despite these factors makes his findings all the more robust. The impact of the experiment can't be overstated. The study, although small, was so well conducted that it provided tantalising evidence that Monteiro's theory may indeed explain the rise in obesity across populations. Hall's work gave a scientific heft to the NOVA classification system, and many scientists started to see it as a legitimate way of defining the category of food associated with obesity. It seemed like it might have the power to resolve the contradictory observations that had dogged nutrition research for so long: the confusion over fat and sugar, the failure of diet products to help with weight loss, the relentless increase in obesity around the globe. Hall's findings catalysed a massive new research effort and have been cited by hundreds of other scientific papers and dozens of policy documents.

Clinical studies like Hall's cost millions of dollars and can only be conducted in a few specialist centres around the world. But 'real world' epidemiological evidence to support Hall's experiment has continued to stack up. Since 2010, more and more evidence has accrued suggesting that UPF is very probably the primary cause of not only the rapid global rise in obesity, but potentially of all sorts of other health problems as well. What was once a trickle of evidence has become a deluge since Hall's study was published in 2019.

I was still on my diet when Rachel Batterham decided to bring someone into her research group specifically to look at this vast and growing body of literature on UPF, a young scientist called Sam Dicken. Sam trained at Cambridge and now has prestigious funding from the Medical Research Council.

I met him one day in Rachel's office at UCL which, by coincidence, looks across a courtyard directly into the clinic room where I treat patients each week. Sam had prepared a presentation of his research for me and, having put up the first slide, he began to talk. In total, he'd looked at around 250 papers – Sam's specific expertise is in these kinds of studies. He systematically addressed all those questions Hall had asked, and which likely occurred to you. As he got going, he spoke faster and faster and without pauses. It was as if he had no need for oxygen.

One of the main criticisms of the NOVA classification is that UPF is simply nutrient-poor food that's high in saturated fat, sodium and added sugar, which is why it causes ill health. Another critique is that, since people who eat lots of UPF eat less minimally processed food like fruit, vegetables, cereals, beans, legumes and seafood,[4] the association between high UPF intake and poor health could be because UPF is displacing good food from the diet. Perhaps if people simply ate UPF with lots of lentils and broccoli the effects would disappear? Or perhaps the UPF could be reformulated, with less sugar and fat and vitamins and minerals added?

There's also the argument that because UPF is, on the whole, pretty cheap, it could be that people who eat it in large quantities are more likely to have lower incomes, which is, tragically, very strongly associated with poor health. Adults and children in the most deprived regions of the UK have almost double the prevalence of obesity than those in the least deprived.[5] Could the real signifi-cance of UPF consumption be that it's a proxy for poverty?

Or could it be that, since unhealthy behaviours tend to go hand in hand, higher UPF consumption is a marker of an overall unhealthy diet or lifestyle? That is, might people who eat lots of UPF drink more or smoke more? In that case, it might look like UPF is the problem, when really it's the smoking and the drinking.

But epidemiologists like Sam are very aware of these problems. Sorting them out is their entire job. And, as Sam pointed out, a lot of work has been done to establish whether there is a real relationship between UPF and the medical problems it seems to cause.

Take, as an example, the large study of more than 100,000 people that was published in the *British Medical Journal*, which suggested a link between UPF and cancer.[6] The teams from France and Brazil looked at the risk of breast, prostate, colorectal and overall cancer, and found that, with a 10 per cent increase in the proportion of UPF in the diet, there was a roughly 10 per cent increase in the overall risk of cancer and the risk of breast cancer. This 'dose-dependent effect' is one factor that gives real strength to the evidence.

But that wasn't all. Because the scientists had access to data about the precise nutritional composition of the participants' diets, they were able to look at whether the increased risk of cancer was merely due to the fact that UPF tends to be high in sugar, salt and fat, and low in fibre. They also looked at whether it was simply that UPF was part of an overall dietary pattern that isn't healthy. In a way, they were answering those same questions that Kevin Hall had posed, but on a massive scale. Their finding was that, even after adjusting for nutritional content in this way, the result remained statistically significant. It looked, once again, like the nutrients were less of a problem than the processing.

'And that study isn't the only one to do that,' Sam told me, pulling up another paper, this one by a Chinese group who analysed data from 92,000 Americans.[7] When the researchers controlled for the usual things – age, sex, and so on (meaning that they took them into account to be sure that the effect of UPF wasn't simply that it is eaten by older people, for example) – they found that increased consumption of UPF is associated with increased death from cardiovascular disease. They then added controls for fat, salt and sugar, and the effect remained. When the researchers added still more controls to see whether UPF simply indicated a poor diet overall, never mind the fat and sugar, still the effect remained the same.

By now Sam was getting into a rhythm. Slide after slide flashed up, covered in such a density of numbers and data that they were almost overwhelming. All showed the same thing, supporting Hall's study: UPF isn't harmful simply because it's fatty, salty and sugary.

Rachel took over to underline the point and to give Sam a chance to breathe: 'Some people think that UPF is just lousy food in terms of nutrition and that it's eaten by people who eat generally poor diets. But when you correct for all that, the effects on death and depression and weight and heart attacks remain the same.' It *is* the ultra-processing, not the nutritional content, that's the problem.

Sam presented in detail on dozens of studies looking at over 50 different health-related outcomes. Even at his pace, it took almost two hours.* He meticulously went through how each study took careful steps to ensure that their findings about UPF were not due to saturated fat, salt, sugar or dietary pattern.

---

* This was in preparation for writing what would be the definitive review of reviews on UPF, to be published a month or so later.

And the data have been tested in lots of ways. Inevitably, most studies focus on obesity, but there is also evidence that increased UPF intake is strongly associated with an increased risk of:

- death – so called all-cause mortality[8–12]
- cardiovascular disease (strokes and heart attacks)[13–15]
- cancers (all cancers overall, as well as breast cancer specifically)[16]
- type 2 diabetes[17, 18]
- high blood pressure[19–21]
- fatty liver disease[22]
- inflammatory bowel disease (ulcerative colitis and Crohn's disease)[23, 24]
- depression[25]
- worse blood fat profile[26]
- frailty (as measured by grip strength)[27]
- irritable bowel syndrome and dyspepsia (indigestion)[28]
- dementia.[29]

This last one may be most alarming for those with a family history of dementia. In 2022, a study published in the journal *Neurology* looked at data from over 72,000 people.[30] Increasing intake of UPF by 10 per cent was associated with a 25 per cent increase in the risk of dementia and a 14 per cent increase in the risk of Alzheimer's disease.

These effects on so many different health outcomes are not slight. In a large Italian study, even after adjustment for dietary pattern, the quarter of participants eating the most UPF had a 26 per cent increased risk of death compared with the quarter eating the lowest.[31] A US study with similar adjustments also reported similar findings.[32] In a study of 60,000 UK patients, the risk of all-cause mortality was increased by 22 per cent.[33] In a Spanish study, the risk of all-cause mortality was increased by 62 per cent.[34] Effect sizes like these were typical across almost all the studies.

Sam pointed out something else important: because processing is not factored into our national guidelines, it's perfectly possible for someone to eat a high-UPF diet that is actually relatively low in fat, salt and sugar. Such a person's diet would be healthy according to the guidance, while according to the evidence it would probably cause health problems.

Take the Nutri-Score system, yet another traffic-light label used widely across Europe on food packaging. It ranks foods from high to low nutritional quality but fully a quarter of the so-called 'high-quality' foods are UPFs;[35] they are often plant based and reformulated to be low in fat, sugar and salt. So, you might be eating healthily according to the packaging and yet consuming huge quantities of UPF. This will be true for many people on diet shakes and drinks that claim to promote weight loss.

From the torrent of studies that Sam presented, together with Hall's clinical study, it seemed to me that the NOVA system explained health effects in a way that the traditional nutritional classification system couldn't. But it's important to note that the NOVA system has not been universally accepted.

There's a handful of papers that are critical. A well-known one, titled 'Ultra-processed foods in human health: a critical appraisal', was published in 2017 by the *American Journal of Clinical Nutrition*.[36]

The authors' main objection is that NOVA is crude and simple. This may be true, although I would argue that describing food in terms of three macronutrients and salt, which is what we currently do, is pretty simplistic as well.

The paper starts by asserting that 'Public health nutrition has been well-served over the past half century by the identification of potential dietary contributors to noncommunicable chronic disease.' I'm not sure that this is true. After all, obesity and metabolic disease rates continue to rise, and the standard nutritional approaches to food have done little to mitigate this situation. Reducing fat and sugar haven't solved the problem.

The authors soon get down to criticising the NOVA system directly, claiming that 'no arguments have been offered as to how, or if, food processing in any way constitutes a risk to consumer health through adverse nutrient intake or chemical or microbiological hazards'. That doesn't seem true to me, either. I have managed to fill several later chapters of this book with evidence about why and how processing affects health adversely. And there were dozens of papers published on this topic before 2017, which a 2021 review article has drawn together.[37]

In fact, the critique of the NOVA system doesn't really address any of the epidemiological literature at all. It's a commentary, not a formal review of the science of the kind that Sam wrote. The authors did manage, however, to dig out the one paper that failed to show a clear link between UPF and obesity.

So, why am I bringing this commentary up in the first place? Because of its 'conflicts of interest' section – the part of scientific papers in which the authors disclose relationships that may bias the results. There is an acknowledgement that one of the authors, Mike J Gibney, 'serves on scientific committees for Nestlé and Cereal Partners Worldwide', but the other authors declared that they had no conflicts of interest. Which is odd, because one author, Ciarán Forde, had previously spent many years in various food industry roles, most recently five years as a senior research scientist at the Nestlé Research Centre. Some of his research on child eating behaviour was partially funded by Nestlé and he sits on the scientific advisory council for Kerry Group plc, a food company with revenue of almost €9 billion that makes lots of UPF like Wall's sausages and thickened yoghurt lolly products called Yollies.* Forde did subsequently submit a correction approximately four months after publication of the article saying that he was, until 2014, 'an employee of the Nestle Research Center' and that he 'has received travel

---

* Wall's sausages: pork, water, rusk (wheat), vegetable protein (soya), potato starch, salt, dextrose, flavourings, stabilisers (diphosphates), spices, herbs, yeast extract, onion powder, herb extract (sage), preservative (sodium metabisulphite), antioxidants (ascorbic acid, alpha-tocopherol), casing (beef collagen). Yollies: cream, yoghurt, whey protein concentrate (milk), dried glucose syrup, sugar, strawberry purée from concentrate, starch, inulin, stabilisers (agar, locust bean gum, guar gum), calcium phosphate, natural flavourings, citric acid, colour (carmine), vitamin D.

reimbursement from Kerry Taste and Nutrition, and [that] some of his research on child eating behavior is partially co-funded by the Nestle Research Center'.[38]

In a way, this is small beer. You don't have to look particularly hard to find out that Forde worked at Nestlé. But the totally clear and transparent declaration of all interests is a bare minimum for credibility, and it's vital to understand whether the industry influences research outcomes (spoiler – it does).

This sort of influence is common. Another paper[39] that opposes the idea of UPF claims that 'NOVA fails to demonstrate the criteria required for dietary guidance: understandability, affordability, workability and practicality.' The paper is officially credited to Julie Miller Jones, but there's a statement tucked at the end about how the article was actually written: 'The concept and much background for the present paper resulted from work of the Ad Hoc Joint Food and Nutrition Science Solutions Task Force.'

It turns out that this 'Task Force' represented the Academy of Nutrition and Dietetics (whose sponsors include major nutrition companies like Abbott and BENEO, a subsidiary of the largest sugar company in the world), the American Society for Nutrition (whose 'sustaining partners' include Abbott, Danone, Mars, Mondelēz, Nestlé, PepsiCo and General Mills) and many more institutions with funding from companies that make UPF.

And, even if Jones had been the sole author, it wouldn't have been above reproach. She's a scientific adviser to companies like the Quaker Oats and the Campbell Soup Company and has written papers or given speeches for *CIMMYT* (the International Maize and Wheat Improvement Center in Mexico) and Tate & Lyle, the sugar giant.

Yet another paper critical of UPF and the NOVA definition, which argues that terms like UPF are more misleading than explanatory, was written by Heribert Watzke, who set up the department of food material science at Nestlé in Switzerland.[40] A paper that suggested that diets lacking UPF could also exceed the recommended number of calories was authored by Christina Sadler and colleagues.[41] Sadler and one of the other authors are employed by the European Food Information Council, which receives a third of its funding from the food and drink industry. Sadler's research is partially funded by Mondelēz and McCain Foods.

The involvement of UPF companies in challenging the association between UPF and poor health is unsurprising. But there is a wealth of data about the pharmaceutical industry, as well as other industries, showing that, when an industry funds science, it biases the results in favour of that industry.[42-47]

Of course, not every single paper critical of NOVA has identifiable conflicts of interest. But all the papers that are critical cite evidence from those written by authors with conflicts of interest, and none of them presents an explanation that begins to undermine the strong evidence that UPF is associated with poor health.

I'd been eating my diet for a week when I spoke to Rachel and Sam, and it already seemed clear to me that there is this category of food – never mind the individual items; I'm happy to acknowledge a huge grey area around the margin – that three robust sources of evidence link to ill health.

First, there is fundamental biological evidence giving plausibility to the connection. A growing weight of evidence suggests that some specific ingredients routinely used to manufacture UPF may be harmful, and that some of the peculiar characteristics of UPF (like its softness and its energy density) are associated with weight gain and ill health. We're coming to all this.

Then there is Kevin Hall's clinical study – small but watertight and conducted by a sceptic who is known for rigour. Finally, there is all the epidemiological evidence: dozens of well-conducted studies carried out independently of industry funding showing convincing links between UPF and a range of health conditions, including early death.

I now understood the evidence for the harms of UPF and, following my discussion with Paul Hart, the logic of why it has taken over our food system. But something Paul had said about the history of making synthetic fat sent me on a detour that I want to take you on too. I was in search of what would prove to be the definitive UPF, a substance that helped me to understand something entirely new about the universe of products on our shelves. I'll tell the story backwards.

4.

(I can't believe it's not) coal butter: the ultimate UPF

If you'd picked up a copy of the *New York Times* on 21 February 1989, you would have been met with what has to be one of the most arresting openers in the history of business journalism: 'A West German company suspected of playing a key role in building a poison-gas factory in Libya confirmed today that it produced and shipped an illegal drug known as ecstasy to the United States.'

The company in question was a German company by the name of Imhausen-Chemie. A spokesman confirmed that they had indeed manufactured and shipped the drug, but that they hadn't been aware that the substance was covered by West Germany's drug laws.

Of course, chemical companies make a range of molecules for other companies without necessarily being fully aware of their intended purpose, and ecstasy didn't enter the public imagination as a dangerous drug until the mid 1990s, so you might be inclined to give Imhausen-Chemie the benefit of the doubt. Or perhaps you would have been, but for the troubling mention of that poison-gas factory.

Just a month earlier, the same paper had run another story about the same company with this headline: 'Germans accused of helping Libya build nerve gas plant'. Imhausen-Chemie's president, Jürgen Hippenstiel-Imhausen (known as Hippi to friends and colleagues), acknowledged in an interview about *that* controversy that the company had sought a contract in Libya to manufacture plastic bags, but he denied any connection to what he called 'the plant presumed to be making chemical weapons in Libya'. (It turned out to be one of the largest chemical-weapons factories in the world, with a daily estimated output of between 22,000 and 84,000 pounds of mustard gas and nerve agent.)

Hippi was not the type to back down, and certainly not the type to make things easy for his communications team. He declared that the company name had been misused: 'Everything has been based on suspicion and rumours. Libyans don't have money to pay for things like that. We totally deny any involvement. The Libyans are much too stupid to run a plant like this. All the Arabs are lazy and they call in foreign slaves to do the work.'[1] The following year, he was sentenced to five years in prison. The prosecution depicted Hippi as 'the supreme salesman of death'.

And yet, remarkably, this episode wasn't the ugliest in the company's history. Not by a long way. For that we need to go back to 1912, when Hippi's wife's grandfather, Arthur Imhausen, took over a soap company and began making chemicals,[2] including explosives, during World War 1. After the war, the company's new soap, improbably named Warta, became popular throughout Germany.

At the same time that Warta was flying off the shelves, two scientists at the Kaiser Wilhelm Institute, Franz Fisher and Hans Tropsch, were working on a process to free Germany from reliance on foreign oil, which it needed for tanks, planes and cars.[3] Germany lacked its own oil but it did have vast deposits of low-quality coal – stuff called lignite that was only around 30 per cent carbon.

The Fisher-Tropsch idea was simple enough: they'd smash coal with steam and oxygen to turn it into carbon monoxide and hydrogen, because those are the basic ingredients you need for making a near-limitless range of useful molecules. Next, they'd pass the gases over a catalyst which would cause the carbon, hydrogen and oxygen to recombine into liquid fuel. They gradually perfected the method*

---

* In 1925, they made a breakthrough. Using zinc oxide (the same stuff you find in sunblock and nappy rash cream) they made methanol, the simplest alcohol. Then, with the simple addition of some iron and cobalt, more complex molecules could be made.

so that by the early 1940s, nine production sites were producing 600,000 tons of fuel per year from coal. This process left behind a by-product, something called 'slack wax' or 'Gatsch', the substance we know as paraffin.[4]

Arthur Imhausen, who was still doing great business with Warta, heard about the paraffin waste and thought he might be able to put it to good use for the Nazi party, of which he was a member. His idea was founded on the fact that, as well as fuel, Germany was short of edible fat. By the 1930s, the country was consuming around 1.5 million tons of fat per year but was only able to produce about half that amount domestically. They depended on importing linseed from South America, soybeans from east Asia and whale oil from the Antarctic.[5, 6] Imhausen was working on techniques to turn paraffin into soap and realised that, because soap is chemically a lot like fat, if he could make one, he could make the other.*

He contacted Wilhelm Keppler, a politician, and a key figure in linking German companies up with the Nazi regime.[7] Keppler was in charge of a specific aspect of the plan to make Germany self-sufficient: creating self-sufficiency in industrial fats and oils. He listened eagerly to Imhausen's proposal to make edible fat from the paraffin by-product of turning coal into liquid fuel.[8]

Imhausen partnered with Hugo Henkel, inventor of Persil, and they founded the Deutsche Fettsäure Werke in 1937. This merged with IG Farben, a vast German chemical giant, and by 1938 they were making high-quality fatty acids. From there, it was a simple step to add glycerine, and so produce 'Speisefett' – edible fat.

The Speisefett was white, tasteless and waxy, and still felt a long way from butter. But that was a trivial problem for a chemist like Imhausen. Buttery taste comes from a chemical called diacetyl,

---

* Both start with a molecule called a fatty acid, a long chain of carbons and hydrogens with a couple of oxygens on the end of it. React the fatty acid with an alkali, you get soap. Combine it with glycerine, you get triglyceride – the fat in animals and plants.

which is still used as flavouring in microwave popcorn.* Mixing the
fat with diacetyl, water, salt and a bit of beta-carotene for colour
allowed Imhausen to complete the transformation of German coal
into 'coal butter' – the first totally synthetic food.

Keppler was delighted and wanted to turn the achievement into
confidence-bolstering propaganda. But there were two problems.
First, Imhausen's mother was Jewish. Back in 1937, when the
Deutsche Fettsäure Werke was being put into operation, Keppler
had written to leading Nazi Hermann Göring to ask whether he
was sure he wanted to take part in the inauguration considering
the fact that Imhausen was of 'non-Aryan descent'. Göring asked
Hitler about it, who allegedly replied, 'If the man really made the
stuff then we'll make him an Aryan!'[10, 11]

And so it was that Göring wrote the following to Imhausen: 'In
view of the great merits you have rendered in the development of
synthetic soap and synthetic cooking fat from coal, the Führer, at
my suggestion, approved your recognition as a full Aryan.'[12–15]

So that was the first problem taken care of. The second problem
was the coal butter's safety: if it was going to be food for troops, it
couldn't impair their performance.

In 1943, Imhausen authored an article in *Colloid and Polymer
Science* with the title: 'Fatty acid synthesis and its importance for
securing the German fat supply'.[16] The article described in great
detail the process for the manufacture of synthetic fat, and made
oblique reference to the safety testing: 'Thousands of tests, led by
Director Prof Dr Flössner, confirmed the high value of synthetic
cooking fat and made it the first synthetic food in the world to be
approved for human consumption.'

Otto Flössner was the chief of the Physiological Department of
the Reich Working Group for Public Nutrition. And though it's true

---

* Workers in the factories that manufacture popcorn get a disease that destroys
their lungs, which is officially called bronchiolitis obliterans but is also known
as 'popcorn workers lung'. Diacetyl has also been detected at very low levels in
some vape liquids.[9]

that he did extensive testing on the synthetic fat, what is less well referenced is the context of the experiments, which were conducted on more than 6,000 prisoners in concentration camps.[17-19] *

Ultimately, the regime approved the fat for human consumption, although, after World War 2, British Intelligence uncovered data that the Nazis had not publicised: the fact, for instance, that some studies had shown that chronic ingestion of the synthetic fat caused severe kidney problems and decalcification of bone in animals. Dogs, apparently, refused to eat it.[20, 21] The fat was used by U-boat crews in the North Atlantic, and because, towards the end of the war, the average U-boat crewman lived for only sixty days from boarding the ship, long-term safety data were possibly not considered relevant.

The synthetic butter plant that Imhausen had run in the Ruhr valley was discovered by the Allies after the war. A report in the *Chicago Tribune*[22, 23] shows the giant machinery stopped mid-production, a foot-wide sausage of fat protruding from the mouth of the extrusion machine. Enormous cylinders of synthetic butter lie coiled in an aluminium tub. A British official is quoted: 'It is excellent butter and I doubt that anyone ever would guess it was synthetic.'

The transformation of coal into butter reveals the unavoidable problems of creating synthetic foods. There are inherent dangers in consuming complex mixtures of novel molecules as a source of calories – substances we have never encountered before may have unpredictable effects on our physiology. This means that they require extensive testing in humans and animals which, unless there is no other way of producing food, is, at best, ethically questionable. And to make these synthetic foods appealing to a wide public they seem to require fraudulent marketing, whether it's about the ancestry of the inventor or the health benefits of modern

---

* The results of these tests were presented at a conference held in Berlin in 1944. The participants included nutrition experts like the 1938 Nobel Prize winner for chemistry Richard Kuhn, and of course Flössner. The vote was unanimous in favour of continuing the experiments.

additives. But, most of all, the story of coal butter seemed to me to reveal something about the nature of corporations.

After the war, the occupying Allied powers permitted Imhausen-Chemie to continue operating, and installed Arthur Imhausen as president of the Association of German Chambers of Industry and Commerce.[24] His son Karl-Heinz (Hippi's father-in-law) took over the chemical company, which, in various forms, continues to exist. The original soap company changed hands a few times and is now part of Evonik Industries,* one of the world's leading specialty chemicals companies.[25]

And Evonik isn't the only inheritor of Imhausen's companies. You'll remember that his initial partner was IG Farben, perhaps the most notorious of the German companies. During World War 2, it operated a synthetic rubber factory at Auschwitz, the workforce comprising entirely slave labour. The Zyklon B gas used in the same camp was produced by an IG Farben subsidiary, Degesch.[26–28] † More than any other corporate entity, it was instrumental in supporting the Nazi war effort. Many employees went on to hold positions at the companies that IG Farben was broken into, which are still household names: BASF, Bayer and Hoechst (now part of the French company Sanofi).[29–32]

The breakup of IG Farben left behind a publicly traded shell company that was intended to give victims an entity against which to make reparations claims. After an initial payment of around $17 million in the 1950s, the company never paid any more compensation, refusing to join a national compensation fund that was set up

---

* Evonik have on their website a large section about their involvement in the 'National Socialist era'. Among other things, the company organises trips to Auschwitz for its employees to help them understand holocaust history and come to terms with the roles played by Evonik's predecessor companies.

† It is widely agreed that management and employees knew about these and other activities of the company. After the war, twenty-four IG Farben employees were put on trial. Half were acquitted, and the longest sentence was just eight years.

in 2001 to pay others who had suffered. The company's lawyers blamed former slave workers for holding up the dissolution of the company.[33, 34]

The company's shares were listed on the Frankfurt stock exchange from the end of the war until 2011. So, these companies both do and don't exist depending on whether you are trying to trade the stock to make money (when they do exist) or trying to get compensation for slave labour (when they don't). But the wealth generated by the companies does very much exist somewhere.

Hippi – the snappy-dressing grandson-in-law of Arthur Imhausen – was released from Bruchsal prison on a sunny Monday in spring 1993.[35–37] The public prosecutor calculated that he had earned around 90 million marks in the 1980s from the deal with Libya. He owed German tax authorities around 40 million marks – around $25 million. But Hippi had put his PhD in economics to good use in an arms race against the law. Using what the prosecutors described as a 'giant money carousel', comprising Swiss hub accounts and five shell companies registered in Liechtenstein, the money disappeared.

***

It was while researching all of this that I started to understand these corporations as organisms in an ecosystem powered by money. Railing against the companies that are the direct descendants of the regime feels futile: shame and outrage are clearly inadequate to limit the survival of companies that are complicit in atrocities. And the ecosystem idea seemed to explain why: their behaviour changes only when the flow of energy, the money, is diverted. Shame *may* interrupt the flow of money, but if it doesn't it will serve no practical function to limit corporate behaviour.

It turns out that economists use the same set of equations to describe corporate survival in economic arms races as ecologists use to explain the survival or extinction of species in biological arms races. Companies and groups of living organisms (species, families and so on) are subject to the same laws whether their ecosystem is powered by money or energy.[38-42]

I feel like there is another more slippery idea about the effect of making food from coal, or indeed through any industrial synthetic process. It destroys the meaning of food beyond the ability to sustain life (however temporarily in the case of coal butter and the U-boat sailors). Food must become a technical substance, without cultural or historical meaning – nutritionism at its most extreme.

This certainly seems to be the case judging by a 1949 paper by Hans Kraut. Published (and still available for download) in the *British Journal of Nutrition*,[43] 'The physiological value of synthetic fats' is one of several papers cluttering the scientific literature that cites Flössner's experiments without mentioning they were conducted on concentration camp prisoners. The author goes on to make the case for the ongoing production of synthetic fat:

> Heavy workers cannot take in enough calories unless a fair proportion of them is in the form of fat … This is especially important for those working the long shifts of modern industry without a rest pause for a full meal. The increase of fat consumption in all industrial countries during the last 100 years is, therefore, not a matter of taste only but a necessity of modern life, so I think it a good thing to continue research on synthetic fat.

Here is the inexorable logic of all industrial food: to reduce the time workers require for a meal. I think about this every time I see a lunch-break meal deal. UPF crisps, UPF fizzy pop, UPF sandwich.

When I interviewed the Brazilian team who came up with the definition of UPF and have done so much work on the concept, I asked them about their own eating habits. They all talked specifically about lunch. They laboured the fact that they sit down for lunch every day and eat rice and beans. When I worked in Brazil, I did this too. In the modern world, eating lunch at a table is a sign of health and a good life.

In the past few decades, the replacement of traditional food with UPF has happened at a nearly unimaginable pace in terms of our evolutionary history. This is concerning because, in the hierarchy of biological life's activities, eating (along with reproduction) is right at the very top. Almost everything else we all do is in the service of these projects. To understand the effects of UPF, I had to go back in time and ask questions that had never much bothered me before: what exactly is 'eating' and how exactly have we evolved to do it? Let's head back to the very beginning, when rocks were food, to what I term 'the first age of eating'.

PART TWO

But can't I just control what I eat?

5.

The three ages of eating

I find it helpful to think of eating as something that has happened in three distinct but overlapping ages, all of which are still going on today.

In the first age of eating, living organisms began to eat stuff that has never been alive, like rocks and metal. This process has continued since the dawn of time to the present day. During the second age of eating, living organisms started to eat other living organisms, perhaps after some processing. This has been going on for hundreds of millions of years (and for around 2 million years for humans).

During the third age of eating, a single species (and their pets and livestock) started to eat UPF, which is manufactured using previously unknown industrial techniques and novel molecules. By comparison, this age is just a few decades old. This is why it is useful to consider the effects of UPF by thinking them in the context of the very long history of how we stay alive.

Let's go back to the very beginning.

The Earth is approximately four-and-a-half billion years old. The first 700 million or so of those years were an exciting time – a constant bombardment of asteroids, including one the size of a planet that made the moon. The earth's liquid core constantly turns over the surface, even now, so the evidence of these impacts has been lost, but to get a sense of the totality of the bombardment you only need to look at the moon's cratered surface. Not for nothing are the first half-billion years known as the Hadean period.

However, the term 'Hadean', which conjures images of a hellscape of boiling lava, may not be completely accurate. Not much is left of the early Earth's surface, but a few tiny crystals of zirconium silicate, discovered in Western Australia, give us a clue that conditions may have been milder than previously thought. These 'zircons', dating to around 4.4 billion years ago, betray the presence of liquid water, suggesting that oceans may have formed within 150 million years of the birth of the planet.[1]

They would, admittedly, have been pretty hot. The dense carbon dioxide atmosphere of the early Earth would have created a lid of pressure meaning that, despite being liquid, the oceans might have been superheated to over 200°C. So, Hadean to an extent, but certainly not a sea of liquid rock. And the atmosphere would also have been more benign, too, made up mainly of gases from volcanoes – carbon dioxide, nitrogen and sulphur dioxide. Oxygen was the main thing missing.

Another of those Australian zircons dating to 4 billion years ago contained traces of something even more surprising: carbon with a 'biogenic' signature* – the first indirect evidence of life.[2]

We're confident that single-cell organisms had emerged 3.5 billion years ago. The clues are small but unmistakable: microfossils in a band of iron in northern Canada, the remains of stromatolite microbial colonies with life-like carbon in south-west Greenland, matts of bacterial deposits in Western Australian sandstone.

By 3.2 billion years ago, life was replicating and changing the geology of the earth, creating features the size of counties, huge bands of iron, hundreds of square kilometres in area, deposited as waste by early bacteria.[3-6] The largest of the bands of iron are found in Australia, and they provide clues about the first age of eating, which began with the emergence of this first life.

At the time, the oceans were full of dissolved iron released by underwater volcanoes, and this iron was food for early bacterial life. Whereas we breathe in oxygen, these bacteria took in carbon dioxide. Rust was the waste product released. Those giant striped bands

---

* There are several different types of the element carbon, and these different types are used in particular ratios when proteins are made by cells.

of iron, which provide the metal for so many objects we see around us, are probably vast deposits of bacterial excrement.[7-9]

If you find the idea of metal as food challenging, don't worry. It's all to do with atoms.

Everything is made of atoms, which in turn are made of protons and electrons.[*] Different elements have different numbers of protons and electrons, which gives them their different properties (some elements are clear gases, others are black solids, etc). But each element must always have an equal number of protons and electrons. Oxygen has eight protons and eight electrons. Carbon has six protons and six electrons. But not all atoms are happy with their lot.[†] Carbon, for example, would like to give away electrons, while oxygen is desperate for some more.[‡] These unhappy atoms can get together and share so that both become happier – it's a perfect marriage that forms carbon dioxide. At the ceremony, some energy is given out – this is the chemical reaction that runs a car.

It's easy to imagine that when Lyra becomes tearful in the late afternoon that she is a bit like a car running out of fuel. And the fundamentals are the same. Lyra takes electrons from her food

---

[*] And neutrons, which don't have a charge and so largely don't affect the chemical behaviour of an atom.

[†] Some chemists would rather not use words like 'happy', but others don't mind. At the subatomic level, words have rather fragile meanings. The system behaves as if they have these desires so, as an approximation, I think they are acceptable words.

[‡] This donation of electrons is known as oxidation. Oxygen wants electrons, it turns out, just exactly the right amount for life to exploit. It is not, despite its name, the most powerful oxidant: oxygen will ask politely for an electron, whereas other gases like fluorine or chlorine will tear away an electron of pretty much any other atom without asking. That's why they are such potent toxins – breathe in chlorine or fluorine and they will oxidise (grab electrons from) everything in your body. By a happy accident of chemistry, oxygen can burn all organic matter on the planet, but it needs a spark to do so. In cells, enzymes provide this spark to allow the reaction to happen in a controlled way and energy to be usefully extracted.

(carbon atoms in say a slice of pizza) and passes them to oxygen from the air she inhales, breathing out carbon dioxide. In the car there is a bang produced by this reaction, but 'life' is all about making sure the energy released is extracted more carefully.

Inside nearly all Lyra's cells, electrons are plucked from pizza carbon atoms (in the sugar molecules from the wheat flour) by little proteins. These proteins hand the electrons down a cascade of other proteins in little organs inside her cells called mitochondria. As electrons hop along these proteins, they move like little pumps filling the mitochondria like a balloon with electrical charge. This creates a voltage of 30 million volts per metre, roughly equivalent to the voltage that drives lightning between the sky and earth. At the final protein the electron is handed to oxygen without any fire or smoke.

The balloon of the mitochondria is now full of electrical charge, but it has little pores, tiny mills that allow the charge to escape, driven by that enormous voltage. As it flows out, energy is extracted by these mills to make a new molecule, ATP, which is then used to power every reaction in every cell in your body. Add an ATP to a protein and DNA is replicated, a pore opens, a muscle contracts, a cell moves. A single cell uses around 10 million ATP molecules every second. Per gram, our mitochondria produce 10,000 times more energy than the sun.

And that, as they say, is life. All life. From bacteria living on volcanic vents on the ocean floor to my fingers typing these words on my keyboard, that's what is happening: life captures the energy released by passing electrons from food to breath.* So, food can be anything that wants an electron less than breath does.

Thus, at some point in the first few hundred million years of Earth, geochemistry became biochemistry, and the first age of

---

* You can now say sagely to people, 'Life is nothing but an electron looking for a place to rest,' a quote from the Hungarian Nobel prize winner Albert Szent-Györgyi. If you want to understand this better and don't want to do a degree in biochemistry (or if, like me, you have forgotten the biochemistry you once knew), then read *The Vital Question* by my UCL colleague Nick Lane.

eating began, with single-celled organisms eating rocks to make life. We now neatly separate geochemistry and biochemistry into separate departments, often in different buildings, but there's no exact moment when the chemistry of rocks became the chemistry of life. Yet, like all blurred boundaries, it is still a boundary: life is very different to not life. As with classifying food, there is a line to be drawn.

That first age of eating, in which the food has never been alive, continues today. Bacteria are still eating rocks, and we are still trying to understand the fundamental processes. But at some point, perhaps when access to resources like raw iron became too competitive for comfort, a shortcut evolved: let someone else get the energy from the rock or the sun, and then eat them or their waste products instead. Since that first shortcut, all animals have built their bodies in the same way: by eating other life. That's the second age of eating, the age of eating food.

Exactly when this second age began isn't clear, and the scientific literature is entertainingly rancorous. In a series of papers and published correspondence, dry academic language barely conceals fury over whether markings on rocks half a billion years old are due to active feeding behaviour by an ancient animal or were made instead by stones attached to the holdfasts of kelp in shallow water, or by wrinkled eucalyptus leaves being dragged over sand by wind-generated waves.[10, 11]

But there is general agreement that one day, around 560 million years ago, a little creature did crawl slowly through some mud at the bottom of the sea at the edge of the ancient continent of Rodinia.[12] About as long as your finger, it was flat and oval, with a pattern of ridges radiating away from a central ridge. Enlarged, it would make an attractive design for a rug. Though it lacked a skeleton, limbs, eyes and anything but the most basic nervous system, by the standards of the day it was fabulously complex, the apex of billions of years of evolution. The mud was itself alive, as all mud is: sand bound together by the secreted slime of countless single-celled organisms. As the 'rug', which would later be named

Dickinsonia costata, crawled over this microbial mud, it left a little trail behind it and sometimes little tunnels where it dived in before surfacing again.[13, 14]

Lots of creatures were doing the same thing that day, no doubt. But this one gets all the glory because it was killed suddenly, and something about the circumstances of its death – being covered almost immediately with a layer of preserving dust or ash – and the geological events of the next half a billion years, meant that it was preserved and waiting to be discovered in 1946 by a man called Reg Sprigg, a geologist working in the Ediacara Hills in South Australia.[15]

The movement of the 'rug' through the mud is described in one scientific publication as 'moderately complex interactions with microbial mats to exploit nutrients and oxygen resources'. What it really is, though, is the first recorded trace of eating's second age.

These little *Dickinsonia* rugs remind us that to eat is to be part of an ecosystem. As well as eating, they were preparing other life to be eaten and they were ecosystem engineering – actively changing their relationship with the sediment they lived in, moving it around, ploughing it like soil, fertilising it with waste. These were among the first creatures to be in arms races with each other, competing to extract the energy from the system.

***

There was a whole lot more complexity to come as the second age unfolded. During this period, the evolutionary arms race for energy changed our ancestors from single-cell to multicellular organisms, and from there into primitive fish, and then, via the shrew-like creatures that survived whatever it was that killed off the dinosaurs, into you and me.

Eating evolved into a much more complex process than we tend to credit it with being. It had to fulfil two separate needs at the same time: providing the energy we need to stay alive and providing the construction materials, the elements and molecules, that we need to make our bodies.

All living matter on earth is made up almost entirely of just four elements: oxygen, carbon, hydrogen and nitrogen. In humans and other mammals, they account for around 99 per cent of the atoms in the body. But another twenty or so elements are known to be vital ingredients too. And, since we can't make them ourselves, we need to eat them.

Beyond the big four, my body contains about a kilo of calcium and a kilo of phosphorus.* Then there's around 200g each of sulphur and potassium, 120g each of sodium and chlorine, and about 40g or so of magnesium. Besides those, I contain just under 5g of iron – a small nail's worth to turn my blood red and my snot green – a few milligrams of fluorine to keep my teeth hard, and zinc for making DNA, building proteins and for all sorts of immune functions.

The last few elements keeping me alive weigh less than a gram combined: strontium, found mainly in bones, iodine, essential for making thyroid hormone, copper, for the function of a huge range of enzymes, then almost immeasurably small amounts of manganese, molybdenum and cobalt. Deficiency of any one of these can be deadly, but excess can be just as toxic.

That's a list of very precise requirements, and it shows how tricky the project of eating is for all complex organisms. But whereas humans can try to figure out the science and measure things out precisely, animals just have to get on with it. If you're a carnivore, then another animal has done the hard work for you – cows are made of basically the same stuff as the animals that eat them. But life for a herbivore is very different. Herbivores have to chase the rain, avoid the carnivores and eat the right amount of, for example, selenium. How do they do it?

To understand this, I went to visit Eddie Rixon, a fourth-generation Oxfordshire beef farmer. Eddie lives on a hill in the middle of his farm with three generations of his family and around a

* For the nitpickers – because there is a difference between mass of different atoms, I am about 1.5% calcium by mass but only 0.2% of my atoms are calcium atoms.

hundred cows. If it sounds idyllic, that's because it is – although he did work continuously while we spoke, filling bags with feed and inspecting the cows' feet.

Eddie emphasised the complexity of his cows' eating habits: 'Many of the plants that herbivores, including my cows, eat are full of toxins, as well as energy and nutrients. The cow has to precisely balance the energy intake with the toxin load, as well as getting the right amount of nutrients.'

In their arms race with the plants, cows have had to evolve incredible detoxification mechanisms. Toxins are destroyed by the bugs in their guts or by powerful enzymes in their livers, or are removed entirely by their kidneys. But cows also learn about each of the plants as they eat. They taste a little, remember the taste and smell and link that memory to the effect on their bodies. Eddie's cows constantly add to a memory bank of how plants interact with their bodies – how much energy was released in the form of sugars and protein, whether the toxins made them nauseous, and so on – and they can even learn which plants work well in combination.

Because it's a mistake, as Eddie pointed out, to think that cows and other herbivores just eat grass and not much else. Instead, by copying their mothers and trialling small quantities of different plants, herbivores build up an extraordinarily diverse diet.[16, 17] In some studies, scientists have put holes in the necks and stomachs of free-ranging goats and cattle (this sounds extreme, but animals tolerate this well and the procedure is performed under anaesthetic). This allows the scientists to collect and sample exactly what the animals choose to eat.[18] These studies have indicated that they are often eating between twenty-five and fifty different plants in a day, with all the chemicals in all those plants interacting with each other and memories of the whole lot being recorded for future reference.

As Eddie and I spoke, the cows came over to the edge of the field to greet us, sniffing and blowing, submitting to a scratch behind the ears. Eddie keeps his hedgerows deliberately diverse: 'If you watch the cows, you'll see them eating different plants from the edge of the field. We don't understand exactly what they're doing, but they are making purposeful decisions.'

For example, worms (in the gut, not in the soil) are a big problem for cows. Many of the plants that Eddie grows in the hedges contain tannins that kill gut worms, which means that he can use fewer deworming drugs. This is also good as deworming drugs kill earthworms, thereby reducing the health of the soil.

Tannins don't just kill worms: they can bind and neutralise other toxins. Eat a starter of tannin-rich sainfoin, a perennial with large pink flowers, and the tannins will neutralise the toxic terpenes in a main course of sagebrush. The tannins in a mouthful of bird's-foot trefoil can bind to and inactivate the toxic alkaloids in fungus-infected tall fescue. There are thousands or possibly millions of these combinations. [19, 20]

Perhaps the most remarkable thing about cows is the fact that they can't digest the main source of energy in plants: the structural sugars like cellulose, xylan and pectin. These aren't digestible by any mammals. Instead, we recruit bacteria to do the job for us. I am referring to the microbiome, the trillions of bacteria, fungi and other microorganisms that live on and inside us. Most of these microorganisms are found in our guts where, whether you're a cow or a human, they do pretty much the same thing. (We'll explore the effect that UPF has on the microbiome later, which is potentially one of the ways in which it causes harm.) The cow microbiome is so crucial to its survival that you could invert your idea of a cow and think of it as simply a vehicle for its own microbiome, a four-legged vessel transporting the microorganisms to the plants of their choice. Once you've done that, you can imagine yourself in the same way.

Cows spend a lot of time grinding up plants, before holding the plant material in bacterial fermentation chambers, where bacteria break down the starch and fibre, creating energy and waste molecules called volatile short chain fatty acids. You'll have heard of some of these in other contexts – the bugs in your own gut make most of them too.

Acetate is the main acid in vinegar. Propionate is used as a food preservative. Butyrate is used as a food and perfume additive. Valerate is found in the medicinal plant valerian and used as a food additive to produce meat flavour. The cow can use these fatty acids for energy and to build its body (we can too). Cows and all ruminants live on the waste products of the bacteria in their gut.*

The arms races of the second age, between organisms competing to eat and avoid being eaten drove fabulously complex systems like the microbiome. I left Eddie's farm with a new respect for the complexity of the herbivore project and a head full of thoughts about how humans differ from cows, and every other form of life in terms of our eating habits.

For almost all the second age of eating, across all different species, food has been consumed raw, fresh and often still alive. Then, around two million years ago, a single species started to externally process its food: smashing, grinding, milling and – most importantly – cooking.

Today, it's widely accepted that cooking is crucial to what makes us human. This might seem obvious now, but just a few years ago, a significant number of anthropologists were still claiming that cooking was of purely cultural significance. To my mind, the matter might have been settled with a simple eating contest using a raw steak and potatoes. But it was resolved more scientifically in 2007 when a team including Rachel Carmody and Richard Wrangham at Harvard tested this hypothesis in … pythons. Burmese pythons in fact.[21] (Why they used pythons isn't explained in the article, which is in all other respects almost excessively detailed.) The pythons were fed raw beef, cooked beef, raw ground

---

* The fact that some of these are used as food-processing agents as well as made inside your own body doesn't mean they're harmless. In the human body, these molecules are released in precise places at precise times, and eating lots of them won't have the same effects.

beef, and cooked ground beef. Cooked ground beef made energy 25 per cent more available, which was not all that surprising.* With this experiment, Carmody and Wrangham persuaded almost everyone of their hypothesis that the human digestive tract extends out of the body and into the kitchen.† Heat and mechanical processing are not just a part of our culture – they're a part of our physiology.

This need to cook means that we occupy a unique dietary niche. A 2015 paper proposed that humans were the only cucinivores – animals obliged to cook.[22] In fact, we are the only processivores: we don't just need to *cook* food, we also need to *process* it. Since prehistory, we've been grinding, pounding, fermenting, drying, salting, cooling and burying food. Our bodies bear witness to the long history of food processing.[23] It's evident in the number of genes we have for enzymes to digest starch, milk, sugar and alcohol, and in the size of our eating apparatus: our teeth, jaws and gut are tiny compared to other mammals, around half the size compared to our

---

* Muscle proteins start to break down at just over 40°C – one of the reasons heatstroke is so dangerous. And at around 70°C, all the chewy connective collagen – the sinews and tendons and ligaments – starts to melt into a gel, making the meat easier to shear with teeth. Beyond that, cooking also kills the parasites that infest meat and that can exert a huge energetic cost on their host. There is no other carnivore that can avoid these parasites, which gave the early humans who mastered fire a spectacular advantage over all the other animals wanting to eat herbivores.

† Wrangham hypothesises that *Homo erectus*, with its small molars, mouth, stomach and large intestine, must have had controlled fires more than a million years before the earliest recorded evidence of hearths and controlled fires (200,000–400,000 years ago at the Qesem cave in Israel). Hearths with evidence of cooking of similar age have been found in Africa, France, Spain, China and Britain. But Wrangham's theory is compelling. With its long legs and the shape of the torso, *Homo erectus* was probably not an adept climber. Chimpanzees use tree nests primarily because of leopards, and the predators of the ancient savannah would make a modern leopard look like my cat Winston. Fire would have been essential predator deterrent for non-climbing early hominids.

weight.[24] Processing is necessary for our survival and has made us human,* and so is part of the second age of eating.

The second age continues all around us. You can shop at a supermarket and continue being a second-age organism, by buying meat, fruit and vegetables – although of course it will be expensive and time consuming. Most of the humans in the UK and the US have entered what I call 'the third age of eating', in which most of our calories come from food products containing novel, synthetic molecules, never found in nature.

The Anno Domini is a matter of debate.

1879 is a candidate year. A postdoctoral chemist called Constantin Fahlberg was working in a lab at Johns Hopkins University. A subsequent interview with *Scientific American* in 1886 described him as tall, well-built and handsome. A memorial bust on his cenotaph in Germany seems to bear this out: he looks every inch the nineteenth-century industrialist, with a furrowed brow, immaculate hair, beard and waxed moustache. At the time of the interview, he was a big celebrity but remained, according to the interviewer, 'diffident and reserved'.

Fahlberg was trying to produce medical compounds from coal tar, a black sticky liquid that is the toxic byproduct of coal processing. It's still used in shampoos and soaps to treat psoriasis and fungal infections. I use one to treat my own dandruff, with variable success, although it certainly leaves me smelling like freshly laid tarmac. No one is sure how coal tar works, but its effects are probably due to the fact that it contains huge quantities of toxins: phenols, polycyclic aromatic hydrocarbons and other poisons. In small doses, these kill unwanted human cells and pathogens. In large doses, they are well evidenced to cause cancer.

Versions of the story of Fahlberg's discovery have him licking his hands in the lab, but this isn't quite accurate. I suspect even

---

* There is a fad for raw diets – they don't generally go well according to the evidence, leading to extreme weight loss and fertility problems.[25]

nineteenth-century chemists were more careful than this – although just barely by his own account:[26]

> One evening, I was so interested in my laboratory that I forgot about supper until quite later then rushed off for a meal without stopping to wash my hands. I sat down, broke a piece of bread and put it to my lips. It tasted unspeakably sweet. I did not ask why it was so, probably because I thought it was cake or sweetmeat. I rinsed my mouth with water and dried my mustache, and to my surprise the napkin tasted sweeter than the bread. It flashed upon me that I was the cause of the singular universal sweetness and I accordingly tasted the end of my thumb and found it surpassed any confection-ery I had ever eaten. I saw the whole thing at a glance. I had discovered or made some coal tar substance which out-sugared sugar. I dropped my dinner and ran back to the lab and in my excite-ment tasted the contents of every beaker and evaporating dish on the table. Luckily for me, none contained any poisonous or corro-sive liquid.

Fahlberg had created saccharin, the first artificial sweetener and, because of the sugar shortages caused by World War 1, the first entirely synthetic compound to be added to our diet on a large scale. It is 300 times sweeter than sugar and is a triumph of syn-thetic chemistry. Fahlberg became immensely rich. It's still used today – if you've ever been to a restaurant or motel in the USA, you'll have noticed the familiar pink packets of Sweet'N Low on every table.

The invention of saccharin fell in the middle of a new era of syn-thetic food chemistry. Work on synthetic carbohydrate had been underway for more than half a century. An 1885 paper begins by asserting that the study of modifying starch has attracted more workers than any other area of chemistry.[27] Over the next century, thousands of new molecules entered our food.

And we eat massive quantities of them. In industrialised coun-tries like the UK, each of us ingests 8kg of food additives per year.

When I read this statistic, it didn't seem possible. To put this in perspective, on average we only buy 2kg of flour per year for home baking. But this is all consistent with Carlos Monteiro's observation: that we are purchasing ever fewer raw ingredients, as more and more of our food is industrially prepared and processed.

Clearly, eating 8kg of synthetic molecules per year, not to mention the synthetically modified fats, proteins and carbs, is troubling, but most additive anxiety is misplaced, as I'll come to later. The main point is not that they are themselves harmful, it's that the additives are a proxy for UPF. They signal a method and purpose of food production that we now know is linked to disease. The individual ingredients of UPF may each be harmful, but it is in combination that they do the most harm. I call the consumption of UPF the third age of eating because it is such a recent change from our evolutionary past.[28]

***

Even if you continue to eat whole and minimally processed foods, as humans have for millions of years, you will eat with much more nutritional awareness than people who lived even a few hundred years ago.

Eating has become, in part, an intellectual rather than a purely instinctive project. Many of us consider calories, portion size, good food and bad food, vitamins, etc. Eating purely by instinct, in the way that a cow does, rather than trying to follow the advice of food packaging or nutritionists is an approach nearly unimaginable to many people. The idea that humans might have an internal system just like Eddie's cows that allows us to self-regulate and balance our diets seems unlikely considering how little we are trusted by the authorities to eat without guidance. Could humans really leave eating up to instinct?

The first credible scientific answer to this question was worked out with the help of three infants called Donald, Earl and Abraham in 1928. They were the subjects of one of the most important, and least celebrated, nutritional studies of the twentieth century, which was conducted by a Chicago paediatrician called Clara Davis.

Davis must have been a remarkable person, although we don't know all that much about her. She was one of ten women to graduate from her medical school in 1901 and, by 1926, she was working at the Mount Sinai Hospital in Chicago and worrying about how doctors advised parents to feed their children. For the whole of the second age of eating, children of all mammals had eaten more or less what adults ate. There might have been some extra mashing and softening, and perhaps a little less spice, but there was no 'baby food' – just milk, then food.

However, by the 1920s, feeding a child had morphed into a quasi-science in the USA. 'No one can satisfactorily prescribe food for an infant who does not have knowledge of the composition of that food,' declared an article in the *Journal of the American Medical Association*.[29] American mothers were routinely given eating lists based on the latest nutritional science, but the children did not seem to care about the data and refused to eat the food. It became such a problem that the majority of visits to paediatricians during the 1920s were about fussy eating.[30] The profession responded sensibly … by advising parents to let children go hungry and to treat them 'firmly'. Alan Brown's 1926 book, *The Normal Child, Its Care and Feeding*, provides a good example: 'Force is necessary for children who spit out their food or those who vomit at will. Give such a child a small amount of the food, if he vomits give him more; continue until he keeps the food down.'

Davis disliked this authoritarian trend. She knew that there was no evidence for this approach from history. She also knew that wild animals seemed to maintain their health without being told what to eat by science. She felt that doctors should be listening to what children tried to tell them, instead.

But that wasn't Davis's only concern. She was also worried about the modern food of the 1920s in a way that still feels modern nearly 100 years later. In one paper she describes the 'poor nutrition in infants that were weaned onto the pastries, preserves, gravies, white bread, sugar and canned foods that are commonly found there on the adult table'. She thought such foods were 'incomplete and altered', and observed that they 'formed no considerable part of the diet a hundred years ago'. Indeed, she suspected that those more highly processed foods might be behind many of the eating problems she was seeing as a clinician.[31]

Somehow, Davis managed to persuade a number of mothers to place their children in her laboratory for months at a time – and, in one case, for more than four years – to take part in the longest-running clinical trial of eating that's ever been conducted. The plan was simple but quite revolutionary. Davis would let the infants choose their own food and then measure if they could be as healthy as infants who were fed 'prescribed' diets using the best nutritional advice of the time. She chose children who had been exclusively breastfed up to the very start of the experiment, so that they had 'no experience of the food or of the preconceived prejudices and biases about food'.

Her hypothesis was that, since the human body has internal regulatory mechanisms for water and oxygen intake, heart rate, blood pressure, body temperature and every other physiological variable, the same should be true for body composition and nutritional intake.

Earl Henderson was the first subject whom Davis recruited. Nine months old and the child of a 'thin, undernourished young woman whose diet had not been optimal for lactation', he had spent almost his entire short life indoors. He was poorly on admission, with swollen adenoids, a mucus-y nasal discharge and a ring of bony lumps on his chest wall – the characteristic 'rickety rosary' rib deformity of vitamin D deficiency. Yet this sickly nine-month-old was given total control over what he ate ('The experiment would ask whether he could manage his own gastronomic affairs').

Earl would have thirty-four different food items to choose from each day, all prepared by the kitchen on the ward, that would 'comprise a wide range of animal and vegetable food procured fresh from the market. Only natural whole food. No incomplete or canned food.'

This is the full list (notice that there's hardly any processing of any kind – not even any cheese or butter):

- meats (muscle cuts): beef (raw and cooked), lamb, chicken
- glandular organs: liver, kidney, brains, sweetbreads (thymus)
- seafood: sea fish (haddock)
- cereals: whole wheat (unprocessed), oatmeal (Scotch), barley (whole grains), cornmeal (yellow), rye (Ry-Krisp)
- bone products: bone marrow (beef and veal), bone jelly (soluble bone substances)
- eggs
- milks: grade A raw milk, grade A raw whole lactic milk (similar to yoghurt)
- fruits: apples, oranges, bananas, tomatoes, peaches or pineapple
- vegetables: lettuce, cabbage, spinach, cauliflower, peas, beets, carrots, turnips, potatoes
- incidentals: sea salt.

As I researched Davis, I made a record of what I feed Lyra (three) and Sasha (one). I try to get variety into their diets, but I seldom manage even ten different foods.

For each meal, Earl and the other subjects would be presented with twelve food items, and always milk, fermented sour milk and salt. The individual foods were put in separate bowls, never mixed. The nurses got careful instructions: they couldn't offer the food to the children; they could only give them the food they indicated that they wanted. They were also told not to signal disapproval or approval, and to remove the tray only after the boys stopped eating. If the boys finished a particular food at a meal, then they would be given more of that food at the next.

Earl was admitted to Clara Davis's ward and, for three days, he was exclusively breastfed by his mother. Detailed measurements were made: a physical examination, blood counts, urine, calcium and phosphorus levels. His bones were X-rayed to determine density. 'On the fourth day, breastfeeding was discontinued and the experiment proper begun.'

It's hard to imagine how traumatic it must have been for Earl and his mother at first. Perhaps he was so hungry that having his mother replaced by nurses who were able to give him adequate nutrition meant he didn't mind. None of this is recorded, and this did trouble me as I read about the experiment.

Davis described Earl's first meal – how he 'looked at the tray for a few seconds', then reached 'for a dish of raw carrots, and plumped the whole of a hand into it'. But it seems one handful wasn't enough. 'Back went his hand into the dish,' over and over, 'until most of the carrots had been eaten.'

Davis was pleased. 'Within three days, he had tried almost all the articles,' she wrote. 'He had answered our first question: he could and would indicate his choice of foods ... and would eat an adequate amount.'

A further twelve infants were recruited over the next few years, and they all settled into the diet just as enthusiastically. Almost all of them tried everything they were offered at least once, and their appetites were 'uniformly good': they often greeted the approaching food trays 'by jumping up and down in their beds'. Once they were at the table, they devoted themselves steadily to eating for fifteen or twenty minutes, then ate intermittently, 'playing a little with the food, trying to use the spoon and offering bits to the nurse'.

The night after I read this, I was at the table feeding Sasha and noticed that, just like Davis's kids, she often offers me a chunk of food, even as I feed her. That Davis includes this detail reassures me that she was really there, watching and caring, not just supervising from a distance.

The food in Davis's experiment was unsalted, but each child got a dish of salt with every meal. They would eat this with their hands spluttering, choking or even crying after putting it in their mouth, but frequently went back for more, 'with a repetition of the same spluttering'.

The experiment was an enormous success. There were just two children who wouldn't eat lettuce, and one who wouldn't try spinach. All the infants succeeded in managing their own diets, and all met their nutritional requirements as if they'd been reading all the latest textbooks. Their average calorie intake was found to be within the limits set by nutritional standards of the day, and they were free of all the usual feeding-related problems that are still staples of paediatric practice today. None of the infants had colic, discomfort or abdominal pain after eating. They were never constipated. In fact, no infant went for two consecutive days without a stool. In fifteen children, over many months, that statistic is simply staggering. And there was no fussy eating, either. All had hearty appetites and all, to use Davis's word, 'throve'.

Perhaps the best argument for internal nutritional regulation concerned Earl's rickets. He'd arrived with the condition, in which the bones become soft and weak. There are X-rays of his little hands in the paper, taken when he first arrived, good enough to see the reduced bone density and the loss of the hard outer cortex of the bone.* The growth plates at the ends of the bones are indistinct and fuzzy, and in an accompanying photograph, Earl looks bowlegged and distressed.

So, Davis immediately proposed a treatment for Earl: 'Bound by a promise to do nothing, or leave nothing undone, to his detriment, we put a small glass of cod liver oil on his tray for him to take if he chose.' Cod liver oil was, at the time, the only edible source of vitamin D.† Over the first three months of the experiment, Earl drank the little cup of oil 'irregularly and in varying amounts' until his

---

* Incidentally, you can also see the bones of the hand of the adult holding the child – a reminder of how long ago this was, before anyone knew the hazards of X-rays.

† We get most of our vitamin D from sunlight, which causes it to form in the skin.

blood calcium and phosphorus reached normal levels and his X-rays showed that the rickets were healed, at which point he stopped drinking the stuff entirely. After it went untouched on the tray for more than a fortnight, the nurses stopped offering it.

The other children followed that same pattern, too. Whatever problem they arrived with, once they were allowed control of their nutrition, according to Davis, they all quickly reached optimal health. All ate immense, varied quantities, but in strange and unpredictable ways. They would all go on what the diet kitchen called 'jags' – egg jags, cereal jags, meat jags and so on.

It's a pattern I see in my kids. Lyra loved tomatoes as she was weaning, and would eat a dozen small ones every day for weeks at a time. And then one day she stopped, and inexplicably refused tomatoes for months. I'd cook them and hide them in her food, but she always spat them out. She'd happily eat cat faeces in the flower-bed, or a handful of carpet fluff, so it wasn't conventional disgust. She just didn't want tomatoes – until one day she started up again. Twenty a day. Boom and bust.

When I first started reading about Davis's experiment, I had a few questions about her motivations and her ethics. After all, these were all poor children with mothers in desperate situations – was it in some way exploitative? But, as I read on, a character of sorts emerges far more than it would from modern scientific papers. It seemed clear to me that she cared about the children deeply and she eventually adopted two of the first boys she looked after, Donald and Abraham, who remained close throughout their lives. Donald's widow remembered her mother-in-law as having huge love for both of them.[32]

So, what exactly should we take away from Davis's experiment? There's a danger of misinterpreting it – to take 'Let kids eat what they like' as the conclusion. But Davis was very clear this should not be the verdict – adults need to teach children what to eat to avoid poisoning and so forth – but she did think that, once safe food is established, we should recognise that children should be learning to self-regulate their eating in response to what they need, sending signals back and forth between the brain and the gut. She thought a lot about those food jags, which she felt may be at the root of so much 'fussy' eating, and suggested that this behavioural tendency could be the result of a complex internal juggle. She proposed that, 'as supplies of different food factors are depleted, an increased appetite for foods that will furnish them results.' And she took this reasoning a step further: 'Such an explanation would predicate the existence of a center for appetite and would be wholly theoretical.'

The last line is such an intriguing thought, and Davis expanded on it: 'The accuracy with which selective appetite in the babies of the experiment met known nutritional requirements suggests that appetite is another of the many self-regulatory activities whose functions are preparatory to cellular nutrition, geared to its needs, and require neither nutritional knowledge nor direction from the mind.'

Davis was proposing that humans, like Eddie Rixon's cows, are able to vary their diet precisely, according to what we need – that we too have the apparatus to eat without any knowledge of nutrition in a way that will allow us to construct and maintain our bodies. Perhaps I missed it, but the system that controls this was not mentioned in my six years at medical school.

6.

How our bodies really manage calories

The legacy of the half billion years or more of the second age of eating is an internal system that precisely regulates food intake. Species that eat other life have been solving two simultaneous problems with extraordinary precision for a long time: eating the right amount of all the essential micronutrients while at the same time eating exactly the right amount of energy.

The part of the system that regulates energy intake – and thus body fat – is the part we understand best. Weight is tightly regulated, and each species has a fairly uniform percentage of body fat. It may vary through the year with hibernation, migration and pregnancy, but it is internally controlled like everything else about the bodies of all animals.

Humans have a natural body composition that is fattier than most other land mammals. Male elephants carry around 8.5 per cent body fat and females roughly 10 per cent.[1] Apes, such as chimpanzees and bonobos, have less than 10 per cent body fat.[2] By contrast, even hunter-gatherer human populations have body fat percentages of around 21 per cent in women and 14 per cent in men.[3] Obesity is rare in human populations that still live in the second age of eating, even when food is abundant, and wild animals (also part of the second age of eating) don't seem to develop obesity either.*

* While I was writing this book, various friends sent me articles that proposed varied causes of obesity: several of them reported that animals are also gaining weight. Two of the pieces referenced a paper by David Allison: 'Canaries in the coal mine: a cross-species analysis of the plurality of obesity epidemics'.[4]

In fact, this study examined groups of animals from eight species that don't represent wild populations. The paper provides no evidence to suggest that

Of course, human obesity did exist during the second age, and it *is* ancient. So, before we go any further, let me clear this up. The Venus of Willendorf is a figurine representing a female body with a high percentage of body fat, carved some 20,000–30,000 years ago. There is evidence that the sculptor was not working from imagination, but may have been depicting themselves.[7]

Several members of the Ptolemaic dynasty, which ruled Egypt from 305 to 30 BC, were purported to be obese to such an extent that their breathing was disrupted at night. Alexandrians gave Ptolemy VIII the nickname 'Physcon', meaning 'large bubble'.[8] The writings of ancient Greece, Egypt and India all acknowledge the presence of obesity and metabolic disease. And the Old Testament, the New Testament, early Christian writings and the Talmud all reference obesity – almost always negatively.[9] Portraits and paintings from the last few hundred years often have representations of obesity. In 1727, the British physician Thomas Short wrote that 'No age did ever afford more instances of corpulency than our own.'[10]

All these instances pre-date the advent of UPF. But increased body weight was extremely rare, and all but unheard of in children. In many contemporary human societies in the third age of eating,

---

widespread human obesity is directly caused by anything other than the rise of UPF. David Allison is an academic at the University of Alabama which has been widely reported as having extensive links with Coca-Cola. In 2008 and 2011, both the *New York Times* and *ABC News* reported on David Allison's funding by Coca-Cola, Kraft, PepsiCo, McDonald's and the American Beverage Association.[5, 6]

This funding may have no influence on what he publishes, but a recent publication of his 'French-fried potatoes consumption and energy balance: a randomized controlled trial' is an example of how industry-funded science frequently makes discoveries that align with the interests of the funder. The study was supported by a grant from the Alliance for Potato Research and Education (APRE). This is from the conclusion: 'Results do not support a causal relationship between increased French-fried potato consumption and the negative health outcomes studied.'

most of us have body-fat percentages on par with those of famously fatty sea mammals. Blue whales have one of the highest percentages of any wild animal at around 35 per cent, and – spoiler alert – by the end of my diet I was getting close to this proportion. So, while there has been some human obesity for a long time, it is the rapid increase in body weight in the vast majority of countries between 1900 and the present day, especially since the 1970s, and the increasing prevalence of children with obesity, that is the focus of much of this book.

But, despite the fact obesity has been rare until relatively recently, the idea that there is a system that regulates body weight for humans, or for any creature, is a relatively new idea. For a long time, many doctors and scientists, myself included, had assumed that humans' percentage body fat had previously been lower because food had generally been hard to get hold of. In this model, we have evolved to find food rewarding and desirable, and so we are driven to consume as much as we can. So, in an age of abundant, safe and delicious food, weight gain is an inevitability.

But this idea – that weight is regulated externally by the supply of food – would make weight an exception among physiological parameters. Consider, for example, the amount of water in your body. It may feel like it's under your conscious control and indeed you *can* choose to have or delay a drink, but over the course of your life the amount of water in your body, and thus the concentration of the hundreds of thousands of dissolved chemicals that make you up, is precisely controlled internally, even as you drink, sweat and pee. The conscious control of fluid balance is temporary at best and largely an illusion. And the case of breathing is more obvious still if you try to stop doing it. Food intake is under little more conscious control than breathing or drinking, and this is why it is nearly as hard to limit food intake as it is to limit water or oxygen intake. What, when and how we eat is determined by complex systems that operate far below our conscious level.

***

There is a dizzying complexity to how wild animals maintain a healthy body weight while balancing nutritional needs. We owe rats a heavy debt for their role in helping us to figure it out.

In 1864, a German physiologist named Paul Bert joined two rats together so that they shared a common blood circulation. It didn't involve great technical skill. He simply removed strips of skin from the flanks of each animal and stitched the rats together. As the wound healed, blood vessels naturally grew from one rat to another so that they became a 'parabiotic pair'.

Grim, yes, but it did allow scientists to tease out the effect of things in the blood. In an early experiment, one rat of a parabiotic pair was fed sugar, while the other wasn't. Both developed high blood sugar – although only one developed tooth decay, showing that it was sugar in the mouth, not the blood, that rots teeth. In other experiments, old mice were joined to young mice, which extended the life of the older and shortened the life of the younger.*

Nearly a century later, in 1959, an English physiologist called G. R. Hervey began a series of experiments using the parabiotic pair technique to understand weight control. The study is tough reading. Ninety-three pairs of rats were sewn together, only thirty-two of which survived long enough to be used in the experiment.[13] These rats then had a small electric probe inserted into their skulls, which was used to specifically damage a part of the brain called the hypothalamus. If you were to stick a finger directly into your nose and push it through the bone at the back there, you'd end up touching your hypothalamus. The hypothalamus maintains homeostasis in the body, controlling temperature, water intake, how much you sweat and so on.

Hervey found that the rats with a damaged hypothalamus lost control of their eating and often developed obesity. So, he started damaging the hypothalamus of just one rat in each parabiotic pair

* Those experiments ultimately gave rise to a number of Silicon Valley start-ups that tried – unsuccessfully – to extend the lives of ageing billionaires by giving them the blood of young people.[11, 12]

and, if anything, the results got even more horrifying. The rats with the damaged hypothalamus ate so much so quickly that they sometimes died by choking on their food: they were no longer able to detect the 'stop eating' signals coming from their bodies. Meanwhile the other rat – entirely normal apart from being attached to the rat with the hypothalamus lesion – started wasting away. It *was* getting a signal through the shared circulatory system telling it to stop eating.

This was the first strong evidence that there is a feedback mechanism for weight, just as there is for every other system in the body. Hervey's findings suggested that animals have a 'correct' physiological weight and body-fat percentage, just as they have a 'correct' blood pressure, temperature, sodium levels and so on.

We now know that one of the signals that told the rats to stop eating is a hormone called leptin, which is produced in the fat tissue and detected by the hypothalamus in the brain.[14] Leptin is also a hormone that should subtly alter how we think about the fat on our bodies. There's a tendency to consider fat almost as dead tissue – a layer of lard, an expandable tank of fuel – but really it's a sophisticated endocrine organ, producing a range of hormones that act on the brain to regulate body weight.

Leptin is one of several hormones involved in long-term control of weight. It lets the brain know how much fat there is on the body. When leptin secretion falls, it's a starvation signal, causing wide-ranging effects on different parts of the brain that drive increased food intake. If a person has a high body-fat percentage, then leptin should tell the brain: 'Lots of fat to be going on with, here. No need to be too food-focused.'

Leptin and other hormones are involved in the long-term control of food intake, but there's also a system for short-term control. Your liver, pancreas, stomach, small intestine, large intestine, microbiome, fat tissue and many other organs all detect sugars, fat, protein and other molecules in the gut and the blood after you've eaten. They send signals to – and receive signals from – the brain via a network of nerves, blood vessels and hormones. There is a dialogue between organs, which constantly chatter away inside you about what you should eat, when to eat it, and when to stop.*

These long-term and short-term systems are about the somewhat mechanical regulation of food and energy, the amounts of fuel and nutrients required for basic function. But their descriptions in the scientific literature often omit the conscious experience of eating. It's only fairly recently that scientific papers have begun to describe eating as a process that involves pleasure, or using words like 'reward', 'delicious' and so on. These are terms associated with another system, after all – the hedonic system, mixed up with the ancient circuits that drive us to want and like and enjoy things.

Understanding how the regulation of fuel and energy interacts with pleasure brings us to the emotional interface between our conscious experience of the world and the workings of our body as a machine. It's at the border between philosophy and science.

We know that these two systems – the one that guides eating for pleasure and the one overseeing eating to gain nutrition and fuel – are intimately linked through a chain of evolutionary pressures extending back hundreds of millions of years. The primitive fish that were our distant ancestors 300 million years ago seem to have already had a version of the same reward circuits that motivate so much of our behaviour today.[15]

For a long time, even the scientists studying these systems felt that the two were in competition with each other: hunger and

---

* Before you even start to eat, your stomach secretes a hormone called ghrelin – the 'hunger hormone' – which flows in the blood to a part of the brain called the hypothalamus and tells it to start eating. Ghrelin stimulates the 'wanting' neurons, too – the dopamine ones in the limbic system. As the food makes its way into your intestine, still more hormones get released. There's cholecystokinin, which sends a nerve signal to the unconscious centres of the brain at the top of the spinal cord, which in turn pass the message on to the hypothalamus, making you feel physically full. Then there's peptide YY and glucagon-like peptide 1, which flow in the blood to the hypothalamus and reduce the joy of eating, and a whole host of other catchily named hormones and neurotransmitters that act in concert to determine food intake. And that's before we get to the hormones secreted when you fast or starve.

reward increase intake, while the feeling of fullness reduces intake. This way of thinking quickly leads to the assumption I had always made – that, if food is delicious enough, it simply overrides the system that's desperately trying to tell us we're full. It's the 'I'll-actually-puke-if-I-eat-one-more-slice-oh-go-on-then' problem.

But is that *really* the problem? Unbelievably delicious food?

Kevin Hall – he of Bethesda, Maryland, and the Monteiro-proving experiment – previously felt like I did – that it was just a case of deliciousness triumphing over fullness. Hall suspected that ultra-processed, highly rewarding or addictive foods simply override the homeostatic system inside us. He doesn't think that anymore. He explained his former thinking to me with an analogy – a beautiful and appealing explanation of how we can't cope with UPF, but one that he now thinks is wrong.

'Imagine a small house in northern California. It will have a small heater, suitable for the mild winters, and a thermostat. The temperature rises and falls from summer to winter,' Hall said. 'The thermostat and the furnace work together, switching on and off according to the outside temperature. The house stays the same temperature all year round.'

This house with a heater suitable for the climate is like a human body, or any body, during the second age of eating. Food is sometimes plentiful and sometimes in short supply. The system maintains the necessary intake.

'But then,' Hall continued, 'let's say I pick this house up and move it to Edmonton in northern Canada.' Edmonton has notoriously grim winters and has particular significance for Hall – he lived here during a tough few years, flying frequently and working remotely for a company that seemed to be going under. 'In Edmonton, the furnace is still working perfectly well and the thermostat is set to a comfortable temperature, but there's just no way it can compete with the environment. The furnace is on all the time, but the temperature outside is so extreme and so cold that the house can't help but get cold too.'

The weather is too cold, so the house gets cold.

In this analogy, when we're surrounded by extremely delicious food, we gain weight, just as when our houses are surrounded by extremely cold weather, they become cold. It's an argument that certainly makes some intuitive sense, but Hall is no longer happy with it: 'I don't think that's how it works anymore.' He didn't have an elegant analogy about how he thinks UPF *does* disrupt our energy intake system. 'Now, I think that somehow the food environment – the UPF – somehow resets the thermostat, or bypasses it, or perhaps just breaks it completely.'

Hall's theory is not simply that UPF food is delicious and so creates 'hedonic overdrive', where we enjoy eating more than we hate being full. Instead, it's that the new UPF food environment is affecting our ability to self-regulate.

And indeed, while exactly *how* our current food system breaks or bypasses our evolved method of regulating weight is unknown, an increasing number of studies are showing that every aspect of UPF disrupts our multi-million-year-old network of regulatory neurons and hormones.

Hall's theoretical-physics instincts have led him to start joining up the thinking. Along with others (like Sadaf Farooqi and Stephen O'Rahilly at Cambridge), he has brought a number of the ideas and studies into something that gets near a grand unified model of weight regulation: the energy balance model. In a 2022 paper,[16] Hall and his co-authors start to describe the connections between the hedonic areas of the brain and the nutrient-detection areas, where our emotional conscious experience meets our internal physiology.

Perhaps this connection can be best understood by the almost daily sensation for many of us of being unable to stop eating even though we want to. Something in the food, or in the signals in the blood or in the brain is in conflict with another area. Frequently the physical and nutritional fullness don't seem adequate to override the circuitry of desire.

It's not just the food itself that influences these processes. We know that all those external cues to eat – advertisements, shop fronts, price, packaging, smells – have significant effects on our brains and bodies that we're only just beginning to understand.

The model emphasises that powerful signals inside and outside the body influence food intake and energy balance far, far below the level of consciousness, involving slippery related ideas like salience, wanting, motivation and reward. We smear a conscious layer over all this, but eating is far less of a choice than it appears.

This is one of the many reasons why simple advice like 'Eat less and move more!' is ineffective for sustained weight loss. It's as crazy as saying 'Drink less water!' to someone who's feeling thirsty.

We don't just get hungry and eat. We're controlled by ancient neuroendocrine feedback systems, which evolved to ensure we consume everything we need to pass on a few genes. The system is intricate, complex and in some senses extraordinarily robust. But for many of us, it is unable to cope with novel food presented constantly in a novel way. The system didn't evolve to handle the concoctions that arrived with the third age of eating.

And yet I still had some lingering doubts about whether UPF really was the *main* cause of rising obesity levels. There are so many other possible causes that many of us have come to accept as obvious, such as individual responsibility or our increasingly sedentary lifestyles. And of course, sugar. Surely the fact that we eat so much more sugar than we used to must have something to do with global weight gain?

7

Why it isn't about sugar ...

How UPF subverts this system of weight control in lots of ways is coming up in part three. But for the last 20 years there has been another culprit blamed for the rise in the number of people gaining weight: sugar. This chapter is about why sugar and carbohydrates are not to blame.

Gary Taubes is probably why you're aware of the idea that carbs are the problem. He's also probably why you've heard of keto diets (high in fat, low in carbs) and might even have tried to cut down on sugar and other carbohydrates (like starches which quickly become sugar in the body).

When I first read his work as a medical student, Taubes seemed to me like the Galileo of nutrition – the archetypal genius heretic. In a movie of his life, Taubes could play himself. Now in his fifties, he has the same physique that he had on the Harvard football team as a physics undergraduate. He went from there to Stanford to study aerospace engineering – literal rocket science – because he wanted to be an astronaut, but his height and self-professed difficulty with authority diverted him into journalism.

For someone who became one of the most influential voices in nutrition this century, he had a decidedly slow start. By 1997, age forty-one, he'd written two well-received books about the history of science, but was still working freelance and struggling to pay his rent. Then he started writing about public health with a piece on salt and blood pressure. This harnessed his full range of character traits, from his desire to push against authority to his obsessiveness about detail and data, and robustly challenged one of the mainstays of conventional medical advice – that salt is bad for blood pressure.

He won a Science in Society Journalism Award for the piece. At the time it inspired me to use as much salt as I wanted (more or less), and its success inspired Taubes to turn his attention to dietary fat.

He spent a whole year writing an article called 'What if it's all been a big fat lie?' for the *New York Times*, which became one of the most-read articles of 2002. It arrived at a moment when people seemed ready for a new take on their weight. Perhaps it's always that moment, but Taubes had the charisma and credentials to catalyse a movement. Obesity levels had been growing year on year, and the previous four decades of global dietary advice – to avoid fat, especially saturated fat – didn't seem to have made any difference. During the 1980s, the number of US children with overweight tripled, and there were a growing number of reports of type 2 (diet-related) diabetes in children, especially among Indigenous communities.

According to Taubes, the establishment believed that eating fat was making people fat. And, although the extent to which that's true is debatable,* there is something intuitively satisfying about that argument. Fat, for one thing, does contain more calories per gram than protein or carbohydrate. And the diets of those with obesity did seem to contain large quantities of fatty food. Yet even as the idea that fat was to blame became more widely publicised during the eighties and fat was increasingly replaced by sugar in people's diets, still the population continued getting larger. It seemed the advice was all wrong.

---

* Many people felt that Taubes had overplayed the strength of the orthodox belief. It's not really clear that nutritional advice was ever given in the way he asserted. The US surgeon general's report, which advised cutting down on fat, was edited by Marion Nestle, one of the most important, thorough and respected figures in global nutrition for the past five decades. She was clear that the report never said to avoid fat – it simply acknowledged that fat contains more calories than protein or carbs and so fat will be fattening unless you limit other sources of calories. Whether or not the 'low fat is good' dogma was in fact the orthodoxy, Taubes is right that, by the turn of the century, it was widely acknowledged that, in both clinical and real-world trials, low-fat diets had broadly failed to have a significant impact on participants' long-term weight.

Taubes proposed an alternative – what he still calls the 'heretic' low-carb hypothesis:* Robert Atkins had been right all along.

You'll likely have heard of Atkins, who published *Dr Atkins' Diet Revolution* in 1972, recommending a virtually zero-carb diet.†

Taubes' alternative hypothesis runs something like this: Americans (and everyone else) are eating more because they're hungrier, and they're hungrier because of the hormone insulin. Insulin is secreted into the blood by the pancreas, and removes sugar from blood and allows it to enter cells as fuel. If you eat carbs, your blood sugar starts to rise, but insulin brings it back down to normal. When insulin is high, like after a meal, it reduces appetite and turns sugar into fat for storage. When insulin's low, like when you haven't eaten in a while, you start burning fat instead.

The idea is that, when we eat lots of carbs, they cause a rapid spike in our insulin levels to cope with the sugar. The spike not only promotes the storage of fat, but it drops sugar levels to lower than they were before the meal. This starves our muscles of energy, meaning that we're less active as well. Moreover, the fact that the muscles feel starved sends signals to the brain to consume more food. And when it's high, insulin suppresses appetite but when it crashes down after the spike you also feel hungry. Taubes suggests that, if we avoid carbs, the opposite will happen: our insulin won't spike, we'll store less fat, our energy expenditure will go up and our appetite will go down. But insulin has a huge range of other functions in multiple body tissues, and there are many other

---

* Again, how heretical this stance really was is debatable. For example, even Taubes acknowledges that Walter Willett, who was then the chair of the Department of Nutrition at the Harvard School of Public Health – hardly a counter-culture figure in the diet world – had undertaken a $100 million study on nearly 300,000 people which contradicted the 'low fat is good' message.

† Atkins was a controversial figure, not least because he seems to have had at least one heart attack and when he died after a fall he weighed 117kg (more than 18 stone) according to the *Wall Street Journal* and a leaked medical examiner's report.

hormones in the mix that help determine whether we store fat or whether we burn fat or protein or carbs for our fuel.[1]

There were always huge holes in the evidence that sugar might be the sole cause of overweight and obesity. Taubes' theory depended on the idea that, since a low-fat diet had been recommended, everyone had not only been eating more sugar, but also been eating less fat. Taubes used low-fat yoghurts as an example, because they were often sweetened with sugar and thickened with carbs to make them palatable. He quoted US Department of Agriculture economist, Judith Putnam, about increases in carb consumption: that, between 1980 and 2000, the average person increased their annual grain consumption by 27kg and their annual sugar consumption by around 14kg.

However, although it was true that Americans had been eating more refined carbohydrates, they had not been eating less fat. They'd been eating more. According to the US Department of Agriculture, consumption of fats had increased between the late 1970s and the publication of Taubes' article in 2002. In a report on Taubes' piece published by the Center for Science in the Public Interest, Putnam stated that she had explained all this to Taubes, but he had selectively quoted her.[2]

Taubes presented the possible causes of obesity as a dichotomy: fat or carbs. Other possible explanations – exercise, the role of industry, processing, air quality, or some combination of all these things – were brushed aside.

Before long, the idea of sugar as *the* dietary problem had become practically orthodox, and Taubes was determined to prove it. He devised an experiment that would become one of the most influential in the recent history of nutrition, although not in the way Taubes expected. In 2012, he partnered with a charismatic Canadian physician called Peter Attia and together they set up NuSI – the Nutrition Science Initiative – and raised millions in funding. The plan was to solve the problem of obesity in the USA. They would conduct a series of experiments to demonstrate, once and for all, that calories from sugar promote weight gain more than calories from fat.

To their credit they recruited excellent scientists who were sceptical of the whole hypothesis. One of these scientists was Kevin
Hall. The NuSI approach was an adversarial one, somewhat like a
court case. The funders expected different outcomes to the experimental scientists, but they all agreed on the methodology to test
them.

Hall's first experiment was a pilot study of seventeen volunteers.
NuSI and Hall's team all agreed that, if this study showed a significant result, then they'd follow up with a larger study. Volunteers
would start on a four-week high-carb diet, before switching to an
ultra-low-carb diet for another four weeks. Calories would remain
the same on both diets. Everything about their bodies would be
monitored in a highly controlled lab environment. Everyone agreed
on the diets and the protocols.

The low-carb diet did result in decreased insulin in all volunteers
which meant that the experimental conditions were adequate to
test Taubes' hypothesis that insulin levels were important. But
when the overall data were analysed, there was a surprise: there
was no difference between the groups in terms of the effect of fat
or sugar on metabolism. A calorie was a calorie, regardless of
whether it came from carbs or fat. It was a small study, but a rigorously conducted small study can still disprove a hypothesis. Hall
published his findings[3] and reviewed them in the *European Journal
of Clinical Nutrition*.[4]

This article was as much about the philosophy of science as it
was about nutrition. Hall drew on his physics background to show
the principle of falsification, recalling how, in the late nineteenth
century, scientists had proposed that light was a wave in something
called the 'luminiferous ether'. The model made intuitive sense, but
it was wrong, and several experiments proved this.

Hall reiterated that we can't definitively *prove* any scientific
model. Instead, scientists run a series of experiments and make
observations. Only if the model stands up to these tests does it
become widely accepted. But the most important part of any model
or theory is that it should make predictions that, if wrong, will

invalidate the model. As much as we all like to be right, good science is about trying to prove yourself wrong. Hall felt that, whether NuSI could admit it or not, important aspects of Taubes' carbohydrate–insulin model had been shown to be incorrect – the model was too simplistic.

NuSI started to collapse and finally closed in 2021. I called Gary Taubes to get his view on what had happened and the state of the carb debate. We spoke one evening on a video call. It was late for me and early for him. He was bathed in bright California sunshine in a wood-panelled room and somehow not as I expected. He's quiet, humble and funny. I'd messed up the timing of the call due to the eight-hour time difference and a clock change, but he reassured me: 'Don't worry. A dear friend of mine is a math professor at Harvard and whenever he calls me he gets the time difference wrong.'

My first and lasting impression was a warm one. People have said horrible things about Taubes online, but I found him decent and sincere. We spoke for three hours and he was nice about everyone, seemingly without effort. It was really cool.*

I asked if he was bored of writing about carbs. 'My wife says if I saw someone hit by a car crossing the road I'd find a way to blame carbs,' he replied. 'But I just think a terrible injustice has been done. I feel like a whistle blower. Hundreds of millions of people are getting the wrong advice about how to eat. It's hard to walk away from.'

We got into a lot of long grass about experimental details and his disagreement with Hall. The protocols and the stats were agreed to, but in Taubes' mind it was just a pilot study. It was only when

---

* The critiques have, however, sometimes kept him awake at night. I'm always curious about why people are up at 4am, because I'm often awake at this hour, fretting. 'In the small hours I try to say to myself, "Don't take any of this too seriously,"' Taubes told me. 'I like to joke that some Jews evolved to be awake at 4am worrying. Many in Europe who survived the twentieth century, after all, would have been the ones who were awake, ready to leave in the middle of the night, when the knock came on the door …'

the data were in that it became clear, in his view, that the method was flawed.

I understand this. Until an experiment has actually been done, it's impossible to see all the ways it might go wrong. When I was a lab scientist, I worked on experiments with dozens, even hundreds of stages, all invisible, even under a microscope – invisible molecules modified in invisible ways. We'd account for as many variables as we could, but sometimes a negative result just meant we'd screwed up, not necessarily that our hypothesis was wrong.

Part of being a good experimental scientist is finding the balance between being paranoid enough at every stage to think of everything and do it right, without being so paranoid that you can't trust your result. At some point you need to say: 'I did this experiment. This is the result. This is what I think it means.' Then you need to be big enough to have others tear it to pieces, and then figure out whether they're doing that because you were wrong or because you've just shown their life's work to be wrong.

But it wasn't just Hall's pilot study that seemed to have contradicted significant parts of the carbohydrate–insulin hypothesis. There's no shortage of *other* evidence that contradicts it too. The hypothesis has been tested many times, and the longest-running study in people living in the real world found no sustained differences in calorie intake between low-carb and high-carb diets.[5]

In another experiment, volunteers ate two diets in a random order – one 10 per cent carbs and 75 per cent fat, the other 75 per cent carbs and 10 per cent fat. Contrary to what the carbohydrate–insulin hypothesis would have predicted, it was found that participants actually ate 700 *fewer* calories per day on the high-carb diet, and that only the high-carb dieters reported a significant loss of body fat.[6, 7]

Out in the real world, people seem to find that really low-carb diets are very difficult to stick to and that they don't work well. As far back as 2003, there was a year-long dietary study, published in the *New England Journal of Medicine*, that put a low-carb diet head-to-head with a low-fat diet. The results showed that, although after three months the low-carb group had lost more weight, after twelve months there was no significant difference. Both diets decreased blood pressure and improved insulin responses to eating sugar, but lots of people didn't stick to either diet.[8]

There was one NuSI study, undertaken by researchers at Harvard and published in 2018, that did seem to confirm the carbohydrate–insulin hypothesis.[9] In the study, 164 college students, faculty and staff living with overweight were put on a low-carb diet, which had a beneficial effect on metabolism. Kevin Hall was the first to identify a significant problem in the data analysis: the Harvard team appeared to have analysed a slightly different outcome from the one they set out to investigate.

When you design a study, you have to decide what you're going to measure and how you're going to report it *before* you conduct the study. If you change the thing you're measuring, it is somewhat like moving the dartboard after you have thrown the dart. As Hall mildly put it in a commentary, 'Reporting study outcomes according to prespecified analysis plans helps reduce bias.'[10]

When Hall reanalysed the data according to the Harvard team's own original plan, their claimed effect disappeared. In fact, the study seemed to support the generally held belief that varying fat and carbs in the diet doesn't significantly change energy expenditure.

I've tried a keto diet myself. I found that I could eat lots of things that I enjoyed, that I could feel full and also that I did lose weight. But I eventually craved spaghetti with Bolognese sauce, rice with my chicken and chips with my steak, so I gave up. My experience is borne out by extensive studies of people on ketogenic diets for epilepsy (which do seem to reduce seizure frequency, particularly in children). You might imagine that adults following low-carb diets to reduce seizures would be very incentivised to stick to the diet. But they are around five times more likely to drop out of studies compared with people in studies of standard drug treatment.[11] We should, however, note that these diets sometimes differ from the standard Atkins diet in ways that might make them harder to stick to.

I don't wish to suggest that low-carb diets don't help some people lose weight or that they don't have any health benefits. I'm also not suggesting that insulin isn't an important regulator of body fat. But I am saying that, looking at the full spectrum of evidence available, provided you keep consuming the same number of calories, the fall in insulin that comes from cutting carbs doesn't seem to make you store less fat or burn more energy.

Indeed, for people who can stick to them, I suspect that low-carb diets do work* – it's just that humans have evolved to eat carbs as the foundation of our diet, and carb-free food is harder to eat. Protein and fat fill you up before you can eat lots of calories. But the problem, common to all diets, is that *we don't really choose what to eat*. We are guided by that internal system. You can avoid carbs in the same way you can hold your breath, but eventually most people will crack.

In the end, Taubes wasn't Galileo. But he does seem a little like Pope Urban VIII, Galileo's friend and sponsor. It was Urban, after all, who invited Galileo to compare the geocentric and heliocentric models of the solar system, just as Taubes invited Hall to investigate the carb-centric model of obesity, only to discover in both cases that the results didn't match what they'd hoped to find.

So, it would seem that sugar doesn't drive weight gain because it increases insulin levels. But how *does* it figure in the story of human health and UPF?

✳✳✳

Humans have for a long time eaten enormous quantities of carbohydrates in the form of sugars and starches. A diet binds us to the people around us – or at least it should – and those bonds,

---

* There are (largely anecdotal) reports of people who have sustained significant weight loss on a low-carb diet. I wonder if this is less due to the low insulin levels than to the fact that a keto diet rules out almost all UPF, which is typically based on carbohydrates and sugar.

historically and prehistorically, have typically been formed with a small number of starchy plants, basically one per society: maize, potatoes, rice, millet, wheat. We are really good at eating starch and sugar (in the context of fruit or sugar cane or honey), and it seems to be something that the human body can handle and enjoy, even in reasonably large amounts.[12, 13]

Honey is a really interesting example, because it's one of the most energy-dense foods in nature. But chemically it's nearly indistinguishable from high-fructose corn syrup (both are mixtures of glucose and fructose in varying ratios) and table sugar (both are crystallised pairs of glucose and fructose molecules).* But throughout pre-history, humans have gained a substantial proportion of their calories from honey – up to 16 per cent on average in some communities, and, according to one study done with the Mbuti of the Congo forests, during the rainy season up to 80 per cent of the calories in their diet come from honey.† There are no reports of widespread overweight in these communities (and many contemporary foraging and hunter-gatherer societies still consume large amounts of honey).[16]

And then there's the fact that Carlos Monteiro found a bag of sugar on the table to be a sign of health in his research, because it signified a household that cooked. That doesn't, however, mean that sugar is healthy. It simply means that our diets are so terrible that

---

* Maple syrup, agave nectar, table sugar, golden syrup – the body treats them all largely the same. People argue about glucose versus fructose, but honey and high-fructose corn syrup are so similar that adulteration of the former with the latter can be hard to detect.[14] There's also a long history in commercial honey manufacturing of feeding bees high-fructose corn syrup if the hives are in a place without enough wild nectar.[15] This raises the question of whether much – or even most – commercial honey is in fact UPF made by bees.

† In studies of the Hadza people in Tanzania, hunters obtained between 8 and 16 per cent of daily calories from honey. Meat provided 30–40 per cent, baobab fruit 35 per cent and tubers 6–22 per cent. That honey comes with comb, which is full of semi-digestible fats and huge quantities of soft protein from the bee larvae and eggs living in the comb. It's a nutritionally complete food.

buying your own sugar to make your own sweet food at home is healthier than buying pre-made industrial UPF with sugar added at source.

I know it seems like I want this both ways, saying that sugar is both a sign of healthiness *and* unhealthiness. But this is how I see it: sugar (including honey) can harm the body, not because it increases your insulin levels, but because it rots your teeth and makes you eat more food.

I tested this second idea* on Lyra and Sasha over breakfast one morning. You can do the test as well if you have a child handy, or someone who will eat without restraint. You'll need sugar, milk, a bowl and some Rice Krispies. First, pour out two equal bowls – say 30g each. Then remove one spoonful of cereal from one bowl and add a spoonful of sugar in its place. Finally, add the milk.

In nutritional terms, the sugar-sweetened bowl and the bowl with no added sugar are almost identical. There is the same amount of carbohydrate, fat and protein in each bowl, and each bowl will have the same effect on blood sugar.†

Yet the girls responded very differently to the two bowls: they ate the entire bowl with added sugar and then asked for more. They didn't mind the unsweetened bowl, but neither finished it. The sugar made the girls eat more of the fat and protein calories from

---

* Geoffrey Cannon was the first person to frame sugar in this way for me. He's a friend and long-time collaborator of Carlos Monteiro and was crucial in bringing an understanding of the role of industry to the NOVA classification.

† Rice Krispies themselves increase blood sugar more than table sugar. On a scale of impact on blood sugar, if glucose is 100, then white bread is also 100, Rice Krispies are 95, Kellogg's Corn Flakes (as sold in the USA) are 92, Alpen is 55, Special K (as sold in France) is 54 – the same, roughly, as porridge – Special K (as sold in the USA) is 70. Skittles are 70. A Snickers is only 41. Carrots range from 32 to 92. Table sugar is around 60. It's hard to know what to make of this variation, other than it shows the limitations of thinking about food in terms of glycaemic index. It may be that sweet things affect blood sugar less because the instant they arrive in the mouth they stimulate the release of insulin, which drops the blood sugar level.

milk and more of the starch calories from the cereal. Sugar and salt are the two greatest food additives in terms of driving appetite, which is why they are nearly universal in UPF, whether it's beans or pizza. So, high sugar content is one of the properties of UPF that drives weight gain.

The other obvious problem with sugar is that it destroys your teeth. Tooth enamel ranks somewhere between steel and titanium in terms of hardness, but its strength comes from the mineral content, especially the calcium, and this is leeched out by acids. The main source of dietary acids are now fizzy drinks, which also supply the sugars that feed bacteria living in the mouth. These bacteria crap out acids directly onto the the surface of teeth, dissolving them.

Almost all juices and fizzy drinks are acidic enough to dissolve a tooth. Ocean Spray cranberry juice is approximately pH 2.56, while Coca-Cola Classic is 2.37, Coke Zero is 2.96, and Pepsi is 2.39.[17] Immediately after an acidic drink, the mouth is so acidic that, if you brush your teeth, you are literally brushing away a slurry of tooth enamel. You need to rinse your mouth out thoroughly, then wait for at least half an hour for the pH to readjust to normal levels.

We all know this, and yet it remains an ongoing public health catastrophe. Even in the UK, where we have a huge and relatively well funded public health infrastructure and labelling about sugar content, tooth decay is the most common reason that children in the UK have a general anaesthetic.[18] Let that sink in. In England, more than 10 per cent of three-year-olds, and a quarter of five-year-olds, have tooth decay. Almost 90 per cent of hospital tooth extractions among children younger than five are due to preventable tooth decay, and tooth extraction is the most common hospital procedure in children aged six to ten.[19] The most common operation we do in children – ahead of fixing bones broken on trampolines, hernia repairs and appendix removals – is for rotten teeth. The statistics in the USA are even worse.[20]

This dental crisis is almost entirely due to UPF. Table sugar is consumed in small quantities at meals. The sugar that really rots teeth is the stuff we consume with acids between meals: fizzy drinks, sweets and so on.* These UPF products damage our teeth because we eat them constantly. They're marketed as treats and snacks. UPF is why dental caries cause suffering in up to 90 per cent of school-aged children in industrialised countries.[27]

Nowhere on any can of fizzy drink anywhere in the world is there a warning about the risks of oral disease and the risk of early death. I can't see any argument why Nestlé, Coca-Cola, Pepsi or any of the others selling sugar-sweetened beverages (or anything with a high proportion of added sugar) should not be forced to put a warning on the packet about tooth decay.

---

* Tooth decay, like obesity, precedes the invention of UPF. It has even been found in wild primates, but at very low rates.[21] Some of the earliest evidence of hominid tooth decay is from australopithecines living 1.5–1.8 million years ago, but dental caries was present in less than 3 per cent of the roughly 125 skeletons found in a single location – lower than the rate in *Homo erectus* skeletons found at the same site.[22] In general though, pre-agricultural populations have low rates of tooth decay and relatively shallow cavities. We know this partly because of the low rates of dental decay on ancient skeletons, but also because there is no evidence of dentistry until the neolithic age roughly 10,000 years ago. This was when humans started to make permanent homes rather than just wandering from cave to cave. It was also when we started to domesticate and farm cereal crops like wheat and barley in the Middle East. The presence of caries in human skeletal remains starts to increase in this age. Anyone who has experienced tooth ache (which is sadly most of us) can understand how a neolithic human might be driven to extremes to get rid of the pain. In Pakistan 9,000 years ago, some bold person – with know-how originally developed by skilled artisans for bead production – made one of the first attempts at dental drilling in a form of presumably agonising proto-dentistry.[23] As we started to eat more refined fermentable carbohydrates and sugars, rates of tooth decay soared. Cuneiform tablets carved 4,000 years ago defined special incantations to request the Babylonian god Ea to 'get hold of the worm and pull it from the offending tooth'. Ancient folklore thought that the tooth worm caused tooth decay. This belief either arose in different places or spread around the world until the middle ages and beyond.[24–26]

8.

... or about exercise

There's a three-step escalator in the Oracle Shopping Centre in Reading. As a medical student I had a rotation there, and my boss at the time, a doctor with an interest in obesity, talked constantly about that escalator in lectures he gave. It was, he said, 'a monument to the obesity crisis'. He had a little slide deck all about it, with a photo he'd surreptitiously taken of someone with a high percentage of body fat 'riding' it in a 'slothful' bid to avoid the stairs.

Of course, these kinds of escalators exist to make places more accessible – not because people are lazy. But the perception that obesity is due to a lack of exercise (and, by extension, that people living with obesity are slothful) is pervasive, even among the physicians treating the disease.

In a way, this is unsurprising. It seems obvious that we burn fewer calories today than we did historically and that inactivity is thus a major driver of weight gain. There are large numbers of papers in respectable journals that contradict the hypothesis that UPF is a significant contributor. These papers claim to show that inactivity is a primary driver of weight gain, and that increased calorie intake is less important.[1–12]

There are a few authors that come up repeatedly in these papers, including Steven Blair, Peter Katzmarzyk and James Hill. A 2012 study by Hill proposed that increasing physical activity would 'reduce the need for dramatic food restriction'[13] – great news for people like me, who love to eat.

Blair co-authored a 2014 paper, 'What is causing the worldwide rise in body weight?', which stated that, 'Although most people think [the obesity epidemic] is due to people eating more, there is scant evidence to support this hypothesis.'[14] It also proposed that increasing physical activity might be easier than reducing calorie intake, and that it could 'offset excess intake'. In other words, you *can* outrun a bad diet. Blair set up a new institute to study this theory: the Global Energy Balance Network. In a press release, he said that when it came to blaming fast food and sugary drinks for increases in weight, there was 'virtually no compelling evidence that that, in fact, is the cause'.

Katzmarzyk co-authored a 2015 study of 6,025 children, the results of which showed clearly that a lack of physical activity is a major predictor of childhood obesity.[15]

The conclusion that exercise is important for preventing and treating weight gain seems inescapable. After all, it's an iron law of metabolism – and one I'm not looking to overturn – that if you eat more calories than you burn, you'll gain weight. It's been demonstrated many times, using different methods, in different laboratories. So, logically inactivity must – surely – contribute to weight gain, especially since we're doing a lot less than we used to throughout the industrialised world.*

And indeed, a large US study showed that the reduction in energy expenditure between 1960 and 2006 nearly perfectly accounted for weight gain over the same period.[19] According to a 2011 paper, physical jobs of the type that many more people used to do (like coal

---

* In the UK and the USA at the turn of the twentieth century, around half of workers were doing jobs that demanded physical labour, such as agriculture or manufacturing. There was more manual labour to be done at home too, because washing machines, tumble dryers and vacuum cleaners were either not yet invented or not widely available.[16, 17] By contrast, at the beginning of the twenty-first century, around 75 per cent of UK and US workers were employed in service jobs, and even those who still worked in manufacturing or agriculture did far less physical work per day, partly due to increasing automation and partly due to the items being produced (e.g. less shipbuilding and more microchip-making). Cars and public transport have made commutes less physically demanding. The British Heart Foundation estimates that the distance the average person walks per year shrunk from 250 miles in the 1970s to 180 in 2010.[18]

mining) are around five times more strenuous than sitting at a desk.* Not only that, I found another paper suggesting that inactivity must be to blame because people in the UK are collectively eating fewer calories than they used to.[22] If people are eating fewer calories but still gaining weight then they must be far more inactive than before. This paper was by Christopher Snowdon, the journalist (and 'head of lifestyle economics') at the Institute for Economic Affairs (who also derided the very idea of UPF in Chapter 2). Its title, riffing off Gary Taubes perhaps, was 'The fat lie'.

Snowdon took a strong position: 'All the evidence indicates that per capita consumption of sugar, salt, fat and calories has been falling in Britain for decades.' If this is true, and our calorie intake has truly been falling for decades, then the whole idea that UPF – or any kind of food for that matter – is a significant driver of our increasing weight has to be wrong.

I read on. According to Snowdon, the conventional wisdom that Britain's obesity epidemic is caused by the increased availability of high calorie foods and drinks 'has no basis in fact'. The paper claimed that, since 2002, the average body weight of English adults has increased by 2kg, adding that, over the same period, there had been a decline in calorie consumption of 4.1 per cent and a decline in sugar consumption of 7.4 per cent. The piece concludes: 'The rise in obesity has been primarily caused by a decline in physical activity at home and in the workplace, not an increase in sugar, fat or calorie consumption.'

Snowdon used official UK government sources, like the Department for Environment, Food & Rural Affairs, who have carried out annual surveys of the British diet since 1974.[23] I checked their data and it did seem to show that, per person, calorie

---

* The Institute for Fiscal Studies used these data to do some modelling and produced a simple example. If an average-sized man in a sedentary job works a forty-hour week, he'll burn about 30kg fat per year. If he worked in a strenuous job, he'd burn almost 70kg of fat. To compensate for the sedentary job, this man would have to jog an extra 10.6 hours a week, not far off the time commitment to exercise of Olympic marathon runners.[20, 21]

consumption had gone from around 2,500 per day in 1974 to just 1,990 in 1990 – a staggering drop of 21 per cent. Snowdon's graphs of calorie intake looked like stock charts from the Wall Street Crash.*

If we are eating less in the USA and the UK, then it would have to be increased inactivity that's making us heavier. This chimes with things like the rise in screen use, reductions in manual labour, children spending more time indoors and the proliferation of three-step escalators.

This explanation would have major policy implications: if calorie intake is falling without government activity, there would be no justification for policies aimed at reducing consumption. And it struck me as surprising the food industry could still be profitable with a 21 per cent reduction in calories.

***

That Snowdon article had enormous influence, and was featured on *Channel 4 News*, in the *Sun* and on BBC Radio 2, among other places. Allister Heath, now editor of the *Sunday Telegraph*, wrote a piece in 2016 in the *Telegraph* with the title 'We are far too fat, but a sin tax on sugar would do nothing to help'.

Snowdon's data would make Monteiro wrong, and they would make a lot of other people wrong too. Giles Yeo, for instance. Yeo is an internationally respected Cambridge geneticist who studies obesity. I'd spoken with him endlessly about weight, but he'd never mentioned this fall in calorie intake. I had, however, previously asked him how we were sure it was what we were eating that was driving weight gain, and he had given two reasons.

* Snowdon confirmed this with data from other sources, including the UK National Diet and Nutrition Survey Data, the UK Living Costs and Food Survey, and the British Heart Foundation. The United States National Health and Nutrition Examination Survey also showed the same thing, namely that average calories purchased and consumed had fallen since the 1970s – i.e. we're eating *less*.

First, he said, there's a dosage effect: 'Let's take a chocolate bar, which is roughly 240 calories.' (Yeo knows his way around confectionery.) 'If I were motivated, which I very often am, I could finish a chocolate bar in less than a minute. But it will always take me twenty or thirty minutes on a treadmill to burn those calories off.' The consumption of calories is quick, but the burning of calories is slow. That's why we don't need to eat continuously. But quick consumption also opens up the possibility of eating more than we need.

The second reason was related to our genes: 'All the genetic influences on obesity that we understand so far affect eating behaviour.' In other words, if obesity were due to doing too little, we'd expect that the genes discovered related to obesity would be associated with things like 'activity behaviours' or metabolism, but they're not.

Then I looked again at the numbers in Snowdon's paper, and it struck me that there was something weird about them. It's this: average calorie expenditure for people in the UK is around 2,500 calories. Yet the survey data Snowdon quoted suggested that we're eating fewer than 2,000 calories per day, which would mean an average daily deficit of around 500 calories. We are gaining weight when, according to the data, our calorie consumption is now so low that we should be losing weight as a nation – even if we did nothing. And by nothing, I really mean *nothing*.

I could live for a long time on 2,000 calories per day, but not without losing weight. To consume so few calories and maintain or gain weight, I would have to reduce my activity levels so much that I couldn't even get out of bed to pee. In fact, I wouldn't just have to be bedbound: I'd need to cease some of the energy-intensive bodily functions necessary to sustain life, including handing my kidney function to a dialysis machine and using a ventilator to breathe for me.[24]

So, what is going on? I found the answer in appendix 10 of the National Diet and Nutrition Survey,[25] which detailed a sub-sample of people who also took part in something called a 'doubly labelled water sub-study'.

This technique was invented in the fifties. Participants drink water in which the hydrogen and oxygen atoms have been 'labelled' – the nuclei of the atoms have extra neutrons in them, which means that the atoms can be traced. You may have heard of 'heavy water' – this is that. The body gets rid of the oxygen and the hydrogen at different rates according to calorific expenditure.* It's not perfect, but it's very consistent from one year to the next and it's widely agreed to be the best way of measuring how much energy people are expending.

These doubly labelled water data showed people burning around 2,500 calories per day, exactly as expected. We simply *cannot* be gaining weight as a nation if we're eating fewer than 2,000 calories per day but burning more than 2,500. It breaks rules of physics that everyone agrees on.

What the doubly labelled water study showed is that people in surveys were underestimating their calorie consumption by more than 30 per cent. US studies back this up. A comparison of the US National Health and Nutrition Examination Survey's doubly labelled water data with the actual survey data showed consistent under-reporting of how much people eat and over-reporting of how much they move.[26]

Snowdon's argument might have been valid if people had been consistent over time in underestimating what they eat. If we had always underestimated our calorie intake, then it might still be the case that inactivity could be the main problem leading to weight gain. But the doubly labelled water experiments show that we're actually underestimating how much we eat to a much greater extent today than we did a few decades ago.

---

* When people drink the heavy water, it becomes diluted throughout their bodies and they gradually pee it out. The labelled hydrogen can only leave the body as water loss – mostly urine and sweat. The labelled oxygen leaves the body in two ways: with the hydrogen as water loss, and in breath as carbon dioxide. The more calories you burn, the more carbon dioxide you breathe out. By looking at the differential rate at which the oxygen and the hydrogen leave the body, you can get an estimate of calorific expenditure.

There are several explanations for this under-reporting, and they're all very well evidenced. First, studies show that people living with obesity misreport on questionnaires, and then, if they lose weight, they stop misreporting and admit to their previous inaccurate responses.[27] It doesn't take too much empathy to imagine why respondents living with obesity might provide underestimates when answering food questionnaires. People regularly under-report things they find shameful.*

Second, studies have shown that a desire to lose weight increases under-reporting, and there has been a huge increase of diet-awareness, dieting and the desire to lose weight since the 1990s. We know, for example, that the number of men who want to lose weight nearly doubled between 2003 and 2013.[28]

Third, people are eating more snack food outside the home than previously, and this food is easily forgotten and harder to capture. Snacking has grown into a $400 billion industry.[29, 30] Fourth, we're getting worse at responding to surveys in general. Economists are upset about this, so they've studied it.[31-35]

Fifth, the portion sizes of our foods are bigger, and their energy higher, than the reference databases say they are. The British Heart Foundation found that, in the twenty years between 1993 and 2013, individual shepherd's pie ready meals have doubled in size, while a portion of crisps from a family pack has increased by 50 per cent.[36] This means that if someone responds to a survey saying they had a ready-made chicken pie or a portion of nuts, the reference data may well underestimate the number of calories they have consumed.

Sixth, people are wasting less food. A report from 2012 estimated that household food waste had declined by around 20 per cent since 2007.[37, 38] If food waste is declining, then people will be consuming a larger proportion of the food they report purchasing.

---

* For example, comparisons suggest that reported alcohol consumption could be 40–60 per cent lower than the reality.

Seventh, while there has been a fall in official calorie intake figures, data from a commercial source – the Kantar Worldpanel, a continuously reporting panel of 30,000 British households – shows a rise in calorie purchases over the past ten years.[39]

Snowdon's 'Fat lie' article misunderstood the data: calorie consumption isn't in decline – it has been increasing for a long time. The papers by other authors pointing out these errors didn't receive any publicity though, which is a shame because policies about weight and diet (and human suffering) are affected by what's covered and written about in the press.

***

So, the doubly labelled water studies (and lots of other data) tell us that we *are* eating more. But what about that modelling by the Institute for Fiscal Studies showing that coal mining is (unsurprisingly) eight times more strenuous than office work? After all, it could be that, thanks to our sedentary lives, we are in a situation of double jeopardy: doing less while eating more, meaning that what we eat is only half the story.

To understand how exercise and activity affect our body weight we need to turn to the work of, among others, Herman Pontzer. He's an associate professor of evolutionary anthropology at Duke University whose research is transforming how we think about diet and metabolism. Pontzer wanted to work out the difference in daily calorific expenditure between hunter-gatherers, farmers and sedentary office workers. To do it, he spent time with the Hadza, a population of hunter-gatherers living in savannah woodland in northern Tanzania. The Hadza hunt and gather on foot with bows, small axes and digging sticks. Men hunt game and gather honey, women gather plants. Wild foods, including tubers, berries, small and large game, honey and baobab fruit, provide 95 per cent of the Hadza's calories.

Pontzer measured total daily energy expenditure over eleven days in thirty adults.[40] His team used the doubly labelled water method and a portable respirometry system, whereby the participant wears a hood device that measures how much oxygen they consume and how much carbon dioxide they produce. The team also gave participants GPS devices to gather accurate travel data.

The results were so surprising that the team recalculated them again and again, in many different ways and controlling for different factors, convinced they had to be wrong. Because, very much contrary to expectations, the number of calories that Hadza adults burn was found to be very similar to that of American and European populations. Even breastfeeding or being pregnant made no difference.

In fact, these results are supported by other studies. Amy Luke and Kara Ebersole of Loyola University showed that there was no difference in total energy expenditure between a cohort of women in rural Nigeria and another in suburban Chicago.[41] In fact, this pattern holds true for all human populations ever studied. And the same thing has been reported in non-human primates like monkeys and apes: captive populations burn the same number of calories as their counterparts in the wild.[42-51]

These findings challenge everything about our understanding of how the body uses calories. It seems that people burn the same amount of energy each day whether they walk ten miles or sit at a desk. The significance of this can't be missed: it means that we *cannot* lose weight just by increasing activity. Variation in body-fat percentage is unrelated to physical activity level or energy expenditure.

So, how do we square this with those data that showed that coal mining burned eight times as many calories as office work? Well, it turned out that no one actually measured coal miners in those studies. The data were all based on surveys and assumptions about time use. When a team from the USA and Turkey actually *measured* coal miners with heart-rate monitors, they found that the miners burned ... between 2,100 and 2,800 calories per day – the same as the rest of us.[52]

And yet it seems impossible that I wouldn't burn more calories if, rather than sitting at my desk, I laboured in a mine. How could that possibly work?

I'd always imagined that I burn around 2,000 calories just loafing around breathing and maintaining basic cellular functions, and that any physical activity, whether it's jogging or mining, gets added to the total number of calories I burn in a day. But it turns out that, if we are active, our bodies compensate by using less energy on other things, so that our overall energy expenditure stays the same.

This is especially true when we look at longer timeframes of several days or weeks. In the case of the Hadza, when they rest, they *really* rest. And it's true for athletes and everyone else who is active too. We can be very active for a period of time, but we claw back that energy debt later. It's this reduction of energy usage in other ways inside the body that may explain why exercise is associated with improved physical health, even if it doesn't lead to weight loss.

Pontzer's model posits that going for a long walk or run results in simply scaling back on routine non-essential bodily processes, reducing the amount of energy spent on your immune, endocrine, reproductive and stress systems. That may sound bad, but a bit of downtime actually seems to help to restore those systems to a healthier level of function. And it makes sense evolutionarily: throughout hominid history, there will have been significant periods during which food was scarce. Under the conventional model of calorie burning, that would mean using the most calories when food was least available because you would inevitably work harder to hunt or gather those calories. The fixed energy model means that energy use is consistent even if we do have to walk further to get food. And in a time of scarcity, it makes sense to borrow from – for example – the reproductive system to reduce fertility.

According to Ponzter's data, we burn around 2,500 calories per day at desk jobs, the same number of calories as if we were walking a long distance. Since we're not spending that energy on walking, we spend it elsewhere, on things like being stressed. The hypothesis says that office workers will likely have increased levels of adrenaline, cortisol and white blood cells, all of which make us anxious and inflamed.[53, 54] A sedentary life (of the kind you probably live if you're reading this – although not necessarily) leads to higher levels of testosterone and oestrogen, which might sound good to some people, but which can increase risks of cancers. By contrast, the Hadza – who do around two hours of moderate and vigorous physical activity every day, many times more than typical people in the UK and the USA – have morning salivary testosterone concentrations that are roughly half those of western populations.[55]

This is a good thing, and it may explain why exercise is such an important treatment for many chronic conditions and seems to reduce depression and anxiety.[56]

Once you wrap your head around the idea that you wouldn't burn any more calories even if you moved to Tanzania and became a hunter-gatherer, it explains why (as lots of studies have shown) exercise doesn't help weight loss. Energy balance is not something we can consciously alter, and this makes sense: we couldn't leave something so important up to the vagaries of conscious control, any more than we would with oxygen levels.

The evidence is clear that we are eating more calories than ever and that trying to change our energy expenditure is not going to make a significant difference to weight. Obesity is caused by increased food intake, not inactivity, and the best evidence (as Kevin Hall and Sam Dicken demonstrated) shows that, by food, we mean UPF.

But why is the scientific literature so confused about an issue that seems fairly easy to resolve?

In Christopher Snowdon's case, he is paid a salary by the Institute of Economic Affairs, a free-market think-tank. Their finances are largely opaque, but they have received funding from sugar giant Tate & Lyle.[57, 58] The sugar industry has an interest in promoting the narrative that inactivity, rather than food, is the problem. How much this arrangement informed Chris Snowdon directly isn't clear, but we know from research in other areas that people are often unaware of how they are influenced. Doctors consistently deny that drug company funding affects our practice or our research, but the data show it clearly does.

Of course, Snowdon's paper made an impact, but it wasn't published in a proper academic journal with expert, independent peer reviewers. What about those papers that were though? The ones by professors Steven Blair, Peter Katzmarzyk and James Hill, among others, that emphasise the role of inactivity? Remember Blair saying that there was 'virtually no compelling evidence' that fast food and sugary drinks are to blame?

I went back to papers by these authors to look for conflicts of interest and found papers from 2011 and 2012 that stated clearly that there were none to declare.[59-61] But in 2015, some scientists sent freedom of information requests to the universities that employed these and other scientists.[62] In response they received 36,931 pages of documents, including emails between the scientists and Rhona Applebaum, then chief science officer of the Coca-Cola corporation. Thanks to these requests, and a huge amount of subsequent journalism and research, we now understand the depth of Coke's influence on the discourse around obesity and exercise.

Coke helped Blair establish that non-profit group, the Global Energy Balance Network,[63] which promoted the message that there was no compelling evidence of a significant link between sugar-sweetened beverages and obesity.[64] Coke funded all those papers I listed earlier, by Blair, Hill and Katzmarzyk.[65, 66] Coke even funded an entire national programme, run by the American College of Sports Medicine, called 'Exercise is Medicine'. Steven Blair has served as the vice president and the president of the American College of Sports Medicine.

In 2015, Coca-Cola published a 'transparency' list of experts and projects it funded, but it proved to be less than transparent. For every author Coke disclosed, there were another four whom they didn't.[67]

A team from Oxford and the London School of Hygiene & Tropical Medicine mapped the universe of Coca-Cola's research funding, which involves almost 1,500 different researchers (probably not all direct grant recipients), corresponding to 461 publications funded by the brand. The researcher who has published the most articles (eighty-nine) with Coca-Cola funding is Steven Blair. His research institution received a total of around $5.4 million of research funding to study the role of energy balance at high levels of energy intake.[68]

There are two problems here.

Coke began funding Blair, Hill and Katzmarzyk and others in 2010, but in 2011 and 2012 they were publishing papers saying they had no conflicts of interest.[69] Funding from Coke for research on health constitutes a conflict of interest, and it has been argued in the academic literature that failure to disclose a conflict of interest should be viewed as serious research misconduct.[70, 71]

But disclosure would not solve everything. From around 2013, many articles did disclose funding from Coke, yet the influence the company had was still vast. When Georgia Governor Sonny Perdue signed a proclamation in 2009 recognising May as 'Exercise is Medicine Month' in the state, he did it with pride: 'especially as it is supported by a local organization, the Coca-Cola Company'.[72]

When any industry funds research, the findings are typically biased in favour of the funder[73-78] – not in every single study, but overall this pattern is very consistent. This is true even for the pharmaceutical industry, which operates in an extraordinarily regulated research environment in which regulators have absolute power over how products are sold and can inspect every data point from every experiment. Compared with the pharma industry, the regulation of food company research, including the studies and papers cited here, is virtually non-existent. Manufacturers of soft drinks have been very successful at exploiting this lack of regulation. A review of the relationship between sugar-sweetened beverages (like Coke) and weight gain found that industry-sponsored studies were five times more likely to produce results favourable to the companies.[79]

Coke is not a public health agency. They aggressively sell drinks that, when consumed in excess, harm children and adults (although what constitutes excess is not written on the can, or anywhere else that I have been able to find). I don't want to shut Coke down, but it seems uncontroversial to suggest that respectable health journals shouldn't publish research funded by Coca-Cola any more than they should publish health research funded by the tobacco industry.[80, 81] Whatever work has been funded by them should be disregarded. Coke should not fund public health programmes, and should have no influence over public health policy. The relationship between Coke and health policymakers should be adversarial – not collaborative.

You might think that the controversy around those hundreds of papers funded by Coca-Cola solved the problem. But in May 2021, Coca-Cola funded the Latin American Nutrition and Health Study,[82] which published results showing that inactivity was associated with weight status and in which the authors claimed that they had no conflict of interest to declare.

Discovering the truth in any area of science is like assembling a jigsaw. The pieces are observations, papers, data points. As you fit pieces together, the jigsaw becomes easier and easier as the picture – the truth – emerges.

In the case of obesity, the completed jigsaw will show that inactivity is not a significant contributor, and that the primary cause is ultra-processed food and drink. This is an existential threat to the companies whose existence depends on sales of these products.

The tactic of Coca-Cola, and other UPF companies, has been to create jigsaw pieces that look like they might fit, but in fact they aren't part of the puzzle at all. The jigsaw box fills up with thousands of misleading pieces, papers and data points, which make it nearly impossible to assemble. Too many pieces just don't fit together.

If, like me, you're surprised by the idea that doing more won't allow you to eat more calories, it may be because the opposite idea, that you can burn off excess calories, has been promoted by companies like Coke all the way from the scientific papers through to policy initiatives like Exercise is Medicine. It took me some time to accept that, despite having a medical degree, part of the way that I have understood my body and its energy requirements has come from the Coca-Cola Company.

9.

... or about willpower

Just as we think we can consciously modify energy expenditure by doing more exercise, there is a nearly universal idea that you can consciously override the internal system that regulates food intake using willpower. It's pervasive, and it's linked to a lot of stigma. For some reason, in medicine at least, this idea is very specific to weight gain. You never hear it about people with other diet-related disease like cancer or cardiovascular disease.

Linked to the idea that weight gain could be reversed by the exertion of will is another discomfiting idea – that there might be two categories of people with obesity, those who have a biological or genetic condition, and who are therefore not to blame, and those who have simply made bad choices. This idea is routinely promoted in the press,* so let's inspect it.

Obesity is somewhat heritable. Almost everyone living with obesity will have genes that drive it. There are two broad kinds of genetic obesity. There are rare defects in single genes, which lead to cases in which weight gain is essentially unavoidable no matter the environment.† But the vast majority of people who live with

---

* To take only one example, in February 2021, Matthew Syed, a columnist for the *Times*, wrote an article about a new obesity drug and posted it on Twitter with this message: 'Here I say that some obese people could lose weight with willpower – more exercise, less food. I explicitly exclude those with thyroid & other conditions. That this has caused offence underlines my point: we've seen a collapse in individual responsibility.'[1]

† Sometimes a single mutation means that the condition is treatable. Around 100 families globally have been discovered to have a mutation that affects leptin (the hormone that seems to be the main way the brain senses the amount of fat

obesity have many minor genetic differences compared with people with lower BMI. Most of these differences are in genes that work in the brain and that affect eating behaviour.

Giles Yeo had told me that genes affect eating behaviour, including the speed at which people eat and the foods they choose. The work done to discover this was done at UCL by Jane Wardle and Clare Llewellyn, who show that genetic variation affects eating behaviour in children and contributes to obesity. The fact that genes can affect eating behaviour creates confusion because it seems counter-intuitive – it feels after all like we make conscious choices, amenable to the exertion of will. And even the people who have genes that make them eat more will still have the experience that they cannot control their intake, which might feel to them like a failure of willpower. I say this as someone with many of the genetic risk factors for obesity.

While almost everyone living with obesity will have genetic risks, some people who live at a so-called 'healthy weight'* also have genes for obesity, which could suggest that they are exerting willpower over their genes. However, that is not the case. The difference between people with the same genes and differing weights is the environment they live in, not their willpower. Again, I know this from personal experience.

on the body) and they typically have severe obesity (i.e. a BMI of over 40). There are also more common mutations, such as mutations in the *MC4R* gene. New drugs are being developed the entire time, including setmalanotide. Drug companies are being cautious (or rather they are required to be cautious by their various regulators). They start with trials on children who are very severely affected to ensure benefit will outweigh risk, and then move on to trials in more and more people.

* 'Healthy' corresponds to a BMI of between 18.5 and 24.9. 'Overweight' refers to BMIs from 25.0 to 29.9, and 'obese' to BMIs of 30.0 or higher. There are many problems with this, and it is of course absurd to label someone unhealthy or healthy according to a single measurement – or perhaps at all. But this is the way it is discussed in science, so please forgive some clumsiness here.

My twin brother, Xand, is also my big brother. He's literally seven minutes older, but he has also been up to 20kg heavier than me, the biggest weight difference of any pair of twins studied in the UK.

We share a genetic code,* meaning we have identical genes, and I know – because I did a test with Giles Yeo – that we both have many of the major genetic risk factors for obesity. If you are a food-obsessed person, then you probably have these genes too regardless of your weight.

Xand gained weight when he moved to the USA. He got a scholarship to an American university to do a master's degree. Around the same time he found out that he was going to have a child with someone he didn't know well, in a way that was totally unplanned. Now, it could not be a happier situation (Xand's son Julian, his mum Tamara, her husband Ken and their son Harrison are much-loved family), but at the time it was stressful. Xand also lived in Boston in a food swamp.

You may have heard of food deserts – places where shops simply don't sell fresh food and healthy groceries and only UPF is available. There are over 6,500 food deserts in the USA according to the US Department of Agriculture. They're found in areas with higher levels of poverty and higher percentages of ethnic minority populations.[2] In the UK, over 3 million people do not have a shop selling raw ingredients within 15 minutes of their homes by public transport.[3] This means it is difficult to source real food – let alone cook it.

Anyway, food swamps of the type Xand found himself in are similar to food deserts. Fresh food may be available, but it is submerged in a swamp of fast-food outlets selling UPF. Filming a BBC1 documentary about UPF, I went to Leicester to meet a group of teenagers to understand their food environment. They showed me exactly how food swamps work. When it came to food they were passionate, angry and cheerful, often at the same time.

---

* In a sense, we share a body. People think that we're the same person, and a paternity test would show that my children are his, and vice versa.

They took me to the Clock Tower, the central landmark where all the young people go to hang out, and pointed out the shops in the immediate vicinity: McDonald's, Five Guys, Burger King, KFC, Greggs, Tim Hortons, Taco Bell, another Greggs, Pizza Hut, a chicken shop, Costa, Awesome Chips – and there's yet another Greggs just out of sight next to a Subway. McDonald's has the prime location, right at the foot of the Clock Tower.

Leicester is a food swamp. UPF is everywhere but real food is harder to reach, both geographically and financially. There is a clear correlation between poverty and the density of fast-food outlets, with almost twice as many in the most deprived areas compared with the least. In one deprived area in northwest England, there are 230 fast-food outlets for every 100,000 people, compared with an England-wide average of ninety-six per 100,000.[4]

The swamp isn't just the density of restaurants. It's also the total immersion in marketing. The teenagers showed me their bus tickets, which are also vouchers for McDonald's. Their social media feeds are crammed with ads for these same brands and so are their games. They don't have Spotify Premium, so songs are interspersed with ads, largely for fast-food chains. All the media they consume is funded by the fast-food industry. They're soaked in the advertising that we know works.

You will often hear those in favour of deregulation argue that advertising doesn't promote excess eating, that kids are already buying a burger and the advertising merely suggests to them which one they should buy. This argument is incorrect, and there is a lot of data to prove it.

A Dutch research group studied children playing an 'advergame' – a new advertising technique that involves creating entire games dedicated to increasing consumption.[5] One such game is KFC's '*Snack! In the Face*', which was developed to solve the problem of low KFC snack sales and awareness among Australian teens.

The game was number one on both the Apple and Google app stores. It plays an insistently catchy theme song while you fire blobs of chicken into the mouth of a miniature bandy-legged Colonel

Sanders. If the Colonel eats enough chicken, you win vouchers that can be converted into real chicken blobs. As you might expect, games like this one succeed in getting children to eat more chicken, as the Dutch team showed. Additionally, after playing advergames promoting UPF, children consumed more nutrient-poor snack foods and fewer fruits and vegetables.[6] Even if you advertise fruit in the game, they eat more UPF. The simple reminder to eat will drive children to eat more junk if it's available.[7]

In a study at Yale, primary school children watched a cartoon that contained either food advertising or advertising for other products and received a snack while watching. Children consumed 45 per cent more food when exposed to food advertising.[8]

Perhaps the most definitive evidence showing that advertising food, and especially junk food, makes children eat more comes from a paper by Emma Boyland, a professor of food marketing and child health. Boyland did a comprehensive review, commissioned by the World Health Organization, to inform the development of updated recommendations to restrict food marketing to children. She looked at data from nearly 20,000 participants across eighty different studies and showed, beyond all doubt, that food marketing is associated with very significant increases in children's food choices, food intake, and food purchase requests.[9]

The only products advertised to young people like the ones I met in Leicester are UPF. This is for a simple reason: UPF is proprietary, so its manufacturers can generate a lot of money. People will pay a lot for a KitKat relative to its cost of production. No one else can really make KitKats, because Nestlé owns the recipe and the trademark and everything that creates the KitKat's unique barcode that keeps bringing us back.

By contrast, for companies selling beef or milk or red peppers, there's a massive cost of production, especially for the high-end stuff, and all of us treat the different types available as pretty much the same. Sure, we might *say* that we care that our red peppers are organic, or our beef grass-fed. Indeed, people *will* say this as they go into a supermarket. But when researchers have looked in the bags of those same customers as they leave the store, they've usually bought the cheapest of each item.

So, it's much trickier to make lots of money from NOVA groups 1–3, especially at small scale. Huge food companies like Cargill can make money from beef because they're so big, but they still rely on supplying that beef to manufacturers of UPF. There aren't any start-ups making great milk or beef. There's little growth to be had in these areas. Growth is UPF. And a lot of that growth comes from advertising.

In Leicester, I saw the extent to which the fast-food industry has a grip on our lives, and especially on children. McDonald's has become the de-facto community hub. As one teenager put it: 'It's where we have to hang out, because all the youth clubs have been shut down. Where else are we going to go?'

Christina Adane is a young food activist who grew up in south London and qualified for free school meals as a kid. She was behind the UK petition for free school meals over the summer holidays in 2020, which footballer Marcus Rashford supported. We met in the rain in a park near where she grew up and she passionately explained her view on the responsibility of government to protect children and ensure they have access not just to food but to healthy food. She pointed to the food environment around us, chicken shops lining the road across from the park. 'I don't want any child to live in a food desert,' she told me. 'Young people have a right to grow up in environments where healthy food is the default option, where it's attractive, accessible and affordable.'

Like the teenagers I met in Leicester, Adane is acutely aware of how much influence the food industry has over her and her friends: 'It is deeply scary how successful junk-food companies have been in infiltrating youth culture. It's everywhere I go. Celebrities go on chicken-shop dates to promote new albums, energy drinks are advertised at every event celebrating up-and-coming young artists.' When I ask where she was able to hang out after school, the story was the same as that in Leicester: fast-food companies have capitalised on young people having no safe and dry place to social-ise after school.

'Not enough of us realise that these fast-food companies are not our friends,' Adane said. 'We are living in a world where one in three children by the age of eleven are at risk of diet-related dis-ease. One in three. We shouldn't see these companies as relatable or sexy.'

Adane and the teens in Leicester gave me a fantastic picture of their 'food environments', the physical, economic, political, social and cultural contexts that affect what they end up buying and eating – it includes all the advertisements. Food environments determine what we eat far more than conscious choice.

Xand and I have the same genes for obesity but, living in Boston, Xand was far more immersed in UPF than he had been in the UK. He was also stressed, far from home and undergoing huge changes in his life. Stress, from any source, but especially the chronic stress of poverty, has dramatic impacts on those hormones that regulate appetite, increasing the drive to eat. The exact mechanisms aren't clear, but when you're stressed you secrete more of the hormone cortisol; this seems to drive increased intake of calorie-dense UPF through effects on many of those hormones involved in the energy-intake regulation system. Cortisol may also lead to fat accumulation around organs, known as visceral fat, which is associated with worse health outcomes. Chronic stress in low-income settings com-bined with the extreme marketing and availability of UPF creates a double jeopardy.[10, 11]

The 20kg weight difference between Xand and me was not an exertion of will on my part. Put either of us in a food swamp and stress us out and we'll gain weight. But because the idea of will-power is so pervasive, it prevents us looking at possible solutions, like regulation, food pricing, etc. Xand didn't feel like his genes were to blame in this new UPF-rich environment. Rather, he felt like a failure every day, all the more so because I worried about him and started to nag. He said the same thing that many people who live with obesity say, that he felt like he was eating 'because of his emotions', the stress of his situation, and this is superficially true. But that some people solve emotional problems with food – that's genetic.

Clare Llewellyn made a remarkable discovery about how the same genes behave very differently in different environments, which helps to explain this difference between Xand and me. She studies the heritability of obesity using twins and leads the Gemini twin study, one of the largest twin studies ever set up.

Most of what we know about the varying influence of nature and nurture on obesity, and on a vast range of other human traits, has been worked out in similar twin studies.* They have shown that body-fat percentage is highly heritable – up to 90 per cent.[12] But, depending on the group you study, heritability can also be as low as 30 per cent. What's going on?

In a 2018 study of 925 twin pairs, Llewellyn demonstrated that heritability is dependent on that *food environment*.[13] She and her colleagues found that, in families with secure incomes and high levels of food security, the heritability of their body weight was around the 40 per cent mark. But in households with the lowest incomes and the highest levels of food insecurity, it jumped to over 80 per cent. The genes that cause obesity are found equally in high-income and low-income households, but being in a high-income household is protective. Being born into a lower-income

---

* The studies work because there are two types of twins: identical twins like Xand and I, who are genetic clones of each other and share 100 per cent of our genetic material, and non-identical twins, who share only about half their genetic material – around the same as normal siblings. Since identical and non-identical twins have (give or take) equally similar environments, it's possible to tease out the genetic influence on any characteristic you like. For characteristics that are 100 per cent genetic, such as eye colour or blood type, *all* identical twin pairs will share the trait but only some of the non-identical twin pairs will share it. By contrast, characteristics that are more environmentally determined, such as whether or not you've broken your right arm, occur with the same frequency in both identical and non-identical twins. Twin studies allow us to work out if a particular trait is heritable.

household can double the risk of obesity. So, by alleviating (or more properly 'curing') poverty, especially childhood poverty, we could cut the risk of obesity in half without any other intervention.

We know that low-income households tend to eat more UPF, for many often-sensible reasons: it's cheap, it's quick to prepare, children generally eat it readily and it lasts for a long time. It's also regularly the only food that's available and affordable. Almost a million people in the UK lack a fridge, almost 2 million people have no cooker, and almost 3 million lack a freezer. The price of energy is now so high that, even if people own the equipment, many can't afford to run it. This makes UPF indispensable, and it will mean that if, like me, these people have genetic risk factors for weight gain, then those genes will be allowed to exert their effects.[14-16] Llewellyn's findings rightly shift much of the blame onto the more proximate cause of obesity: poverty.

***

About halfway through my diet, I went for lunch with Rachel Batterham. We were ostensibly celebrating a successful grant application. I'd pressed Rachel on where we should eat, but it was clear that she simply didn't care. Even though I know that genetics influences how much we think about food, I still find indifference to food hard to understand. I plan dinner at breakfast. When I'm at a wedding, my whole focus is the canapés. My holiday itineraries are just lists of restaurants and markets.

I was feeling exhausted after a disrupted night – Lyra had had a nightmare that woke me, and I couldn't get back to sleep. Perhaps I was feeling unusually blunt when I asked Rachel if she thought that the fact that she is slimmer than me and her patients was because she can exert more power over her desire to eat. She dismissed the idea without hesitation: 'Some of my patients have lost your entire body weight many times over.' She was right that such weight loss takes incredible willpower (increasing amounts with each effort), but could Rachel have even *more* willpower still? She is, after all, a high achiever.

She rejected that idea too. 'I exert no willpower not eating a biscuit,' she explained. 'I might be able to imagine it would be nice, but I basically don't want it.' She picked at her lunch indifferently. 'If you made me eat the biscuit, I'd be less happy. Food simply doesn't motivate me. It's just my genetics.'

I was half-listening, half-wondering if I knew her well enough to ask to finish the food on her plate. Because my genetic make-up is different to hers. It's obvious how the palaeolithic van Tullekens survived, but what were the Batterhams up to, unmotivated by food: declining mouthfuls of mammoth? When it comes to complex behaviours like eating, which are influenced by hundreds of different genes, we don't understand the advantage of one particular set of genes historically. Certainly, whether a particular behaviour is advantageous will be highly context specific, and that context will include the genetic make-up of those around you. If you live in a food-obsessed community where your fellow humans obsessively gather and hunt food, then being someone who pursues other tasks may make you more useful to the community than if you too were food-obsessed.

***

Rachel is probably someone who could move to the USA or switch to an 80 per cent UPF diet and still not gain weight (although she would still be vulnerable to the many other harmful effects of UPF), just as there are people with a genetic make-up that allows them to smoke twenty cigarettes a day for sixty years without getting cancer. Rachel has the lived experience of not being motivated by food, but I also wanted to speak with an expert in obesity with lived experience in the other direction. So, I turned to my friend Sharon Newson.

Sharon and I met filming a documentary. At the time, Sharon weighed 149kg (over 23 stone), and I used to give her advice about weight loss in a way I am now ashamed of. Over the course of our friendship, Sharon managed to ignore my unhelpful comments and tips and began working as a personal trainer and accumulating qualifications. Then she quietly got accepted to do a PhD in sports science. She built up a network of obesity specialists around her and became one of my most trusted sources of advice about weight and personal change. Despite her expertise, Sharon still struggles to accept that weight gain was not her fault. Intellectually, she understands the genetic and environmental vulnerabilities, but her experience, like Xand's, is that she is to blame: 'It feels like I am lazy, that it is my fault. And that's what I'm told every day in the press. I feel like I eat because of my emotions.'

But while it may be superficially true that many people, like Xand and Sharon, solve emotional problems with food, the fact that they do is an 'eating behaviour' – and such behaviour has been shown by Llewellyn (among others) to be genetic. But knowing things intellectually doesn't help shift what Sharon calls 'decades of internalised stigma and blame'. As a society, we constantly judge and criticise people who live with increased weight and it soaks in. 'It's like having a newspaper columnist living inside my head.'

Over the years, Sharon has transformed how I think about the experience of people who live with increased weight, especially my brother. Just as I had advised Sharon, so too had I been nagging Xand for a decade, contributing to a cycle of shame, stress and frustration that drove further weight gain. He always knew I was judging him. 'If I was eating a burger on the other side of the world to you, I would still feel your judgment radiating out, and it would make me furious, so I'd eat more,' he told me.

Xand put on weight, but I took ownership of it. For a decade, I felt like his weight was my problem. I was embarrassed by him, but I learned to dress my embarrassment up as concern for his wellbeing. And I was truly concerned as well. He'd had Covid much more severely than I had, probably because of his weight, and it had damaged his heart to the extent he needed surgery.

Eventually, to force him to lose weight, I demanded an intervention of sorts, that he see a behaviour-change expert called Alasdair Cant. Alasdair trains social workers and police to help the most vulnerable families, many of whom are at risk of having their children put into foster homes because of violence or substance misuse. Alasdair wanted to speak with me first. I told him all about how I wanted Xand to lose weight, and why. 'As you start to talk about what you want for Xand,' Alasdair said, 'it makes me wonder what he might want.'

Alasdair suggested that I ask Xand about what he wanted and that I try letting go of Xand's problem. A lot of Sharon's words about shame and stigma over the years fell into place. Xand's problem was, it turned out, mainly a problem with me. I was doing to Xand what online bullying, doctors in their clinics, columnists and the government do on a vast scale when they all nag people to lose weight.

Alasdair was done in about twenty minutes. I stopped hassling Xand and, unsurprisingly, things got a lot better. But I didn't realise how much better until I specifically asked him a year later. 'I didn't dread seeing you anymore,' he told me. Every aspect of our relationship changed for the better: 'It wasn't just that you stopped hassling me; it's that I *knew* you actually stopped caring. It allowed me to grasp hold of my own problems.'

This was true. I hadn't just stopped hassling him. Alasdair had persuaded me that I really shouldn't think about my brother in the way I had been: as a shape or a weight. 'When I finally decided to get fit and eat well, I wasn't losing an argument with you,' Xand said. 'I was just running my own life.'

The difference in people's weight has nothing to do with willpower. It's simply a collision of genes and the constraints of the food environment. The most famous test of willpower showed exactly this.

The original experiment, better known as the marshmallow experiment, was devised by Stanford's Walter Mischel in the 1970s. It's a simple enough idea: leave a child alone in a room with a marshmallow for fifteen minutes and tell them that, if they can resist eating it, you'll come back with another one. The child has a choice: enjoy the treat now, or delay gratification for double the reward. Mischel followed ninety of the test participants for the next two decades, and found that those who had been able to delay gratification had lower BMIs and higher educational attainment.[17, 18]

But the study has since been repeated with a much larger number of subjects – 918 children from a range of backgrounds.[19] And this new analysis seemed to show that the biggest predictor of whether a child could delay gratification was socioeconomic background: the children were more likely to take the instant reward if they came from disadvantaged households.

There's good sense in this from the children's perspective. Living in poverty creates uncertainty, so taking an opportunity when you get it might well be a better strategy than waiting on a future reward that may not arrive. Revealingly, when scientists compared children from mothers without degrees, they found that it made no difference to life outcomes whether or not the child had held off eating that marshmallow. It is the child's social and economic background, not whether they can resist a marshmallow, that determines children's long-term success. So, the marshmallow test may well be simply a test for poverty.*

---

* As is often the case in psychology studies, the conclusion that the experiment simply tests for poverty is not a firm one. The study I discussed that revisited Mischel's marshmallow test[20] was itself re-revisited in another paper,[21] which questioned some of the methods used. My reading of the wider evidence is that using a simple test at a moment in time in a child's life to make predictions about their individual life outcomes is fraught with risks and requires extraordinary evidence. There is a lot of evidence that poverty alters decision making in rational ways. It's not hard to imagine that promised food may sometimes never arrive in a context of extreme poverty, for example. Mischel himself went to some lengths to refute the idea that willpower is an innate trait that you either have or don't have, and showed that children with absent fathers were prone to opt for immediate rewards, again for rational reasons. And a 2020 follow-up study (which Mischel himself was an author on!) found that children

So much of who we are is determined by the structure of the world around us. You can't exert willpower over the system of weight regulation produced by the half a billion years of the second age of eating, any more than you can exert it over your long-term oxygen or water intake. But there may be a way of treating UPF that will allow some people to escape its spell: it may best be thought of as an addictive substance.

who quickly gave in to the marshmallow temptation are generally no more or less financially secure, educated or physically healthy than their peers who resisted temptation. So, don't sweat too much if your kids eat sweets when you leave the room ... but do hide the sweets.[22-27]

10

How UPF hacks our brains

At the end of week two of my diet, I was still enjoying products like the Morrisons All Day Breakfast. A classic frozen meal, it comes in a three-compartment plastic tray with a film lid – 768 calories of baked beans, hash browns, pork sausages, omelette and bacon, oven-ready in 20 minutes. It reminded me of the unbearable excitement of long-haul flights to visit my cousins in Canada when I was a child. My brothers and I could often persuade the crew to give us extra meals and we'd lick the trays clean. Air Canada's 1986 macaroni cheese would be my last meal if I could arrange it.

The first complete frozen meals were, in fact, airline food: Maxson Food Systems' 'Strato-Plates', so called because they were developed to be reheated on the new airliners of the day – Boeing's Stratocruiser, introduced in 1947.

A few frozen meals were developed during the late 1940s, but it was Swanson's 'TV Dinners' that took off in 1954. By then, more than half of American households had televisions, and this was the perfect hook. The dinners cost ninety-eight cents and were ready in twenty-five minutes. Over the next three decades they would become ubiquitous. A 1981 picture shows Ronald and Nancy Reagan in the White House wearing matching red jumpers over matching white shirts, sitting in matching red armchairs on a matching red carpet, and eating TV dinners.[1]

In the UK, we lagged behind on both purchases of household appliances – it wasn't until the 1960s that TVs and freezers became common in UK households – and consumption of ready meals. But now we eat more of these ready meals than any other country in Europe. According to *The Grocer*, the UK's ready meals category was worth approximately £3.9 billion in 2019. Almost 90 per cent of us eat ready meals regularly.[2]

While my All Day Breakfast sat in the oven, Dinah and I made some salmon, rice and broccoli for her and the kids. Twenty minutes of continuous preparation, using nearly unconscious skills handed down from our parents, as well as knives, three pans and a chopping board, resulting in dinner, yes, but also a big pile of washing-up and fishy hands.

As we ate, Dinah read my meal's ingredients out loud: 'dextrose, stabiliser (diphosphates), beef collagen casing, capsicum extract, sodium ascorbate, sodium nitrite, stabilisers (xanthan gum and diphosphates), flavourings. Why are you eating diphosphates?'

The diphosphate stabilisers hold everything together through the freezing process so the water doesn't end up in crystals on the surface. They're just one aspect of what makes the All Day Breakfast such an enjoyable product, with the hash browns a little crispy and just the right level of salt and pepper.

Above all, it's easy. While Dinah was still chewing her second mouthful, I was licking the container like I used to on those transatlantic flights.[*]

Things started to change during the third week of my diet. I was working with Sam and Rachel designing a UK study to test whether it was possible to follow UK nutritional guidance while still eating lots of UPF and whether this would have any measurable effects. There is a vast amount of planning before a study like this: finding the money to do it and working out the details of study design. I was speaking with dozens of experts around the globe, asking them about the effects of UPF and the things that we should measure in our volunteers.

I've never learned about a potentially harmful substance while deliberately exposing myself to it, and before my diet I'd never even

---

[*] It's rare to leave anything behind in UPF packaging. I'm sure I've never left a crisp or a bite of sandwich in a packet.

read an ingredients list. UPF is perhaps the type of food we inspect the least as it passes our lips.

I would come off a phone call to an expert in France or Brazil and then sit down to a banquet of UPF. I'd often eat during the call. It was like reading about lung cancer while smoking a cigarette, the basis for that remarkably well-evidenced self-help book I mentioned in the Introduction, *The Easy Way to Stop Smoking*,[3-5] (which is even included in the World Health Organization's 'quitting toolkit').[6] Like many of the smokers who've used Allen Carr's method, my relationship with UPF began to change.

By that third week, I was struggling to eat the UPF without thinking of things the experts had told me. Two comments in particular kept coming back to me.

The first was made by Nicole Avena. She's an associate professor at Mount Sinai in New York and a visiting professor at Princeton. Her research focuses on food addiction and obesity. She told me how UPF, especially products with particular combinations of salt, fat, sugar and protein, can drive our ancient evolved systems for 'wanting': 'Some ultra-processed foods may activate the brain reward system in a way that is similar to what happens when people use drugs like alcohol, or even nicotine or morphine.'

This neuroscience is persuasive, if still in its early stages.[7] There is a growing body of brain-scan data showing that energy-dense, hyperpalatable food (ultra-processed but probably also something a really good chef might be able to make) can stimulate changes in many of the same brain circuits and structures affected by addictive drugs.[8] We have this 'reward system' to ensure we get what we need from the world around us: mates, food, water, friends. It makes us want things, frequently things with which we have previously had pleasurable experiences. With many positive experiences of a particular food, in an environment in which reminders of that food are all around us, wanting, or craving, can be nearly constant. We even start to attach the wanting to the things that surround the food, like the package, the smell or the sight of the place where you can buy it[9, 10].

But the part of the discussion with Avena that stuck with me most was a casual aside about the food itself. Paul Hart had explained how most UPF is reconstructed from whole food that has been reduced to its basic molecular constituents which are then modified and re-assembled into food-like shapes and textures and then heavily salted, sweetened, coloured and flavoured. Avena speculated that without additives these base industrial ingredients would probably not be recognisable as food by your tongue and brain: 'It would be almost like eating dirt.' I don't know if she was being serious, but I started to notice that much of what I was eating had little more than a veneer of food. This was especially true of the snacks and cereals manufactured from pastes of raw materials, which had been fried or baked or puffed.

For example, I'd come to quite enjoy a Grenade Carb Killa Chocolate Chip Salted Caramel Bar as a mid-morning snack. It seemed a little healthier than a simple chocolate bar. I was doing the experiment because I was curious, after all, not because I wanted to deliberately harm myself in the name of science.

I inspected the ingredients after speaking with Avena. These bars, like many others, are constructed from very modified carbohydrates (the first ingredient is something called maltitol, a modified sugar, itself made from a modified starch, which is less calorific but almost as sweet as table sugar), protein isolates from milk and beef (calcium caseinate, whey protein isolate, hydrolysed beef gelatine) and industrially processed palm fat, all bound together with emulsifiers. On its own, as Avena says, it would likely be unpleasant. It's made palatable with salt, sweetener (sucralose) and flavouring.* As I ate these snack bars made from cow tendons, her words started

---

* Many biscuits and bars have a similar basic formula. Maryland Minis Chocolate Chip Cookies are a favourite in the tearoom at work. Again, they comprise modified carbs (refined flour and invert sugar syrup), plus industrial fats (palm, sal, shea), plus added protein (whey), glued together with soy lecithin emulsifier. This blend is made palatable with salt, sugar and flavouring.

to resonate in a way that stopped me enjoying the food quite as much as I had been.

The expert who made the deepest impression was Fernanda Rauber, a member of Carlos Monteiro's team. Her work and ideas permeate this entire book. She told me at length about how the plastics from UPF packaging, especially when heated, significantly decrease fertility (and according to some experts, may even cause penile shrinkage). She also told me about how the preservatives and emulsifiers in UPF disrupt the microbiome, how the gut is further damaged by processing that removes the fibre from food, and how high levels of fat, salt and sugar each cause their own specific harms. And there was one small comment that stuck. Whenever I talked about the 'food' I was eating, she corrected me: 'Most UPF is not food, Chris. It's an industrially produced edible substance.'

These words began to haunt my every meal. They echoed and underlined Avena's idea that without the colouring and flavouring it would most likely be inedible.

I spoke to Rauber just before a family meal of Turkey Twizzlers, a notorious product that was banned from school meals in the UK more than a decade ago because it seemed so unhealthy to food activists. The original version had up to forty ingredients – only a third of a Twizzler was actual turkey meat. The new version is still less than two-thirds turkey, and the manufacturers have managed to get it down to a mere thirty-seven ingredients.

The formulation is remarkably similar to that Carb Killa bar. A paste of turkey protein, modified carbohydrates (pea starch, rice and gram flours, maize starch, dextrose), industrial oils (coconut and rapeseed) and emulsifiers, is combined with acidity regulators, antioxidants, salt, flavours and sugar and then moulded into a helix. In the oven they un-twizzle into springs made of 63 per cent turkey. Dinah, the kids and I all gathered to watch the spectacle through the oven window: a rare moment of family calm.

As I ate, there was a tussle in my brain. I still wanted this food that, according to Rauber, wasn't really food, but at the same time

I was no longer enjoying it.* Meals took on a uniformity: everything seemed similar, regardless of whether it was sweet† or savoury. I was never hungry, but I was also never satisfied. The food developed an uncanny aspect, like a doll that looks just the wrong degree of realistic and ends up seeming corpselike.

By the final, fourth week, the diet had started to have very noticeable physical effects, too. I didn't weigh myself, but I had to loosen my belt by two notches. And, as I gained weight, so did my family. It was impossible to stop the kids from eating my Coco Pops, slices of pizza, oven chips, lasagne, chocolate. If I went to eat secretly, Lyra would hunt me down and demand whatever I was having.

It's hard to tease out the effects of UPF from the general living of life. I was having a lot of anxiety dreams, usually about the death of the girls. It's not like I had never had these sorts of dreams before, but I didn't remember them from the washout period when I wasn't eating UPF.

I was now eating a lot more salt, which meant drinking more water and having to pee a lot. Maybe this was causing the dreams? I'd frequently wake up at 3 am or 4 am from a nightmare or because I needed to pee or both. Unable to sleep, I'd go to the kitchen and have a snack, more out of boredom than anything else.

* Wanting and liking were first separated in an experiment using rats, conducted by Roy Wise and Kent Berridge. Rats share much of our brain circuitry, especially for things like motivation. Wise and Berridge first suppressed dopamine in the rats with a drug and then destroyed the dopamine pathway with a neurotoxin. They were expecting the rats to experience less pleasure from sugar (Berridge was an expert in detecting pleasure in rats). Instead, they found that, although the rats wouldn't move to eat and were no longer motivated, when sugar was placed on their tongues they seemed to like it just as much as before.

† After the Twizzlers, I had a Gü Hot Pud Chocolate Melting Middle dessert: pasteurised whole egg (egg, preservative (potassium sorbate), acidity regulator (citric acid)), sugar, dark chocolate (20%) (cocoa mass, sugar, fat-reduced cocoa powder, emulsifier (soya lecithin)), butter, wheat flour (wheat flour, calcium carbonate, iron, niacin, thiamin), vegetable oil (palm oil, rapeseed oil), glucose syrup, water, preservative (potassium sorbate).

I was eating it at 7 pm, but the Gü website says 'If you're ever wondering if a Gü dessert is acceptable at 11 am, just know that somewhere, somebody is tucking into a Gü every single second.'

I had become very constipated because UPF is low in fibre and water and high in salt. Constipation led to piles and an anal fissure. Most people experience this because most people eat UPF. Straining at the hard dry stool drags a little bit of the soft lining of the anal canal to the outside and it feels like you've got a peanut stuck in your bum. The discomfort led to even worse sleep, which increased my anxiety more and reduced work productivity, leading to even more anxiety – a vortex of physical and mental effects that started to impact every aspect of our family life.

In just a few weeks, I felt like I aged ten years. I was aching, exhausted, miserable and angry. Ironically, food often felt like the solution rather than the problem.

As my diet went on, I became obsessed with what is and isn't UPF. So did everyone around me. Friends started sending me ingredients lists. 'Does "fruit concentrate" mean this is UPF?' (Yes, it does, btw.)

I met Bee Wilson at a food festival at which we spoke on a panel together. She's a food journalist and author who has written about UPF. She asked whether I would classify baked beans as UPF. She didn't think that they were. 'It might be quite an important dividing line for much of the British public,' she said.

Canned baked beans, comprising white beans in tomato sauce, are a staple in the British diet. As Wilson put it, although they're obviously not the healthiest food in the world, 'in the context of so much else that's in the average diet, there's quite a lot of real food in the can'. This is true: most of a tin of baked beans is actually beans and tomatoes.

In fact, Wilson had gone straight to the source and asked Carlos Monteiro: 'I don't think he actually understood what I was asking. They don't have an equivalent in Brazil. But he strongly emphasised that canned beans in general are processed not ultra-processed.'

This may seem like a small point, but it isn't. The foods around the margin of UPF are used by the UPF industry to rubbish the whole concept. First, a harmless-seeming common food is found that contains a single additive that means it technically meets the definition of UPF. Then the argument is made that this means the

UPF definition must be rubbish, or that those who think the NOVA system is useful want to treat Special K or baked beans like cigarettes or heroin.

In the specific case of Heinz baked beans, they are actually both NOVA 3 and NOVA 4. There are different varieties with different ingredients. The organic ones contain 'beans (52%), tomatoes (33%), water, sugar, cornflour, salt, spirit vinegar' – not UPF. But the original variety are UPF because they also contain *modified cornflour, spice extracts and herb extracts*. The difference in nutritional terms is zero, but there are reasons to think that those few ingredients may drive excess consumption, as we will see.

However, for many of us, baked beans, even with some modified corn starch, are a healthy, affordable and easy way to make a main course. This is where we meet the limitations of NOVA, a system designed to look at dietary patterns rather than to evaluate individual foods. There is almost certainly a spectrum of UPF, yet exactly how or whether any one product will be harmful is impossible to tell because we don't eat just one food – we eat a range of foods. Stuck on a desert island, you'd live longer on a diet of nothing but chicken nuggets than a diet of nothing but broccoli; the nuggets do contain more protein and calories. But you'll live much longer on a dietary pattern which includes broccoli in the context of a Mediterranean diet than you would on a dietary pattern based around chicken nuggets.

As I started to feel more unwell, and more anxious about the health consequences, I searched harder and harder for 'healthier' UPF. I switched from full-sugar Coke to Diet Coke.* Instead of

---

* I started with a can for breakfast but gradually began craving Diet Coke with every meal and between meals. In the end, I was drinking about six cans per day. I have no way of explaining how addictive these felt. We think that food addiction is mediated at some level by physiological reward, but Diet Coke is just sweetener, acid and caffeine. As we'll see, it may be that I had become addicted to the flavour and the can, but I never craved real Coke as much as Diet Coke. This is widely reported by many people and I've never seen a satisfying explanation.[11]

reformed chicken nuggets, I would buy oven-ready lasagne – at least until Dinah pointed out that my Sainsbury's beef lasagne, which I had assumed was UPF, contains only normal kitchen ingredients. It turned out that the same is true of the Tesco, Co-Op, M&S and Waitrose lasagnes. The Morrisons version is also pretty benign, with just plain caramel colour and onion concentrate. But Asda and Aldi's formulations are less debatably UPF. Asda's has modified maize starch and colours (paprika extract, annatto norbixin), while Aldi's has lactose, maltodextrin, modified maize starch, dextrose, olive extract and xanthan gum.

I called another of Monteiro's collaborators to see whether the Sainsbury's lasagne, my personal favourite, counted as UPF. Maria Laura da Costa Louzada is a young assistant professor of nutritional epidemiology in São Paolo. She speaks with the steely, passionate optimism of a revolutionary and is comfortable getting deep into the mathematics of the data she draws on for evidence. She studied in Brazil where she helped to write the national nutrition guidelines, and then went to Harvard for a year before coming home.

I asked her about these lasagnes, the sort of high-end quasi-UPF that is ubiquitous in the UK. It's almost homemade, but still seems like UPF: wrapped in plastic and with huge numbers of admittedly normal ingredients.

Da Costa Louzada was entertained by the question: 'NOVA is an epidemiological tool that tells us about the health effects of dietary patterns. It's a very good way to understand the food system.' But to understand an individual food, we need to think beyond NOVA. 'Some products are not technically UPF,' she explained, 'but they use the same plastics, the same marketing and development processes and they're made by the same companies as UPF. The additives are part of the definition, but they are not the only problem with the food.'

Some additives are harmless, whereas others cause direct harms. But in either case, as we'll see, their presence indicates that a product probably has lots of other properties that may cause harmful effects. According to da Costa Louzada, the Sainsbury's lasagne is not UPF if you apply the technical classification, 'But these foods are like a fantasy. They are not home-made foods.'

The argument around what is and isn't UPF is important when it comes to government interventions and labelling. My personal rule of thumb is: if I'm struggling with whether to call a food UPF, then it probably is UPF. For reasons that will become clearer when we look at the effects on the body, it will have been developed in a way that promotes overconsumption even if it lacks the specific harms of, say, emulsifiers.

For the purposes of my diet, however, I was sticking strictly to the NOVA classification, which meant switching to the Aldi lasagne.

When I went back to UCL for testing at the end of the diet, the results were spectacular. I had gained 6kg. If this rate had continued for a year, I would have nearly doubled my body weight. Additionally, my appetite hormones were totally deranged. The hormone that signals fullness barely responded to a large meal, while the hunger hormone was sky high just moments after eating. There was a five-fold increase in leptin, the hormone that comes from fat, while my levels of C-reactive protein, a marker that indicates inflammation, had doubled. I had taken my obesity genes and exposed them to an environment in which they could be maxed out, just as had happened to Xand in Boston.

But the most terrifying result was that MRI scan, which I'd been expecting to be a waste of time and money.

Claudia Gandini Wheeler-Kingshott is one of my collaborators and ran this part of the experiment. She's a professor of magnetic resonance physics at the UCL Institute of Neurology, where I met her to go through my results. Her soft Italian accent brings a warmth to discussions of magnetic resonance imaging which might otherwise tend to be dry. MRI scanning is notoriously complex, but Claudia had experience of simplifying it: 'My ninety-year-old grandmother in Italy, who's not a physicist, called me every day of my PhD wanting me to explain my research.'

From the scans, which you'll recall I had thought would be pointless, Claudia had built up a map of how different parts of my brain were connected to each other, as well as of their microstructure and physiological properties. One of the scans was what's called a resting-state scan. I just lay in the scanner gently daydreaming and they took 5,000 images of my brain every few seconds, building up a picture of how much oxygen and blood flow there is going to each part of the brain. Areas of the brain that are connected are synchronised in terms of oxygen consumption, so they 'light up' together on the scan at the same time. 'Imagine,' Claudia explained, 'recording phone calls all over a city – you'd be able to identify those houses which were connected, speaking to each other. You map their locations and the strength of the connection between them. Do they phone every day? Or perhaps just once a month? Or never?'*

After my diet, the connectivity between several regions increased, especially the areas involved in the hormonal control of food intake, and the areas involved in desire and reward. Interpreting this isn't easy, but it seemed to represent something of my experience, which was a tussle between the parts of my brain wanting the food more or less subconsciously and the parts that consciously understood the harms.

As my knowledge about the harms of UPF grew, it became less enjoyable but not less desirable. I had two conflicting analytical thoughts: the desire to complete the experiment versus my increasing knowledge about UPF and how it was harming me. On top of all that, my body was getting very real physiological rewards from consuming all the fat and sugar. I looked forward to dinner, but struggled to like it. Claudia put it like this: 'It's as if one part of your brain, your cerebellum, the part that deals with habits and automatic behaviours, was saying this is all an error, but your frontal cortex was saying it was OK.'

* For instance, the parts of the brain that control movements are constantly checking in with the parts of the brain that initiate movements, even when you're not moving. These connections are called 'resting-state networks'. We know that people with neurological conditions like multiple sclerosis or Parkinson's disease have very different resting-state networks of connectivity, but we understand much less about the effect of diet on such networks.

The changes on my MRI were physiological not morphological – the actual wiring in my brain hadn't changed, but the information flowing through the wires had. Claudia explained that, over time, such changes in information flow are what cause the structural changes: 'If traffic starts to flow down a side road it will eventually become enlarged to become a main trunk road. New permanent connections grow.'

I pressed Claudia about whether it could all be noise – I am after all just one patient. Perhaps I was more stressed at work or got less sleep before the second scan? She was clear: 'No, you don't see these big changes unless you do something significant to the physiology of the brain. It's not random.' She also did something called brain-stem spectroscopy, which looks at the breakdown products of neurotransmitters, and these data were all consistent with the same changes noted in the MRI.

As I absorbed these findings, I started to think of Lyra and Sasha. The impact on children and teenagers is a real concern. They will be eating UPF at the dose I was, only they'll be doing so for years, and while their brains are still developing. We have no idea what that means. We do know that messing about with the reward pathways isn't a good idea. That's what all addictive drugs do, after all. Claudia described it as the million-dollar question: 'Will UPF affect their IQ, their social performance? We just don't know what's happening to children's brains.'

Claudia was optimistic about quitting UPF though, which was nice, and a bit reassuring, suggesting that it might be the case that if we could scan people living with overweight as they quit UPF, we would eventually see beneficial changes in their brains. 'People think they are going to lose fat,' she said, 'but it may actually modify the brain in a very positive way that affects other areas of life. I suspect that we might see people's concentration and memory improve, though we'd need to prove that.' I found this helpful to imagine: that healthy food might rewire the brain in a positive way.

After the scan, the diet was over, and I stopped eating UPF immediately and completely.

Rauber had flicked some switch, and I was able to quit cold turkey.* I use the language of addiction for a reason. I had come to think that I had been somewhat addicted to UPF before, and that my brother Xand certainly was.

Within forty-eight hours I was sleeping at night, my bowels began to function and work became easier. Of course, life has its own ebbs and flows, but nothing else seemed to have changed apart from the end of the diet.

There was a lot of UPF that I had never been tempted by, but there were certain types – mainly savoury, fried, spicy and laden with monosodium glutamate (MSG) – that I would occasionally eat to the point of vomiting. This had never struck me as disordered so much as practical: it made a good night's sleep easier if, having massively overeaten, I wasn't bursting with food. Disorder or not, at the end of my diet all this stuff – stuff I had previously struggled to stop eating – became inedible.

Food addiction is, scientifically, very unfashionable, and with good reason. There are two problems. For a start, because food contains such a wide range of molecules, how could any single combination be identified as addictive? And the briefest thought experiment about individual macronutrients like pure fat or sugar tells you they're not addictive.† But the biggest problem with considering food an addictive substance is that, logically, it leads to a strategy of abstinence when, of course, you can't be abstinent from

---

* Dinah amused herself when she pointed out that cold turkey was in fact something I didn't need to quit.

† A 2018 paper – 'Food addiction: a valid concept?' – by Paul Fletcher (against) and Paul Kenny (for) is readable and free.[12] They're both heavyweights. I side a little more with Kenny in his conclusion, but Fletcher is mainly advising caution to scientists about extending beliefs beyond what the evidence clearly shows. Kenny frames what he thinks are the addictive substances: 'combinations of macronutrients in palatable high-calorie food items that do not occur naturally, but that when combined can pack a supraphysiological punch to brain motivation circuits that is sufficient to modify subsequent consummatory behaviors'.

food. And addicts can't be moderate with addictive substances. Food just can't be addictive.

So, as a solution, some scientists have proposed that food addiction is 'behavioural'.[13] This is one of the two broad categories of addiction. There's substance addiction – defined as a 'neuropsychiatric disorder characterized by a recurring desire to take a drug despite harmful consequences' – which covers tobacco, alcohol, cocaine and so on. And then there's behavioural or non-substance addiction, which covers things like eating, pathological gambling, internet addiction and mobile phone addiction.

The behavioural explanation just doesn't ring true to me. Just as smokers have cigarette addiction, I, along with many others, have felt very strongly addicted to food itself – or more specifically to particular types of UPF. I've tried a number of traditionally addictive substances – cigarettes during a strange few years in the army, alcohol in immense binges as a medical student, heroin, also known as diamorphine, after an operation on my right testicle – but nothing has ever drawn me in like the food I love, the stuff that really tickles those ancient parts of my brain, the reward centres that motivate so much behaviour, good and bad.

This impasse between reality and science is partly responsible for the confused way we conceive of obesity: we tend to locate the problem in the individual, not the food, despite the mounting evidence that the food itself is the problem for obesity and perhaps for many eating disorders. Together with Xand, I read through the defining criteria of addiction in the latest version of the US *Diagnostic and Statistical Manual of Mental Disorders*, the psychiatric bible. It classifies problem use of an intoxicating substance as mild, moderate or severe using eleven diagnostic criteria. If you meet more than six of the criteria, you have a severe problem. We both scored a solid nine for the food we love (all of it UPF).

The questions focused on things like 'the substance being taken in increasing amounts' (tick), any 'efforts to control use being unsuccessful' (tick), 'lots of time and effort being spent getting the substance' (tick) and 'the experience of cravings' (tick, tick, tick).

The crux of the matter is the ninth criterion: 'Use of the substance is continued despite knowledge of having a persistent or recurrent physical or psychological problem that is likely to have been caused or exacerbated by the substance.' The psychological effects of the stigma, shame, failure and guilt associated with excess eating are exhaustively documented in the literature, even before we get to the libraries of data that catalogue the physical harms, and Xand and I have both kept eating despite knowing all this.

So, how do we reconcile the impossibility of labelling food as an addictive substance with the fact that some foods for some people do seem to be addictive? By adopting Rauber's idea that UPF is not food, like a banana or a piece of chicken, but rather a separate category of addictive edible substance. It isn't food generally that's addictive – it's UPF. And an increasing amount of mainstream science is backing up this concept.

If you know someone who struggles with substance misuse, it may seem offensive to compare it with excess food consumption, but there is a growing literature suggesting that it's a valid comparison. Ashley Gearhardt is an associate professor of psychology at the University of Michigan and is one of the leading scientists who thinks that considering parallels between UPF and addictive substances can be informative. She has outlined the evidence in a series of papers.[14–16]

First, UPF is consistently associated with higher scores on food addiction scales compared to real food. It's always UPF that people report problems with. Not all UPF obviously – for some it will be donuts, for others ice cream. For me it was cheap takeaway. But when it comes to loss of control of eating and binges, UPF products are almost always the substances used.[17–19] Not all UPF is addictive to everyone, and those who do find they are addicted will likely have a particular range of products. Sharon Newson and I had compared lists of the foods that we struggled with. It was *all* UPF, but there was no overlap between our binge foods.

Second, UPF seems to be more addictive for more people than many addictive drugs. Of course, many people are able to consume UPF in moderation, but that's also true for cocaine, alcohol and cigarettes.[20] Compare the numbers. The transition from trying UPF to being unable to stop using it is extremely high: 40 per cent of the US population live with obesity and we know that the majority of them will try to lose weight in a given year.[21] Cessation rates are so low as to be non-existent. There is no other drug that, having tried it, 40 per cent of people will continue to use regularly despite negative health consequences (a definition of addiction). For example, over 90 per cent of people in the USA consume alcohol but only 14 per cent develop an alcohol-use disorder.[22] Even with illicit drugs like cocaine, only a relatively small subset of users (20 per cent) go on to become addicted.[23]

Third, drugs of abuse and UPF share certain biological properties. Both are modified from natural states so that there is rapid delivery of the rewarding substance. The speed of delivery is strongly linked to addictive potential – cigarettes, snorted cocaine, shots of alcohol. Slowing down delivery transforms the effects – methamphetamine for example becomes a treatment for children who can't concentrate. Nicotine patches are far less addictive than cigarettes. As we'll see, softness and speed of consumption are defining characteristics of UPF compared with real food.

Fourth, drug addiction and food addiction share risk factors like family history of addiction, trauma and depression, indicating that UPF may be performing the same function as the drugs in those people.

Fifth, people report similar addiction symptoms with UPF and other addictive substances, including craving, repeated unsuccessful attempts to cut down and continued use despite negative consequences. And those negative consequences are severe: a poor diet may have worse effects for many people than even very heavy smoking.

Sixth and finally, neuroimaging has shown similar patterns of dysfunction in reward pathways for both food addiction and substance misuse. These foods also appear to engage brain regions related to reward and motivation in a similar manner to addictive drugs.[24, 25]

You may find it hard to consider UPF as equivalent to cigarettes, but poor diet – a high UPF diet – is linked to more deaths globally than tobacco, high blood pressure or any other health risk – 22 per cent of all deaths.[26] Since the risks are so high, there may be advantages to considering UPF as an addictive substance.* It may help to reduce some of the stigma, guilt and blame around obesity and excess consumption, just as campaigners achieved with smoking decades ago. It allows the affected person to focus outwards on the industry causing the harm (something we know is helpful in addiction), rather than inwards on personal failure. And it highlights some useful policy parallels. Tobacco control, for instance, provides a template for the regulation of harmful addictive substances. An addictive behaviour is my problem, hard to regulate or protect against. An addictive substance being marketed with a monkey to my three-year-old is a regulatory failure.

But, above all, considering UPF as an addictive substance solves that problem of abstinence. It's impossible to quit food, but, at least in theory, it's possible to quit UPF. It won't be easy, of course – the contemporary UK is to UPF what the 1950s were to cigarettes.

Having had this revelation, I felt I had to make my brother Xand, living at the low end of clinical obesity at the time, quit UPF too. I went to speak to him with all the evangelism of the new convert, which was probably pretty obnoxious. But now that I was no longer hassling him (having spoken with Alasdair Cant), I proposed that

---

* Nicole Avena thinks that a comparison with cigarettes is fair, although she recognises that there are differences. – primarily that 'people don't *need* cigarettes and they do need food'. Of course, some people need UPF because it is all that is available and affordable, but *physiologically* we do not need UPF. Avena thinks that, in terms of the effects on the brain, cigarettes and a lot of UPF products are comparable: 'Many people will find it easier to quit smoking than UPF.' And the effects on the body may also be similar. 'I think that we need to start paying more attention to the fact that these foods are killing us.'

he try my 80 per cent UPF diet for a bit and he agreed. Not to lose weight but as an (unscientific) experiment. It would be fun. We'd record it for a BBC podcast (*Addicted to Food*) and see what happened. We agreed a week of 80 per cent UPF and I sent him off to speak with Kevin Hall, Fernanda Rauber, Nicole Avena and some of the other experts to see if their words would have the same effect on him as they did on me.

In the meantime, I was convinced from the evidence and my experience that UPF was harmful, but I now wanted to know what exactly it was doing to my body – and how.

PART THREE

Oh, so this is why I'm anxious and my belly aches!

UPF is pre-chewed

Anthony Fardet may not have been the first person to consider what he calls the food 'matrix', the physical structure of food, but he may have thought about it more deeply than anyone else alive. He's serious, with thick, greying hair. I'd guess he's about my age. He's a scientist in the Human Nutrition Unit at Université Clermont Auvergne in France. Everything he says seems profound and important, partly because he uses a lot of long words, and partly because his perfect English comes with a French movie-star accent: 'We eat food, not nutrients. So, from a philosophical point of view, the best thing is to combine holism and reductionism. I am an empiricist and an inductivist.'

I had a feeling I was also an empirical inductivist but wasn't entirely sure and resolved to check later. I was calling him to ask about how ultra-processing affects the physical structure of food and how this in turn affects our bodies. The principle of the matrix is pretty straightforward: that food is not merely the sum of its constituent parts. Anthony explained that the purpose of the digestive system is to destroy the food matrix. He used apples as an example. The fibre that gives an apple crunch and solidity makes up just 2.5 per cent of the apple's weight. The other 97.5 per cent is juice. The way the fibre is arranged around the cells and the fluid – that's the matrix.

With this in mind, a small group of scientists back in 1977 fed ten people apples in three different forms: apple juice without any of the pulp (fibre free), raw whole apple smoothie and whole chunks of apple. They made the participants eat everything at the same speed and then they measured fullness (satiety), blood sugar and insulin in response to the three different apple preparations.[1]

What they found was that both the juice and the puree caused blood sugar and insulin levels to spike higher than the whole apple, before falling to a lower level than they had been in the first place. As a result of the sugar crash all the participants still felt hungry. The whole apple, meanwhile, made blood sugar rise slowly, before it returned to the baseline level – no crash, and the fullness from the whole apples lasted hours. It seems our bodies have evolved to manage the sugar load from an apple precisely, but fruit juice is a relatively new invention.*

Apple juice, which is typically around 15 per cent sugar, behaves much like any soft drink. But so does the apple purée, even though it contains all the constituents of the apple, including the fibre, and was made moments before consumption. Fibre is important, but the matrix, the structure of the apple, is key.

Take Coco Pops. They're branded as being crunchy, and a few do stay crunchy – at least for a while. But each mouthful is predominantly a slick of wet starchy globs. The Coco Pops and milk form a textured liquid. It's *soft*. Softness is one of the characteristics that Kevin Hall identified as a near universal quality of UPF.† The softness is down to the method of construction – industrially modified plant components and mechanically recovered meats are pulverised, ground, milled and extruded until all the fibrous textures of sinew, tendon, cellulose and lignin are destroyed. What remains

---

* Baby food is mainly puréed fruit and for the same reason has very high levels of sugar and is expensive and unnecessary.

† Of course, there are 'real' foods that are as soft or softer than some UPF, like bananas, tomatoes and berries. But these foods all still have a preserved matrix that will be destroyed by processing. When they become UPF ingredients – berry purée, tomato powder and so on – they become even softer than they were before. You never find a whole banana in a yoghurt. Ketchup doesn't contain whole tomatoes. A blueberry, just like an apple, behaves differently depending on whether it's been turned into a smoothie or consumed whole.

can then be reassembled into dinosaurs or letters of the alphabet or the hyperbolic paraboloids of Pringles potato snacks.

The marketing primes us to register an initial crunch of batter, the pop of a puffed rice crisp, the snap of a reformed fried potato powder chip, but these yield to the slightest bite. The foods are cleverly textured – a jelly filling with a dry sponge surround, or chunks of real vegetables in soup – to disguise the fact that, within seconds, we're eating mush.

A McDonald's hamburger (or one from Burger King or any other UPF supplier) is another perfect example of the illusion. The first bite rewards you with a sequence of textural experiences: the sweet bun has a dry crust over a creamy, spongy matrix, the burger is rubbery and seems as salty as seawater, the gherkins and onions provide a crunch, the mustard tickles your trigeminal nerve and the acidity in the ketchup sets off the whole experience. 'Spongy', 'rubbery', 'crunchy' – but really it's all just as soft as down. As a result, I can inhale a burger in well under a minute. And then I'm going to have another because I'm still hungry.*

Why? For the same reason that Lyra was still hungry after one bowl of Coco Pops: the signals that tell you to 'stop eating' haven't evolved to handle food this soft and easily digested, so soft that it's essentially pre-chewed. Rather than being digested slowly along the length of the intestine in a way that stimulates the release of satiety hormones, it may be that UPF is absorbed so quickly that it doesn't reach the parts of the gut that send the 'stop eating' signal to the brain.

While I was on my UPF diet, I began to notice the softness most starkly with bread. As the Real Bread Campaign (which is run by Sustain, a non-profit alliance for better food and farming) have pointed out for a long time, real bread is hard to find and very expensive in the UK. Craft bakeries make up just 5 per cent of the

---

* The softness problem is backed up by evidence suggesting that UPF is eaten far more quickly than whole or minimally processed food, meaning more calories can be consumed per minute.

bread market and in many places no non-UPF bread will be available. Sourdough bread should have just water, salt, wild yeast and flour as the ingredients, but even products claiming to be sourdough in supermarkets are often in fact 'sourfaux', with up to fifteen ingredients, including palm oil and commercial yeast.[2]

If you can find and afford some, then it's worth comparing rye bread or real sourdough to a supermarket loaf. For years I have bought Hovis Multigrain Seed Sensations. Here are the ingredients: 'wheat flour, water, seed mix (13%), wheat protein, yeast, salt, soya flour, malted barley flour, granulated sugar, barley flour, preservative: E282 calcium propionate, emulsifier: E472e (mono- and diacetyltartaric acid esters of mono- and diglycerides of fatty acids), caramelised sugar, barley fibre, flour treatment agent: ascorbic acid'.

Lots of breads like this use low-protein flour and then add separated wheat protein later, because it gives the manufacturer enormous control over the consistency of the product. Many of these ingredients save cost – through cutting time, bakers, etc – and much of that saving is passed onto us. A loaf of genuine sourdough costs £3–5. At the time of writing the cheapest loaf at Sainsbury's is 36p and the Hovis is 95p.

But the various processes and treatment agents mean that I can eat a slice of Hovis even more quickly, gram for gram, than I could put away that UPF burger. The bread disintegrates into a bolus of slime that is easily manipulated down the throat. A slice of Dusty Knuckle Potato Sourdough (£5.99 from one supplier) takes well over a minute to eat, and my jaw gets tired.

However, you won't get jaw fatigue with UPF bread, and the fact that it takes so little chewing may explain many of our contemporary dental problems. In the UK and the USA, around a third of twelve-year-olds have an overbite – a jaw that's too small for their face – which is why so many children today need orthodontic work. I had my right lower wisdom tooth removed for the same reason. Looking through the UPF papers, I realised this is a common problem of modern life. Evidence from skulls shows that pre-industrial farmers who were eating increasing levels of carbohydrate have plenty of cavities and dental abscesses, but fewer than 5 per cent have impacted wisdom teeth, compared with 70 per cent of modern populations.[3, 4]

The reason for this is that our modern faces, especially our jaws, are much smaller than those of our ancestors. This change has happened suddenly: Australian Aboriginal people, many of whom transitioned abruptly to a modern diet in the 1950s, have much smaller jaws than predecessors of even 100 years earlier.[5-7] The jaws of modern Finns are 6 per cent smaller than their ancient (and genetically extremely similar) ancestors.[8]

The reason for this facial shrinkage is the same reason that tennis players have much more bone density in the arm they play with. It's the reason that longbowmen who died on the *Mary Rose* could be identified from the size and density of their arm bones.[9] Bones are not stones: they're living tissues that are constantly being remodelled, broken down and built up according to the stresses applied to them. The face and jaw bones are no exception: if you chew, they'll grow.

Indeed, one study had a group of Greek children chew a hard resinous gum for two hours per day, just to see the effect. At the end of the study, it was found not only that the children who had chewed the gum could produce more force with their bites, but also that they had significantly longer jaws and cheekbones.[10]

I read all this and went to look at Lyra's little jaw and teeth. Her upper incisors protruded far over her lower ones. Was this normal? Would a dentist in twenty-first-century Britain even know what human dentition should look like? Was I already too late? Had she ever really *chewed* anything in her life? I resolved to show her dentist a scientific paper by a Harvard professor called Daniel Lieberman, 'Effects of food processing on masticatory strain and craniofacial growth in a retrognathic face', and I bought some carrots for her to have as a snack.

There's a lot of science that suggests this softness may also be a problem when it comes to calorie intake. In Kevin Hall's unprocessed food versus UPF trial, participants reported that the UPF didn't have an unnaturally high 'sensory appeal': the two diets were equally delicious and satiating. Yet they ate, on average, 500 calories more per day during the UPF portion of the study.

The main difference in the effects of the two diets that Hall observed was that people ate the UPF much more quickly. And, as well as being soft, most UPF is dry, which means that it's calorie-dense. Water dilutes everything, including energy. Meat, fruit and vegetables typically have a very high water content.

This dryness is crucial to UPF. It's one of the key ways of stopping microbes from growing in it, contributing to the absurdly long shelf life that helps make UPF so profitable. The stuff doesn't decompose. There are plenty of newspaper pieces about people who keep McDonald's burgers that don't rot for years. McDonald's Canada broke the first rule of all scandals when they decided to tell their side of one of these stories: 'The reality is that McDonald's hamburgers, fries and chicken are like all foods, and do rot if kept under certain conditions.'[11]

The desperate insistence that the food will rot was a rare instance of corporate marketing doing my job for me. But the statement is correct: lack of rotting is much more to do with the dryness of the UPF than the chemical burden of preservatives.

In Hall's experiment, the softness plus the calorie density meant that participants consumed an average of seventeen calories per minute more when eating UPF compared to the unprocessed diet.* These results are consistent with research by Barbara Rolls that showed that the energy density of food has a crucial role in moderating daily energy intake.[12-14]

Across dozens of carefully controlled experiments, Rolls and colleagues repeatedly demonstrated that higher-energy-density foods and diets promote greater energy intake and increased body weight. This effect appears to be independent of palatability or nutritional content, and is true for men and women, people with overweight

---

* The food was of course processed by cooking and so on, but in the study it's called the 'unprocessed diet'.

and people at a healthy weight, children and adults and in the short-term and long-term. It's one of the most robustly demonstrated facts about nutrition.[15, 16] And, perhaps most importantly, it doesn't seem to matter whether the energy in the food comes from fat or carbs – it's the energy density that is the more important determinant of calorie intake.

There's also a large body of research showing that eating more quickly increases the risk of eating more, gaining weight, and having metabolic disease.[17] The speed at which you eat is partly to do with what you eat: foods that take longer to process in the mouth make you feel fuller.[18–20] But it's also partly determined by genetics. The Growing Up in Singapore Towards healthier Outcomes (GUSTO) study showed that kids who ate more quickly and for longer were more likely to have obesity. The researchers described this as an 'obesogenic eating style'.[21] Clare Llewellyn, the twin scientist at UCL, showed that this eating style is genetic and is associated with higher BMI.[22] Genes for 'fast eating' are likely to make some people especially vulnerable to the softness of UPF.

Another study compared volunteers drinking two chocolate milkshakes, one of which was thick and viscous, the other thin. Both milkshakes were nutritionally identical, with equal energy density and palatability. Volunteers were allowed to consume as much as they liked, and the thin liquid shake was associated with a 47 per cent higher total intake than the thick one. However, if volunteers were forced to drink at the same rate, they ended up drinking the same amount of each shake in total.[23]

The number of chews per bite has a direct effect on slowing and reducing food intake. Chewing each mouthful might seem to be a good way of reducing calorie intake but, of course, this is to confuse cause and effect. Remember our rate of consumption is determined by the food and our genetics – it is not a conscious decision. Anyone who has tried to match the pace of a slow or fast dining companion knows how hard it is.

So, there's a lot of evidence that the rate of UPF consumption is related to its health effects, but what worries me is that some see this as an opportunity to make a different kind of UPF – with textures that would slow down the rate of consumption. A 2020 review analysed the data from five published studies that measured energy intake rates across 327 foods from the UK, Singapore, Switzerland and the Netherlands.[24] The researchers showed that going from unprocessed food to processed food to UPF increased the number of calories consumed per minute from thirty-six to fifty-four to sixty-nine. The researchers concluded:

> Industrial food processing affords an important opportunity to apply wholesale changes to the forms and textures encountered in the food environment, and in combination with reformulation to reduce energy density, can be used to produce widespread improvements in the energy intake rates, palatability, and nutrient densities within the food supply … the future challenge for food processors is to develop products that sustain consumer appeal with optimal satisfaction per kilocalorie consumed, while reducing their potential to promote energy over consumption.

I didn't like this. It felt a bit off. Having established the many ways in which food-processing technologies make food more energy-dense and quicker to eat, and having established that these two aspects of any given food seem central to driving obesity, rather than proposing a shift toward whole food, more processing is proposed instead. This 'hyper-processing' seems an unlikely solution to the problems of ultra-processing.

It's also odd to suggest that this is a 'future challenge', when the food industry has known about the data linking speed of intake to increased calorie consumption since studies conducted in the 1990s.[25]

I also worried that, while the article said very clearly that there were 'no conflicts of interest', one of the authors, Ciarán Forde was on the scientific advisory council for Kerry Group plc (a multi-billion-dollar manufacturer of UPF), and another, Kees de Graaf, was on the board of Sensus (a company that produces food ingredients inulin and oligofructose), and all three authors had received reimbursements for speaking at meetings sponsored by companies that produce food and nutritional products. Being a scientific adviser to a UPF company and writing about food processing must constitute a conflict (unless someone sits on that advisory group for free).

On a paper the following year naming Ciarán G. Forde as an author, there is also a statement saying 'the authors declare no conflict of interest', but at the time he was not just an adviser to Kerry but also (according to the same paper!) part of an academic consortium that received research funding from Abbott Nutrition, Nestec (a Nestlé subsidiary) and Danone.

But mainly, it seems unlikely to me that making UPF harder to eat is going to work. Cigarette manufacturers tried very hard over the years to process their cigarettes to make them less dangerous. They added little ventilation holes, so smokers got less smoke, but then smokers simply sucked harder. We consume addictive products for the sensory hit, and we know that increasing the speed of any drug being delivered into the body is a crucial aspect of making a substance addictive.[26] If you interfere with the rate of consumption, my bet would be you lose a little of that hit and the product won't sell as well. UPF is soft not by accident, but because that's the way to sell the largest amount.

As we'll see, labelling UPF is not going to be trivial because of the opposition from the food industry. But labels that warn about softness and energy density would be very well evidenced.

12.

UPF smells funny

We might think of flavour as frivolous, but there's a school of thought that says artificial flavouring is *the* problem when it comes to obesity and overconsumption. Since I did my diet, it's the word 'flavouring' that I avoid more than any other in food. Flavourings signal that something is UPF, and the need for flavouring tells us a lot about some of the ways UPF does us harm.

The scientific literature on smell is walled away from the papers about health and obesity, confined largely to its own journals. The papers are written by psychologists, with philosophers and chefs often collaborating. Barry Smith is a major contributor to this body of work and is the director of the Centre for the Study of the Senses, as well as a philosopher, wine expert, broadcaster and food scientist.

I met him one day in his office. It looks across at two enormous limestone lions that flank the rear entrance to the British Museum. As soon as I walked in, Barry started challenging my senses with a hyper-real painting of Venice on the wall. The painting is by Patrick Hughes. As I moved past it, I could see around the edges of buildings and down canals, which poked out of the canvas on pyramids. It's an unsettling illusion – the parts of the picture physically closest to the viewer appear to be the farthest away [and appear to move when we move].

'It's called "reverspective",' Barry explained. 'We don't know why it works.' Barry then told me about convergent gaze, subtended visual angles, parallax and the tension between the brain's information about depth perception and what happens to be near or far. The painting is a good representation of his expertise – how little our conscious experience of the world has to do with physical objective reality. Barry himself is constantly creating illusions: he gossips without gossiping, jokes while he's serious, makes you understand things you can't understand. And he used to help companies make UPF. He was an expert ultra-processor, advising food companies on how best to exploit the relationships between our senses (which aren't all as distinct as we once thought) and how we use them to enjoy the food we eat.

Surrounded by wine and chocolates (materials for experiments), Barry explained that hearing influences flavour and smell influences taste. Vanilla, technically a molecule you smell, when added to ice cream will make it seem sweeter, even without adding more sugar. 'Smell even influences touch,' he said. 'Apple-scented shampoo makes your hair feel shinier than other shampoos.'

The fact that taste, smell and flavour are mixed up together in our minds and brains is used by the companies who make our food. Barry gave examples from the field of wine.

In a 2001 paper, 'The color of odors',[1] a team from the Faculty of Oenology at the University of Bordeaux described an experiment performed on fifty-four wine experts. Each was served two glasses of wine – one red, one white – and asked to describe them. The experts found that the white wine had notes of honey, lemon, lychee, white peach and citrus, while for the red they reported blackcurrant, coal, chocolate, cinnamon, red currant, tar, raspberry, prune and cherry.

They were then presented with another pair of red and white wines. But what none of the experts identified was that the white wine was from the same bottle as the *red* they had previously tasted. The only difference was the addition of an odourless red dye. They described the flavours in terms of colours: crimson, black and brown substances for the red, and pale and yellow substances for the white. Anyone who drinks wine would be confident they could tell white from red, but even the experts fall for this illusion because colour exerts a dominant influence over how we perceive the smell and the taste of the wine. This is because our senses interact. This study suggests that colour seems to play a stronger role than odour in determining what we think we are tasting.*

If the wine experts can be fooled, under carefully arranged conditions, then so can you and I. Barry told me about one of his favourite sensory tricks involving ice cream: 'If you go into the freezer for an ice cream bar, as you rip open the packet, it won't smell of anything, because it's too cold. So, lots of companies add a caramel scent in the ribbing of the wrapper we tear open.'

The scent allows our dopamine reward system to respond to the sensory cue of opening the packet, which starts a craving. It also leads us to experience the chocolate and caramel in the bar more intensely. Barry thinks this sort of trick is fine. 'There's an important difference between leading and misleading,' he said. 'In the case of the frozen ice cream bar, the scent is *leading* you to expect real caramel and chocolate. But there are *misleading* sensory experiences: meaty smells in plant products, artificial flavours, gums that replace fats – all of these promising ingredients that aren't there. This is where we start to see the problem.'

Barry started to reveal some of the sensory lies that UPF tells us. But to understand these lies, I first needed him to guide me through the science of smell, taste and flavour because the language, like the senses themselves, is jumbled up. The words 'taste' and 'flavour' are used interchangeably to describe the unified perceptual experience of a food. But in scientific terms, flavour is both taste and smell, and flavour molecules are detected by receptors in the nose as well as by taste receptors in the mouth and throat. So, scientifically speaking, two boiled sweets with the same amount

---

* One of the team, Frédéric Brochet, left academia and now makes wine. In another famous study by Brochet,[2] another panel of experts was served a midrange Bordeaux, but from a bottle with a label that suggested it was a cheap table wine. The following week, the same panel had the same wine, but from a bottle with a label indicating it was a grand cru worth many times more. The tasting notes again reflected that expectation overrides the true sensory experience.

of sugar but different 'flavours' may *taste* identical (sweet), but *smell* distinct.* Confused? Don't worry.

Let's start with flavour. The question of why flavour exists has to start with *where* it exists. Flavour arises when the brain puts together inputs from taste, smell and touch. When we eat, we use information from our eyes, ears, nose, tongue and lips to build up an impression of flavour. The bones and muscles in our face detect vibrations from crunch and resistance from chewiness. Receptors in the mouth detect chemical changes in saliva and alterations in friction from oils and powders. And, of course, we put all this together with our expectations, and our memories (both conscious and unconscious) of the last time we ate the food or the advertisement we saw for it yesterday.

This integrated sensory system is a product of that billion-year arms race to extract energy from our ecosystem.

Smell is all about selecting safe and nutritious food, while avoiding toxic, unsafe food. It's one of the earliest warning systems for whether something is safe to eat. After all, by the time you can taste something, it may already be too late, but there is also the safety net of bitter receptors at the back of the mouth, which we'll come to. Thanks to the global supply chains of modern supermarkets, many of us are used to fruit being ready to eat and ripe all year round, but in a tropical forest this isn't the case. Toxin levels vary, and a piece of fruit may be edible for quite a narrow window, typically determined by exactly when the plant wants the animal to eat it and disperse the seeds. Smell saves the time-consuming trouble of having to put something poisonous in your mouth – although occasionally, as Barry points out, sometimes we only realise something is off once we've started to chew.

---

* If you put food in your mouth and chew, molecules go up your nose from the back of your mouth. This retronasal smell feels like taste, and you experience this kind of smelling as being 'in the mouth' – but it isn't, and it makes a huge contribution to flavour. With a nose clip on, the two sweets will taste the same – sweet. But when you take the nose clip off and odours travel from the mouth to the nose, we can taste their different fruit flavours.

A signature set of volatile molecules evaporates from almost every substance in the world. Smell involves the detection of these molecules using receptors in the nose. And it's fantastically precise.[*] It's often said that we can detect 10,000 different smells, but that's wrong – it's far too low. A 2014 study[3, 4] tested people using a matrix of different smells and estimated that we can distinguish between more than 1 trillion potential compounds, meaning that you could take any two of the trillion and be able to say: 'Yes, those are different.'[†]

This precision requires a lot of genetic information: the olfactory receptor gene family is the largest in the mammalian genome and larger than any other gene family in any other species. Part of the reason we have so many genes is because of a basic problem of the chemistry. Smell molecules are all very different, and have very different properties. There are just a few types of taste receptors because each is detecting similar properties of similar molecules. Our legendarily poor sense of smell is exactly that – a legend.

It does seem like we traded some smell resolution for improved vision, but we still outperform other mammals on some tests. While dogs are almost certainly better at detecting dog urine on

---

[*] How smell works: air inhaled through the nostrils or up from the back of the mouth, passes over long ridges of bone and up towards the olfactory epithelium, where the olfactory nerves – the smell nerves – poke through the bone into the soft mucus-covered skin to touch the inhaled air. The olfactory system is the only example of the brain sending its own neurons into the environment like a probe. These nerves are covered in hundreds of different receptors – proteins with little pockets on them. Odorants (smell molecules) in the air you inhale bind these receptors and send information to the brain to be decoded (using a few hundred receptors to detect a trillion smells is a coding problem). Each smell molecule binds to more than one receptor, and each receptor binds many smell molecules. And they bind with different strengths for different times, thereby encoding a far greater range of possibilities than if it were one receptor per molecule.

[†] The actual number of discriminable olfactory stimuli – i.e. smells – may be much higher than a trillion. You aren't just able to distinguish between individual molecules, but between mixtures of thirty different molecules. You can also distinguish mixtures of identical molecules in slightly different ratios.

lamp posts (though humans haven't been tested), experiments have shown that we're better at fruit and veg discrimination.*

This olfactory precision means we can tolerate similar molecules in cheese and socks.† In fact, faeces, breastmilk, rotting corpses, cheese and aged meat all share molecular signatures, but our olfactory system has evolved to distinguish between them.

There is (probably) no such thing as a good or a bad smell.‡ Smell instead acts like a barcode, which, without effort, we link to our

---

* There are only fifteen odorants for which science has established the lowest detectable threshold for dogs. But humans are better at detecting low doses of five of those molecules, all of which are fruit or flower odours of less significance to a carnivore presumably. But dogs are unsurprisingly good at detecting low levels of the carbolic acids released by their prey in body odours. There's a lot of literature showing humans' sense of smell is similar to or more sensitive than dogs, mice or rabbits for odorants in fruit. Mice are good at detecting the molecules found in the urine of mouse predators (although we aren't bad), and we are better than mice at detecting the smell of human blood. Humans can smell the stinky mercaptan added to gas to alert us to gas leaks, but dogs don't smell it at all. And humans can learn to follow a scent trail like a dog and we improve massively with a little training, indicating that our smell is an underused sense – like our bones and muscles, it has become flabby and inactive.

† It may be that the same molecules may be perceived differently when sniffed compared with when they travel from the mouth to the nose. Barry explained: 'A stinky cheese can smell disgusting – orthonsal olfaction – and pretty much like socks. But it can have a delicious flavour when those odours come from the mouth to the nose – retronasal olfaction.'

‡ We can learn that some smells are sweet, but this seems to be cultural. Ethyl butyrate smells 'sweet' probably because it is a smell usually associated experientially with the sweet taste of fruit juice. If paired with a sweet taste, it can make it taste sweeter and it can mask a sour taste. How we experience any flavour combination depends on how we have experienced it before. We learn that certain tastes and smells are congruent. We build these associations as flavours when we're very young, and they are extremely culturally specific. Cinnamon is nearly always a sweet spice in European cooking, but in Morocco they make a pigeon pie with cinnamon and sugar, and it's also widely used in savoury dishes in many other places. Vanilla is sweet smelling in the West, where it tends to be mixed with sugar, but it smells salty to southeast Asians, in whose cuisine vanilla is often mixed with salt and fish.

previous experience of eating a food. It's a very precise way of labelling something so we can seek it out, or avoid it, next time.

Humans and animals will learn to love almost any flavour with
a smell barcode that is associated with nutritional reward.[5-8] This
was demonstrated in the 1970s in experiments in which rats drank
sweet, zero-calorie, flavoured liquids at the same time as having
either sugar or water infused directly into their stomachs. They
learned to love the flavours they drank while getting the sugar but
not those paired with the water. Broadly speaking, if the last time
you ate a particular flavour–taste combination you got a big nutritional reward and didn't experience nausea, you'll want that food
more in the future. This all happens almost entirely beneath conscious experience, and it's how we learn to love specific food. French
fries smell 'good' because the body and brain have linked the smell
with the huge nutritional load of fat and carbs that follows. These
associations that we learn between smell and taste, odours and
nutrients, are powerful and, of course, easily hacked.

Flavour signatures of particular smells and tastes also allow us
to identify food from our cultures – historically food we would
know to be safe.* This learning process starts before birth. Julie
Mennella at Monell Chemical Senses Centre did an experiment
examining how food choices during pregnancy influence future

---

* I worked briefly in northern Russia in Chukotka. Sergei, the hunter in the family I was staying with, killed a walrus on the first day there, hacked off a flipper
and left it on the ground outside the cabin without explanation. It sat in the dirt
in the grey Arctic autumn at just above fridge temperature for three weeks
before he brought it into the kitchen one day. It was covered in green fuzz, fluids
oozing out of it, with a sickly-sweet smell of rot. Sergei cut away the fuzz,
removed a glob of the fat and presented it to me: 'Snickers'. It had the familiar
tang of fermentation – the acidic breakdown products of the proteins and the
fats – like a cheese that is so mature it's almost spicy. I was there to try to understand the local diet and its effect on blood clotting, so this became a staple food.
It took me about three days to be able to eat even the smallest amount without
retching. Then I remember one day I suddenly found myself craving it. It
seemed to create some sort of incredible internal furnace – I could eat it all day
and stay warm.

flavour choice.[9] During the last trimester of their pregnancies, participants drank a big glass of either carrot juice or water for four days per week for three weeks. They did the same while lactating. Then, as the introduction of solid foods began, Mennella looked at the infants' responses to a mixture of carrot juice and cereal compared with water and cereal. The infants whose mothers had drunk the carrot juice during pregnancy and breastfeeding enjoyed the carrot juice mixture more. Similar findings had previously been reported with garlic and star anise flavours. These early flavour experiences have provided a continuous chain of food knowledge for millennia, but the chain was broken when, for many people, the only food available during pregnancy became UPF.

The body's ability to link calories with a particular smell or flavour barcode is exploitable by UPF manufacturers. They can use complex and entirely secret flavour profiles and pair them with a significant nutritional reward in the form of fats and refined sugars to build brand loyalty. Just as we have evolved a system to detect the infinitesimally small changes in fruit volatiles that occur with ripening, so too can we detect the difference between different types of cola. If a UPF manufacturer can persuade parents to give a child their cola early, then the child will make a link between the sugar, the caffeine buzz and the precise flavour barcode of that specific product, and they'll have that child as a customer for life. All other colas will taste a little 'wrong'. The use of flavourings gives the manufacturer absolute control. I eat the same brands of chocolate bar, yoghurt and ketchup that I did as a child. Food should vary – fruit and whole foods change every day, and crops taste different according to the season and weather. There are good batches, bad batches, odd textures and flavours and differences. Not so with UPF. Adding flavourings (tastes and smells) in precise amounts allows for complete consistency.

As far as Mark Schatzker is concerned, the use of flavourings is one of the main problems with UPF. He wrote such an extraordinary book about flavour, *The Dorito Effect*, that he ended up joining a nutrition research group at Yale and now publishes science papers with them. Kevin Hall specifically mentioned him as a journalist who has moved the field forwards by thinking creatively and speculating usefully beyond the evidence.

Schatzker's idea is that, over the past half century or more, industrial animal and plant breeding has focused on size and looks, such that the flavour has been bred out of meat, tomatoes, strawberries, broccoli, wheat, corn – pretty much everything we eat.* Part of the reason we are consuming so much is in search of missing tastes and flavour, which also indicate missing nutrition.

Schatzker argues that, beyond being a simple barcode, flavour is a signal of particular nutrients, which is what sends us in pursuit of those flavours. He cites research demonstrating that many flavour molecules in tomatoes are the precursors for essential fatty acids and vitamins. Tomatoes for example have a 'rose note' – a really popular smell that's found in food, drink, cigarettes, perfumes and soaps. That rose note is made from a molecule called phenylalanine, which is an essential amino acid (i.e. a molecule that the body needs but cannot make). Another group of tomato flavours is made from carotenoids, such as vitamin A. In fact, we seem particularly sensitive to the flavours made from carotenoids: damascenone, found in tomatoes, berries, apples and grapes, can be detected at concentrations as low as two parts per trillion.

The evidence for this is still being worked out, and there are some gaps. Fruit has many smells, which come from small quantities of essential fatty acids, but you'd need to eat around 2kg of tomatoes every day to get the minimum requirement.† By contrast, one really good source of these fatty acids – oily fish – doesn't smell

---

* Paul Hart pointed out that there is a very clear trend in the UK towards higher sugar varieties, especially of bananas, garden peas, etc.
† Saffron has a desirable smell because of safranal, which comes from vitamin A. Tiny amounts produce strong flavours, but to get your recommended daily allowance of vitamin A from saffron would cost around £2500. So, you can dramatically alter the flavour of something without really changing its nutritional content.

amazing to everyone. And many foods which contain all the amino acids, fatty acids, minerals and vitamins you need to survive, like beef and milk, don't have particularly strong smells compared with, for example, many fruits and vegetables.

But Schatzker's core idea that we are chasing flavours in search of missing nutrition is increasingly well evidenced. A paper by Albert-László Barabási, a Hungarian-American physicist and professor of network science at Northeastern University, attempted to map the chemical complexity of the diet.[10] The paper points out that the US Department of Agriculture quantifies sixty-seven nutritional components in garlic which, while it seems like a lot, is just a fraction of the more than 2,000 distinct chemical components that garlic is known to contain.

Barabási used the FooDB database (a Canadian initiative that holds chemical composition data on common, unprocessed foods) to estimate that there are over 26,000 chemicals in some whole foods. It is these molecules that are stripped out by ultra-processing. Remember, as Nicole Avena and Paul Hart pointed out, the basic construction materials of UPF are industrially modified carbs, fats and proteins, and the processes they are put through remove almost all the chemical complexity. The intensity of ultra-processing means that vitamins are destroyed (or deliberately removed in the case of bleaching), fibre is reduced, and there's a loss of functional molecules like polyphenols. The result is lots of calories but very little other nutrition.

Manufacturers are required by law to supplement their products with a few vitamins and minerals so that we don't develop deficiency diseases. But this doesn't solve the whole problem. Whole foods contain thousands more molecules than manufacturers add back in, and it is these molecules' more subtle health effects that could be responsible for the well-established benefits of eating whole food – protection against cancers, heart disease, dementia and early death.

Those thousands of chemicals bring health benefits, but they also bring flavour. And so, when they're stripped out, flavouring must be added back in. But this added flavour won't contain any of those lost nutrients that it should signal.

Eating more in search of nutrition has certainly been seen in animals. Veterinary surgeon, Richard 'Doc' Holliday, provided a good example.[11] Doc was caring for some cows in Missouri, but late rain had meant that the winter feed store was lacking in nutrition, leaving the cows sick and giving birth to stillborn calves. It seemed like the cows were deficient in nutrients despite the fact they had started to eat huge quantities – up to a kg per day each – of their nutritional supplement, a mix of various minerals. To figure out what was going on, Doc and the farmers decided to let the cows choose from buckets of individual minerals instead. As one of the farmers carried a bag of zinc across the barn to fill one of these buckets, he got mauled by the cows.

Holliday recounts the story in his book: 'Suddenly, several of the normally docile cows surrounded him, tore a bag of mineral from his arms, chewed open the bag, and greedily consumed every bit of the mineral, the bag, and even some mud and muck where the mineral had spilled out.'

Over the next few days, the cows ignored all the other minerals apart from the zinc, before gradually going back to the other feeds too. It turned out that the cows had got into a vicious cycle. Their food lacked zinc, so they'd started eating more and more of that mixed feed, which *did* contain a little zinc, but also calcium. Calcium interferes with zinc absorption, so the more the cows ate, the less they actually got.[*]

Schatzger's proposal is that just like Doc Holliday's cows, we may be eating more food to compensate for becoming increasingly deficient in micronutrients. Ultra-processing reduces micronutrients to

---

[*] These sort of complex mineral and vitamin interactions are seen in human nutritional supplements too, which may be why supplements are generally linked to health problems, including early death. If you take large quantities of calcium, you won't be able to absorb iron. If you take large quantities of iron, you won't be able to absorb zinc. If you take vitamin C, you'll reduce your copper level.

the point that modern diets lead to malnutrition even as they cause obesity.[12-15] For vulnerable groups, like infants and children living on marginal-quality diets, UPF and ultra-processed beverages can cause both obesity *and* stunting.[16] *

This isn't limited to low-income countries. Five-year-old children in the UK don't just have some of the highest rates of obesity in Europe, they are also among the shortest by a very significant amount – more than five centimetres shorter than Danish and Dutch children of the same age who, by the way, also have some of the lowest rates of obesity.[17, 18] In the eighteenth century, American men were five to eight centimetres taller than those in the Netherlands. Now from the age of two onwards, the Dutch are consistently taller. By adulthood the average Dutch man is 182.5cm and the average Dutch woman is 168.7cm. Their American counterparts measure 5.1cm and 5.2cm shorter respectively.[19, 20]

There is also evidence that concentrations of different antioxidants, vitamins and minerals affect weight directly by altering levels of the hormone leptin, which in turn affects appetite and regulation of body weight. When children who previously had obesity and were deficient in vitamin D lost weight, their vitamin D levels improved. Conversely, increasing calcium intake seems to reduce weight gain – though this was quite a specific study, so don't go overdosing on calcium. It's not a weight-loss remedy and you'll end up deficient in other things, just like those cows.[21]

Neither can we supplement our way out of the problem. Micronutrients are way more efficient and beneficial when embedded in the food matrix than they are in supplement form. Whether we're talking about phytochemicals, vitamin E or A or other

---

* Many people express an anxiety about the reduced nutrient content of food produced via industrial farming, with its focus on maximising yields of staple food products while minimising costs. Although there is evidence that even fruit, vegetables and meat may contain fewer micronutrients than in years gone by, most of us are *so* far away from eating a diet of whole food that this is less of a focus for me. In any food-production system though, if good nutritional content isn't an incentive, then good health won't be an outcome.

fat-soluble vitamins, haem iron or methyl folate, they are all more available in their natural form. Remember the paper that influenced Carlos Monteiro so much by Jacobs and Tapsell? It pointed out that, although dietary patterns have benefits to health, no one has ever been able to extract the molecules that confer the benefits. Fish are good – capsules of fish oil not so much.

Flavourings, which is to say molecules that affect the taste and smell of food, are a proxy for the low micronutrient content. This may be one of the reasons that UPF drives obesity and so many of those other health effects that have been seen in the epidemiological data. And, importantly, whether the flavourings are 'natural' or artificial is irrelevant.

If Mark Schatzger is right, then flavours out of context may be messing up the body's ability to make the correct associations between a nutrient and a food. For this to happen the flavours have to be honest and to come from the food itself.

13

UPF tastes odd

While flavours are really smells – molecules detected in the nose – flavour *enhancers* are really tastes. They're detected in the mouth, and include salt, sugar and molecules like MSG.

I went to eat Pringles at Xand's house with a friend called Andrea Sella to try to understand all this. Andrea is an Italian professor of chemistry at UCL. He's tall, erudite, funny and eccentric in the way that very smart people often are. I wanted him to explain why there were flavour enhancers – glutamate, guanylate and inosinate – in Pringles.

You can't hurry Andrea, and neither would you want to. His answer began with the flaws in vegetable-stock risotto before shifting seamlessly into the history of the chemistry of cooking starting in the eighteenth century, eventually arriving back at his mother's risotto recipe: 'If you use beef bones and beef sinew, you get risotto on a completely different level than if you use vegetable stock. Vegetable stock lacks …' Andrea searched disgustedly for the right word. '… it lacks body.'

This lack of body is because vegetable stock is typically missing some of those molecules that I noticed in the Pringles: glutamate, guanylate and inosinate, also recorded as ribonucleotides on various ingredient lists.

Humans have evolved a very sophisticated detection system in our mouths for these molecules because they signify easily digestible protein – not the protein of raw meat, but the protein of perfectly aged, cooked meat. They're the signature of fermented fish and plants, rich meaty broths, vintage cheese. That's why foods with these molecules in them taste great. One such food is Andrea's mother's risotto. The molecules stimulate the receptors in your mouth and signal that there is some real nutrition on its way. When you swallow a bit of the risotto, your gut is primed to handle some rich meaty goodness, free amino acids. With the Pringles, it's a different story.

Andrea wrapped up the risotto lecture and placed a Pringle theatrically on his tongue. To understand what is about to happen to Andrea and the Pringle and why he will find it hard to stop eating them, we need to understand taste properly. It starts with the tongue.

The moon's surface is mapped more precisely than the surface of the mouth, and it has less confusing geography.

Examine your tongue and you'll see little buds. These are *not* taste buds. They are papillae. Taste buds are invisibly small, don't look like buds (they're more like pits), and are found on the papillae – hundreds of them per papilla. Within each taste bud, there are around 100 specialised cells that have specialised receptors on them to detect molecules in your food, turn those molecules into a signal and send it to the brain. You taste all over your mouth and a bit at the back of your throat and, contrary to popular belief, there don't seem to be particular areas for each taste.[1-4]

In fact, taste receptors are found throughout the body in the larynx, the testes and in the gut. There are bitter receptors in the lungs and sweet receptors in the brain, heart, kidneys and bladder.*

Exactly how many tastes there are is a matter of debate. When physiologists talk about a taste, they really mean: 'Is there a specific receptor to detect a specific molecule?' We're pretty sure we have at

---

* The artificial sweetener saccharin makes rat bladders contract. Detecting glucose in the urine might well be important, because it should never be there. One could imagine a system in which the bladder responds to the presence of glucose by signalling to the pancreas to stimulate insulin secretion, although this hasn't been studied. Neither has the effect of sweeteners on the bladder or any onward signalling from the bladder.[5]

least five types of receptors for five distinct tastes in our mouths: sweet, umami (savoury), sour, salt and bitter.* We may also have specific tastes for water, starch, maltodextrins, calcium, various other metals and fatty acids, but it's remarkably difficult to be sure if we are truly detecting taste. The mouth is also assessing chewing resistance, pastiness, gumminess, gelatinousness, and so on. Fatty taste may in fact be the alteration of the friction of the tongue against the mouth and teeth: oil is slippery in a different way from saliva.

Sweet taste is stimulated by all simple sugar molecules that we can use for energy. The sweetest naturally occurring carbohydrate is fructose – almost unpleasantly sweet. Glucose is a much milder experience. We also seem able to detect the breakdown sugars from starches that are similar to maltodextrin. We don't exactly taste them as sweet, but they do seem to activate brain areas associated with reward.

Salt taste comes from sodium salts and a few other compounds. 'Low-salt' products often used by people with high blood pressure are made of potassium chloride, which does have a saltiness but doesn't taste exactly right. We are now fairly sure that there's a specific sodium channel in the skin of the mouth that detects salt. These sodium channels are found in skin-like tissues all over the body, moving sodium ions around, though how it detects salt concentration and then sends that information to your consciousness is still unclear.[6, 7]

Umami or savoury taste comes from those three molecules familiar from UPF ingredients lists: inosinate, guanylate and glutamate. Glutamate is found in breastmilk, seaweed, tomatoes, scallops, anchovies, cheese, soy sauce, cured ham and many more foods. Inosinate is found mainly in fish – dried bonito and dried sardines.

---

* Even within the agreed tastes, you might argue that the only ones we're sure about are sweet, bitter and umami. The only receptors confirmed (at the time of writing) to exist in living humans are the sweet receptors, the bitter (toxin) receptors and the umami receptors. The others do exist – we can see their signatures in our genes – but our knowledge comes from studies in mice and flies.

It starts to form as soon as a fish dies, reaching a maximum level about ten hours later. Guanylate is found mainly in dried shiitake and other mushrooms, forming from the breakdown of DNA in dying cells.

Sour taste comes from acids. A lot of different receptors for this taste have been proposed, but basically no one knows how we taste vinegar or ascorbic acid (vitamin C). Almost every other animal finds sour tastes aversive – experiments done in other primates show that they spit it out.[8] But for humans the taste may be useful. Sourness is, after all, a sign of fermentation rather than putrefaction. When bacteria ferment food, they produce acids that preserve it. Lactobacilli in milk digest the lactose into lactic acid making yoghurt, which keeps up to ten times longer. Vitamin C is likely the original reason we held onto sour detection, because it's really the only nutritionally important sour taste. Unlike many animals, we can't synthesise vitamin C, and we don't eat enough fresh raw stuff to be guaranteed that we will obtain enough without specifically seeking it out. The combination of sweet and sour reflects ripe, vitamin-C-laden fruit – that may be why we're drawn to that combination.

These four tastes – sweet, salt, sour and umami – are probably handled by basically four receptors. But bitterness is a different story. Bitter signals 'potentially toxic', and a huge number of different chemical structures taste bitterness. We need twenty-five different genes to detect bitterness, which gives us a great ability to detect toxins. But we can learn to love bitterness too. Bitter coffee will make a child gag and retch, but you can learn to associate the bitter taste with the exhilaration of the caffeine such that it becomes essential for making adult life bearable. Edible plants contain toxins inextricably linked to nutrients. These toxins tend to be destroyed by the liver, which handles all the blood coming from the gut. But even a food that contains small doses of multiple bitter compounds will be experienced as intensely bitter – our mouths do a great job of accounting for the total dose of each toxin and whether the liver can handle it all.[9]

Taste is important for omnivorous animals, whereas more specialist eaters have lost tastes. Cats have lost their sweet taste receptor; pandas have lost a savoury receptor. Sea lions seem to have very little taste at all – much of their prey is swallowed whole – but they can still smell. Whales and dolphins meanwhile seem to have lost the sense of smell entirely. Animals get rid of things that are not evolutionarily helpful to them anymore. The fact that we've maintained such elaborate sensory organs, and the neurological tissue to process the information, means that taste and smell are very important to humans.*

The tastes all affect each other too. If you make a cocktail of sucrose, MSG, sodium chloride, citric acid and quinine sulphate, and drink it, you will experience this cocktail as simultaneously sweet, savoury, salty, sour and bitter. You're able to tease apart the individual components, but your enjoyment of each one is affected by the others. We like savoury but only in the context of salt or sugar – MSG on its own is not pleasant. Gorillas will tolerate bitter plant tannins if the sugar content is high. The same is true for human children and almost any food. Likewise, quinine is quintessentially bitter, yet paired with sugar it becomes enjoyable in tonic.

The significance of this is that the manufacturers of UPF can hijack these taste interactions to make us eat their food. They do so in several ways. First, they use a trick that great cooks have been using for centuries: flavour enhancement. At particular concentrations and combinations, sweet, sour, salt and savoury all 'enhance' flavour, making food more delectable. The best traditional foods from many cultures will use sour vinegar, sweet sugar or honey, savoury umami flavours and loads of salt. Think of an Italian pasta dish: tomato and vinegar acids, sugar from the tomatoes, added salt

---

* Birds have lost their sweet taste, but because hummingbirds drink nectar they have repurposed their umami receptors. Barry Smith thinks about this a lot: 'As a philosopher of the senses, I of course want to know if nectar tastes sweet or savoury to a hummingbird.' Hummingbirds hate aspartame but like sugar water. No one knows why toucans like fruit. Not even Barry.

and grated glutamate-rich parmesan. It's the same principle, but UPF companies take it to the next level.

Let's use Coca-Cola as an example, because it's the most popular cola, although any cola would do. When it was invented, the aim was to make a drink to perk people up, and the original formula contained extract of coca leaves – probably a small amount of cocaine, although it's hard to be sure* – and caffeine. Cocaine and caffeine are both extremely bitter, so the company added lots of sugar to mask this. But that initial bitterness was actually an advantage. It was the extreme bitterness that *allowed* the addition of more sugar to the drink than would otherwise have been possible.

It wouldn't have been possible because we have a natural aversion to excess sugar. We can't eat honey by the spoonful or handfuls of table sugar. They are literally sickly sweet. The reason for this is probably simple enough: the body doesn't want to absorb sugar at a rate that exceeds its ability to remove it from the blood. Sweet blood is harmful in lots of different ways – sugar is food for bacteria, for one thing, and having lots of sugar in the blood also causes large shifts of water from cells into the blood. This increases the blood volume and makes the kidneys produce urine, resulting in dehydration – this is why peeing a lot is one of the first signs of diabetes.

Modern Coca-Cola still has caffeine bitterness, enhanced by an extreme sourness that comes from added phosphoric acid. Together, they allow a huge amount of sugar to be smuggled past the tongue.†️ But they don't do it alone. The drink's fizziness contributes, too, as

---

* Coca-Cola themselves don't deny that it used to contain cocaine, but instead say more ambiguously that 'cocaine has never been an added ingredient in Coca-Cola'.[10]

† By the way, the phosphoric acid in your food is not extracted from fruit or vegetables. It's made by burning phosphorus-containing rocks in an arc furnace with coal. It's also used in semiconductor processing and to modify road asphalt. Colas were originally called phosphate sodas. They're early UPF. The phosphoric acid doesn't just rot teeth and disguise the sugar. It also may leach minerals out of bones.[11]

does the suggestion that it be served ice-cold. For reasons that aren't entirely clear, you can suppress sweetness if you make something cold and fizzy. An at-home experiment demonstrates this: warm, flat Coke, despite the bitterness and sourness, is so sweet it's nearly undrinkable.

Good cooks can enhance flavours and tastes by combining them, but I think UPF is the nutritional equivalent of speedballing. In the world of illegal drugs, speedballs are typically a mixture of a sedative, like heroin, with a stimulant, like crack cocaine. One puts you to sleep (opioid overdoses cause death by stopping breathing) while the other wakes you up (crack overdoses cause death by driving the blood pressure so high that patients have strokes). By mixing the two, users can take more of both. People also do this more benignly (but still frequently with deadly consequences) with caffeine and alcohol: an espresso martini or a vodka and Red Bull are entry-level speedballs – the stimulant caffeine offsetting the sedative effects of the alcohol. This wonderland approach to drug use is a theme of UPF tastes.

When drunk as instructed, I'd like us to think of Coca-Cola as harnessing these different tastes in a way that creates sensory confusion similar to speedballing. The sour, bitter, cold and fizz allow multinational beverage corporations to smuggle far more sugar past your child's palate than would otherwise be possible: nine teaspoons of sugar in a can. I served warm, flat Coke to Lyra, who could manage only a couple of swigs (and she *will* eat sugar from the bowl with a spoon given the chance).

But *why* does the Coca-Cola Company want to get us to drink all this sugar? Remember those studies on rats learning to like flavours paired with calories? Well, the same thing is true of humans. Dana Small, a neuroscientist at Yale, did a series of experiments in humans which demonstrated that whether we learn to want a particular flavour seems to depend on how much our blood glucose changes when we consume it.[12] The team gave volunteers randomly flavoured drinks, and after a few exposures they learned to want the flavours that had been paired with a tasteless carbohydrate, maltodextrin. The more their blood sugar went up, the more they wanted the flavour. So it may be that by using fizz, cold, acid and caffeine to give people a huge dose of sugar – and with it a massive calorie load and blood-glucose spike – cola producers are making you want their specific products more and more.

This may also explain a bizarre pricing phenomenon first noticed in Central America but common in low-income countries around the world. Sweet fizzy beverages are nearly as cheap or cheaper than bottled water. Obviously, it's more expensive to make cola, but once people buy one, they will buy more. Water is cheaper to produce, but it's hard to get people to drink lots of it. In San Cristobal in Mexico, residents accused Coca-Cola of causing water shortages in its drive for production, all while its sales increased. The company argued they had been unfairly maligned, telling the *New York Times* that although they were using hundreds of thousands of litres of water per day, this had little impact on the city's water supply, noting that its wells are far deeper than the surface springs that supply local residents and pointing to other factors such as rapid urbanisation and lack of government investment.[13]

By speedballing different tastes and sensations, UPF can force far more calories into us than we could otherwise handle, creating enormous neurological rewards that keep us coming back for more. This is bad, but it's far from the only problem. There are zero-calorie artificial sweeteners to worry about too. What happens when the taste in our mouths doesn't match the calories at all?

***

On 14 October 2012, future US president, Donald Trump, tweeted an observation about Diet Coke: 'I have never seen a thin person drinking Diet Coke.' The next day, he followed it up with what appeared to be a question: 'The more Diet Coke, Diet Pepsi, etc. you drink, the more weight you gain?' By 16 October, he seemed to be resolved in his view of the matter: 'The Coca-Cola company is not happy with me – that's okay, I'll still keep drinking that garbage.'

Then, a week later, perhaps having run some sort of personal experiment, he reached a conclusion about the drink's physiological effect: 'People are going crazy with my comments on Diet Coke (soda). Let's face it – this stuff just doesn't work. It makes you hungry.'

A lot of research on low-calorie sweeteners has been done since that final tweet, but a decade later it's still a reasonable summary of the state of the science. Trump had understood something that a lot of physicians and nutritional scientists had failed to grasp: sweet taste in the mouth affects the body beyond just causing a little pleasure.

It might seem obvious that as artificial sweeteners don't contain calories, they can't cause obesity. But if you can understand why a zero-calorie drink could lead to weight gain and metabolic disease, then you will have understood one of the most fundamental ways that UPF seems to cause health problems.

If food contains an artificial sweetener, it is, by definition, UPF. These sweeteners used to be limited to little sachets and diet soft drinks. Now they're in everything: breads, cereals, granola bars, 'lite' yoghurts, no-added-sugar ice cream, flavoured milk. They're added to condiments like reduced-sugar ketchup, sugar-free jam and sugar-free pancake syrup. They're even in medications, multivitamins and hygiene products like toothpaste and mouthwash. The most commonly consumed are cyclamate and saccharin – the cheapest and oldest – and the global market is worth around $2.2 billion a year.

What exactly artificial sweeteners do to our health isn't clear, but it doesn't look good. There are studies funded by institutions like the Medical Research Council and the National Institutes of Health, which are relatively free of corporate conflicts of interest, showing that artificial sweeteners are associated with weight gain and diabetes.[14–17] While there are also studies that suggest sweeteners don't have any particularly significant effects on health, or that they may be beneficial, many of those studies' authors have declared relationships with food companies like Abbott, Danone and Kellogg's.[18, 19]

One large analysis of the data[20] published in the *American Journal of Clinical Nutrition*, which found no relationship between low-calorie sweeteners and body weight, included the following statement about conflicts of interest: 'We acknowledge the International Life Sciences Institute Low-Calorie Sweetener Committee for providing feedback and review of the study protocol and manuscript.' What the paper didn't mention was that this committee has been funded by Pepsi, Coca-Cola and several other major food corporations.*

When even a statistical analysis undertaken by industry can't find a significant benefit to low-calorie sweeteners, that should be a cause for alarm. My personal reading of the data is that drinks containing low-calorie sweeteners are linked to obesity and type 2 diabetes very slightly more than their sugary equivalents, but don't forget that sugar-sweetened beverages are very strongly linked to these things too – being only as bad as a sugary drink is still terrible.

But what's going on if removing the sugar from food doesn't improve health? Allison Sylvetsky, an associate professor at the Milken Institute School of Public Health, did a study of US children and found that drinking low-calorie soft drinks or sugar-sweetened soft drinks, or both, was associated with an increase in total calorie and sugar consumption compared with drinking water: low-calorie soft drinks may promote general overconsumption.[22]

In other words, Trump was right (not that it translated into any sort of regulation when he became president). When sweeteners are consumed with even a small amount of sugar, insulin levels seem to rise significantly. This will cause a drop in blood sugar and may then cause hunger, driving increased intake of food (again, see

---

* Another study[21] in the same journal looked at weight loss in adults using diet beverages or water. One of the authors was supported by a grant from Nestlé Waters. At the end it says that there are no conflicts of interest, but this is incorrect. If you are funded by a water company (which also makes beverages that are artificially sweetened) and you conduct a trial on water and artificially sweetened drinks, this is, in fact, a conflict of interest. It doesn't mean the study is wrong. But it *is* a conflict.

Trump's tweets). This is one of the mismatches of UPF, one of the lies that Barry explained. Sweet taste in the mouth prepares the body for sugar. If that never arrives, it's a problem.

It may be an even bigger problem when sugar is mixed with artificial sweeteners. Dana Small did another series of studies in which she gave volunteers drinks of varying sweetness (using different doses of sucralose) and calories (using tasteless maltodextrin). Some drinks had lots of calories but no sweetness; others were sweet but had no calories. Her papers are not the easiest to read – 'starting to eat' is phrased as 'initiation of consummatory acts' – and the conclusions in the lab are hard to draw out to the real world. But her findings are intriguing, nonetheless. She showed that the degree to which people would learn to want a flavour was affected not just by calories in the drink but by whether the sweetness and the calories were matched.[23]

Just as alarming was another study – in which Small gave healthy volunteers drinks containing varying quantities of sucralose, sugar, or both – that seemed to demonstrate that a mixture of sweetener with sugar decreased the body's response to insulin in a similar way to type 2 diabetes.[*]

All this suggests that when sugar is consumed with artificial sweeteners, as it is in the real world, it produces harmful effects on metabolic health. Even if Pepsi and Coke don't directly mix sugar and sweeteners, their customers may well be eating other UPF at the same time.

Aside from their effects on sugar metabolism, insulin and addictive potential, there is also evidence that drinking sweeteners increases preference for other sweet foods.[25, 26] A small study showed that desire for sugar was reduced after a two-week break from all artificial sweeteners. One particular artificial sweetener – Splenda – which contains sucralose and maltodextrin, also seems to alter brain activity in rats in areas that control food intake, obesity and energy control, as well as having effects on the gut itself.[27, 28]

---

[*] This study's findings are consistent with those of studies done in rodents.[24]

Artificial sweeteners may also disrupt the microbiome, the population of bacteria that live on and in us, forming a vital part of our digestive and immune systems. This effect was widely reported because of a very high-profile paper in *Nature*.[29] Evidence from animal studies showed that sucralose disrupts the gut microbiome, even at levels approved by regulatory agencies, and certainly at levels humans frequently eat.*

So, it may be that low-calorie artificial sweeteners are contributing to the rise in metabolic diseases like type 2 diabetes around the world. It remains unproven, but the research does give us some idea that there is at least a plausible mechanism.

All this is worrying because replacing sugar with low-calorie sweeteners is a mainstay of both UK government policy and of the soft drinks industry – which wants to be able to claim that it's benefitting public health.

I hope by now you see that the four green lights on the side of a can of diet drink are a little misplaced.

Many national governments have proposed sugar taxes. These proposals seem sensible, and they do reduce sugar intake, but they also invite reformulation with low-calorie sweeteners. The UK imposed a sugar tax in 2018 because teenagers in the UK were consuming approximately a bathtub full of soft drinks each year.[30] †
The tax led to a dramatic 44.3 per cent reduction in sales of sugary

---

* Other sweeteners may not disrupt the microbiome, but the effects on metabolism through oral taste may be the same: sweet taste in the mouth signalling sugar that never arrives may always be a problem with any low-calorie sweetener. There are other serious concerns about the safety of some artificial sweeteners. For example, the authors of a 2019 paper felt that the European Food Safety Authority had applied lax and forgiving criteria to judge the studies showing harmful effects of aspartame.

† The money from the sugar tax was intended to raise hundreds of millions per year, which would go into dedicated funds to help schools upgrade their sports facilities. I'm uneasy linking the sugar tax to increased funding for sport. I think it suggests that physical activity can somehow offset the health effects of drinking soft drinks.

drinks, a drop of over 40 million kilograms of sugar consumed between 2015 and 2019. This would seem to vindicate the tax. But even as people consumed 10 per cent less sugar per household, the volume of soft drinks consumed didn't change.[31] Instead, people began to drink more artificially sweetened drinks.

The charity First Steps Nutrition found that 65 per cent of toddlers are consuming an average of one can of artificially sweetened drink per day.[32] It's really hard to see this as a public health triumph, especially because current UK regulations prohibit the addition of artificial sweeteners to foods specifically marketed for babies and toddlers. And while artificial sweeteners don't damage teeth directly, many diet drinks are still highly acidic and may cause significant damage to children's dental enamel.

The addition of sweeteners has allowed health claims to be made about many ultra-processed products, and many now have a 'Good Choice Change4Life' thumbs-up logo on them. Change4Life is a Public Health England social marketing campaign that, among other aims, seeks to raise awareness of the sugar levels in foods and encourages consumers to switch to lower-sugar alternatives. This is extraordinary in the total absence of any evidence that they improve health and the very real concerns about harms.*

Despite the worrying data showing possible harm and little benefit, consumption of artificially sweetened beverages continues.† In

---

* There is another absurdity, pointed out by First Steps Nutrition: the Change4Life logo sometimes appears on products that contain artificial colours. Because artificial colours may have an adverse effect on activity and attention in children, products containing them must have a warning on their label. This means that there are some products with both warnings and encouragement labels – not easy for parents to interpret. Also worth mentioning is that the Change4Life obesity campaign in the UK listed the following commercial partners: Tesco, Asda, PepsiCo, Kellogg's, the Co-operative Group, the Fitness Industry Association, the Advertising Association, Spar, Costcutter, Nisa, Premier and Mills Group.

† The British Soft Drinks Association recently reported that, in 2018, 65 per cent of total soft drinks purchased were zero-calorie or low-calorie. A full 88 per cent of all dilutable drinks sold were also zero-calorie or low-calorie.[33]

government and policy circles, there is a sense that any regulatory shift toward things that are healthy is a triumph, because it's so hard to do. I'm not necessarily convinced by this, but then I don't have to try to make policy. Personally, I think that if you want to prevent children developing diet-related disease, then bringing in policies that encourage two-year-olds to drink an average of a whole can of artificially sweetened fizzy pop *every day* doesn't seem like a good way of doing it. It sends a message that these drinks are healthy, and it lets the industry that sells them off the hook.

As I read Dana Small's papers, it occurred to me that those mismatches between tastes and nutrition are found throughout UPF. The gums and pastes that Paul Hart had told me about create a sensation of fat in the mouth. When they do that in the context of a zero-fat yoghurt or a low-fat mayonnaise, what does that do to our internal physiology? No one knows. And no one knows exactly what the flavour enhancers do in that Pringle that Andrea placed on his tongue.

Here's what I suspect happens though (and my suspicions are backed up by quite a lot of data).[34]

The saddle shape of the Pringle, properly known as a hyperbolic paraboloid, is almost exactly congruent with the tongue's curves, meaning that every taste bud in Andrea's mouth was in contact with the Pringle. Then, when he chewed, the shape's double curvature caused the crisp to fracture unevenly, something the engineers call catastrophic failure. Munching away, Andrea began to explain how his umami receptors would be preparing his internal physiology for something like his mother's risotto. 'But,' he swallowed, 'all that will arrive is a sad little ball of potato starch.'

And so, with a physiological confusion that barely makes it to the surface of our conscious experience, we find ourselves reaching for another – searching for that nutrition that never arrived. It's easy to see the Pringle as a piece of malevolent technical genius, as a product deliberately designed to engineer obesity. But it was made in the 1960s, and I don't think anyone set out to make them addictive.* But in the arms race of products available in our shops, it is those with addictive properties that survive.

So, by using additives that affect taste and combining sensory experiences, UPF sneaks more rewards (such as sugar) past our tongues than we would otherwise tolerate. It makes us crave UPF more than we could ever crave home cooking. And, by creating mismatches between the sensations in the mouth and the nutrition in the gut, the companies have (if only accidentally) arrived at a method for driving increased consumption. But what about all the other additives – thousands of them – that you might use to identify UPF. Do they have any specific effects on our health?

---

* My own lawyer suggested that I should probably avoid having a view on whether a specific product is addictive, but in the case of Pringles the marketing team seem comfortable with the implication: 'Once you pop you can't stop.' It's a legal grey area, but nonetheless, in May 2009, an article in the *Guardian* got away with describing Pringles as 'crack in a cardboard tube'.

14.

Additive anxiety

Everyone at my hospital eats Pret. You can see three outlets from the building, and there are two more within a five-minute walk. And surely that's a good thing? The Pret brand is relentlessly natural, ethical and wholesome.

That's why I went there one day during the last week of my diet – for a little respite from UPF. I bought some red Thai soup, but immediately recognised a familiar tang. I looked through the list of forty-nine (!) ingredients, and spotted maltodextrin and spice extracts. I checked the ingredients on the bread in my sandwich, something that in years of eating Pret I had never done before: mono- and diacetyl tartaric acid esters of mono- and diglycerides of fatty acids.

These ingredients seemed to be at odds with the brand I thought I knew. Look at this statement made online by Pret in 2016: 'Pret opened in London in 1986 ... [and] made proper sandwiches, avoiding the obscure chemicals, additives and preservatives common to so much of the "prepared" and "fast" food on the market.'

The web page used the words 'natural' or 'naturally' six more times.

The Real Bread Campaign wrote to the company to check these claims, and discovered that Pret's products contained a 'cocktail of additives', including those I mentioned above as well as E920 (l-cysteine hydrochloride), E472e (diacetyl tartaric acid esters of mono- and diglycerides), E471 (mono- and diglycerides of fatty acids), E422 (glycerol), E330 (citric acid) and E300 (ascorbic acid). The Real Bread Campaign asked Clive Schlee, then CEO of Pret, whether the company would either stop adding the additives or stop making the 'natural' marketing claims. Schlee declined on both counts. So, the campaign wrote to the Advertising Standards Agency, which told Pret to stop making their 'produced by nature' claims. A Pret spokeswoman tried to manage the story: 'We would really like to find a solution, and our food team has been working hard trialling recipes that do not use emulsifiers. They have not yet found one that meets the standards our customers expect.'[1, 2]

It's possible that our expectations would be different if non-emulsified, additive-free bread were more widely available. But consider this from the perspective of the owners of Pret, JAB Holding Company. They're a privately owned Luxembourg-based conglomerate, with a total enterprise value of more than $120 billion as of 2020.[3-7] Making bread without these additives would be much more expensive, and customers, at the moment, don't seem to be very aware that Pret is even using them.

But should we really worry about this? Surely these additives have been through a regulatory bureaucracy that requires lots of safety testing and which ultimately concluded that they're fine? I previously assumed that 'additives', which comprise all those substances added to food for specific technological purposes, were simply indicators of UPF, a sign of all the other processing that does harm but in themselves safe and necessary. And I was reluctant to indulge in any 'additive anxiety', which is often found alongside a general anti-science agenda.

Additive anxiety first emerged, predictably, in 1970s California, when a paediatrician, Ben Feingold, suggested that artificial flavouring and colouring might cause ADHD. He was disparaged by the medical community, and I think I would have dismissed him at the time too. Food is, after all, made of chemicals. *We* are made of chemicals. And, while synthetic chemicals can be toxic, so can naturally produced ones.

Yet, as I spoke with UPF experts, it became clear that these additives may be having a more significant effect on our bodies than I'd imagined. I started to think about how sweeteners and flavour enhancers cause that mismatch between taste and nutrition that may cause harm. And then I found a study published in 2007, twenty-five years after Feingold's death.

It was funded by the UK Food Standards Agency and included around 300 children.[8] They were given either six colourants – all E numbers – and a preservative, or a placebo. The children who drank the additive-enhanced drinks had higher hyperactivity scores than those who consumed placebos. It was published in *The Lancet*, and food and drink containing any of these six artificial colours must now carry a warning on their packaging in the UK: 'May have an adverse effect on activity and attention in children'.* If it's true for colours, are there good reasons to be really concerned about other food additives, too?

It's not clear how much or even how many additives we eat. In the EU, there are more than 2,000 permitted for use. In the US, the number is (terrifyingly) unknown, but is thought to be higher than 10,000.[9] As production has become entirely automated, with computer-controlled robots cutting vegetables, grinding meat, mixing batter, extruding dough and wrapping the final product, many additives are required so that food can withstand the process. If colours or flavours are lost as food is subjected to this robotic mauling, then, as we've seen, they can simply be chemically replaced.

There are so many thousands of these additives that I won't even be able to cover all the major categories. There are flavours, flavour enhancers, colours, emulsifiers, artificial sweeteners, thickeners, humectants, stabilisers, acidity regulators, preservatives, antioxidants, foaming agents, anti-foaming agents, bulking agents, carbonating agents, gelling agents, glazing agents, chelating agents, bleaching agents, leavening agents, clarifying agents and so on. I'm

---

* It wasn't a brilliant study. Both the US Food and Drug Administration (FDA) and the European Food Safety Authority independently reviewed it and concluded that it didn't confirm a link between additives and behavioural effects. But it did open the door to the credible consideration of some of the harms of additives.

going to focus on just a handful, as a way of understanding how they affect our bodies and how they are (or are not) regulated.

One big category of additives is those emulsifiers that are found in bread. In fact, they are nearly universal in UPF.

Almost as much as DNA, emulsifiers are the molecules of life.* Emulsifiers are made up of one part that loves fat and another part that loves water, which means they can glue these two immiscible substances together. The human body is full of these emulsifiers, and they're found throughout nature, as well as in traditional food. The egg yolk in mayonnaise or the mustard in salad dressing are there, in part, as emulsifiers, allowing watery vinegar and fatty oils to mix.

One of the most common emulsifiers you'll notice on ingredients lists is lecithin, which can be derived from egg or soy or other sources. Lecithins are classified as natural, but they're often made up of very unnatural mixtures of naturally occurring chemicals that have been further chemically modified. You'll also notice polysorbate 80, carboxymethylcellulose and the type you find in so much bread in the UK: diacetyl tartaric acid esters of mono- and diglycerides – also known as E472e, or DATEM.

DATEM is produced through the processing of animal or vegetable fats (triglycerides). They don't occur naturally but, like the lecithins, they're similar to biological molecules, and this similarity may be dangerous. In experiments on cells in labs, DATEM seems able to insert itself into cell membranes, which may explain some of the findings you're about to read about how they damage the gut.[10, 11] Exactly how DATEM works in food is also not fully understood. It strengthens and softens and changes the interactions of

---

* All living cells rely on fatty membranes surrounding droplets of water to keep them separate from each other. These membranes are made of molecules with a water-loving head and a water-hating but fat-loving tail – they're emulsifiers. And they naturally arrange themselves into a membrane that surrounds a drop of water: a cell. The membrane separates life from the outside world. They're the boundary between you and not you – the literal edge of life.

bread's protein, water and carbohydrates, and contributes to the moist springiness and long shelf life of many commercial ultra-processed breads.

The American chemical company DuPont makes a range of emulsifiers. Its DATEM is branded Panodan.[12] Then they have another emulsifier that adds an extra creaminess to low-fat products, one that's widely used in chewing gum and PVC, and yet another that can improve cake batter performance and crumb structure – while also working well in plastics as an 'anti-fog' agent.

But the most famous emulsifier-like substance DuPont has worked with is perfluorooctanoic acid or PFOA. This one used to be used to keep Teflon coatings from clumping together during production. It's one of those 'forever chemicals' that accumulate in any organisms that happen to ingest them. According to a 2016 report by the Environmental Protection Agency, it's associated with high cholesterol, increased liver enzymes, decreased vaccination response, birth defects, pregnancy-induced hypertension, and testicular and kidney cancer.[13]

Over several decades after DuPont started using PFOA in the 1950s, the company dumped hundreds of thousands of pounds of PFOA into the Ohio River and 'digestion ponds', from which it entered the local water table, and thus the drinking water of more than 100,000 people near the Washington Works plant in West Virginia.[14] While they were doing the dumping, the company was simultaneously conducting medical studies into the potential harms. They discovered that it caused cancers and birth defects in animals. They then discovered birth defects in the children of some of their employees. According to Rob Bilott, the environmental lawyer who prosecuted the class action case, 'DuPont had for decades been actively trying to conceal their actions. They knew this stuff was harmful, and they put it in the water anyway. These were bad facts.'[15]

Bad facts indeed. According to their own internal standards, the safe upper limit in drinking water was one part per billion. Local drinking water contained three times that level, but DuPont didn't make the finding public. So far, the lawsuits against DuPont have been settled before trial with a total cost to the company of $400 million.[16] The cases are still being litigated, but the DuPont that did all this in some senses may no longer exist.

NBC News reported in 2020 that DuPont had unloaded its clean-up and compensation obligations to smaller companies that don't have any money to pay for them. DuPont denies creating spin-off companies to transfer liabilities away from itself, but one of the companies that DuPont insists wasn't created for this purpose is now suing DuPont, arguing that DuPont intentionally hid the scope of the liabilities when it dumped them.[17]

PFOA isn't a food emulsifier, and it causes harm in very different ways and at different doses than the emulsifiers that are used in some UPF. But I think this story is useful information for two reasons.

First, you might be of a mind to shop as an activist and avoid companies that may have caused significant environmental harms. (Although, admittedly, the tangled supply chain of UPF means that it is nearly impossible to know the names or even the numbers of different companies involved in the construction of a single product. It's all but impossible to find out which company made the DATEM in your bread.)

Second, as we come on to the regulatory aspect of food additives, you'll see that the current system expects you to trust companies like DuPont to self-certify and self-regulate. The story about PFOAs may influence the degree of trust you feel in them.

Beyond being made by companies with controversial legal histories, however, is there evidence that the emulsifiers in UPF are harmful? Well, yes. And most of the harm seems to be brought about by the changes caused to our microbiome.

★★★

The equations that describe a donut and the equations that describe you and me are essentially the same: we're all double-walled cylinders. The tube in the middle is your gut and it has branches to your ears, lungs and a few other places, all of which are coated in mucus, a complex mixture of water, proteins, glycoproteins. It's not fatty, or gelatinous, but intriguingly stringy and extremely variable. It's a living layer full of antibodies and immune cells that help to keep the peace with the other residents of the gut: the microbiome.

A huge amount has been written about the microbiome, but our knowledge of it is still relatively small. However, we are starting to get a toehold on some of the basic science, even if we aren't sure about the implications.

During birth, and in the days and weeks thereafter, a new human is colonised by between 10 and 100 trillion microbes.* For the first few months of life, the infant immune system and its new microbiome test and shape each other in a complex and poorly understood dance. The infant who is breastfed receives their microbiome from their mother as well as specific antibodies in the milk which favour the development of the useful bacteria. There's a frenzied engagement during the first few years of life, until the child and a few hundred species decide to settle down together and the microbiome becomes one of the body's largest immune organs. We provide the microbes with a warm, wet mucus home full of nutrition, and they form biofilms, sheets of slime that limit the ability of harmful bugs to harm either them or us. They are a consortium, a coalition, providing a bulwark against would-be invaders or colonists.

For every one of your cells there are, by some estimates, 100 other organisms living as part of you: viruses, phages, bacteria, protozoans, archaea, fungi, and even a few animals like worms and

---

* The initial colonisation is part faecal but mainly comes from the vaginal flora – these are the pioneer species. And it's important: a review from Denmark of 2 million children born between 1977 and 2012 showed that children born by caesarean delivery had a significantly increased risk of asthma, systemic connective tissue disorders, juvenile arthritis, inflammatory bowel disease, immune deficiencies and leukaemia.[18]

mites. You have 20,000 human genes but many millions of bacterial genes.* The largest number of organisms are in the gut at the end of the small intestine (where food is digested) and throughout the large intestine, or colon, where water is absorbed and fibre is fermented. Human colons have among the highest densities of bacteria of any environment on earth, including rainforest soil. But more important than the actual number is the diversity: between 500 and 1,000 species of bacteria alone exist on and in you. Each of us has a unique set of species, and these change over time. Exactly why is not understood, but caring for the community of creatures that make up our body is intimately linked to good health – and that means eating a good diet.†

The microbes in our gut are an adaptable digestive engine. They make vitamins and turn indigestible food into molecules that have beneficial effects on our hearts and brains. This is why fibre is good for us. Fibre is, broadly speaking, any carbohydrate that we lack the enzymes to digest. We have a very small number of carbohydrate-digesting enzymes encoded in our own genomes, but our bacteria provide us with lots more. The bacteria in the colon ferment fibre to make energy for themselves, which creates waste molecules called volatile short chain fatty acids. We use these fatty acids for energy and for all kinds of other purposes – they help to reduce inflammation, regulate the immune system and are specialist fuels for the heart and brain. In short, like Eddie Rixon's cows, we partly live on the waste products of the bacteria in our guts.

The relationship with our microbiome is one of strictly enforced boundaries, however. We need to keep colon microbes in the colon. If friendly organisms end up in the wrong place, they can quickly become unfriendly. Most urinary tract infections, for example, are

---

* These are really your genes. You can't separate your microbiome from you any more than you can any other organ. It has an unbroken chain of ancestors going back to long before yours were primitive fish.

† In my view, the evidence doesn't support eating lots of other bacteria in the form of probiotics.

caused by faecal bacteria ending up in the urinary system, which can't handle them.

When the gut lining is damaged by food, antibiotics or invaders, the population of the microbiome changes: we get new species that we haven't signed a peace treaty with. They haven't evolved with an obligation to care for our interests: to them, we're simply a niche to exploit. And, like all new colonists, they destroy the local culture and ecosystem both deliberately and accidentally. This is called dysbiosis. We are increasingly sure that dysbiosis is linked to inflammatory bowel disease (i.e. Crohn's disease and ulcerative colitis), necrotising enterocolitis in premature infants (a frequently fatal condition in which the gut dies), severe inflammatory conditions (like rheumatoid arthritis), autoimmune diseases (like multiple sclerosis and type 1 diabetes), allergic diseases (atopic dermatitis and asthma) and metabolic diseases (obesity and type 2 diabetes), as well as cancer and even serious mental illness.[19-22] * Communication between the gut and the brain is not well understood, but the

---

* The microbiome has profound effects on mouse behaviour. Germ-free mice are less social and show a dramatically altered pattern of risk taking compared with mice with microbial passengers. If you give mice antibiotics early in life, they also show changes in anxiety and social behaviours. Introducing microbiota in mice that are raised in a sterile environment around the time of weaning can restore normal behaviours, including perhaps a level of anxiety that is protective. The effects of emulsifiers were elegantly shown in 2019.[23] The mice were given carboxymethylcellulose or polysorbate 80 in their drinking water and became inflamed and gained weight. But, most significantly, they started to exhibit far more anxiety-like behaviours. In case you're curious, the way they measured anxiety in the mice was with an open-field test, one of the most widely used tests in animal psychology. Neither the mouse nor the human conducting the test needs special training to get a result. It's been used in cows, pigs, rabbits, primates, bees and lobsters. It consists simply of a high-sided white box with no lid. The animal feels exposed in the centre and generally spends time at the sides. You can measure how long the animal spends in the open and other things like how much it craps. The emulsifiers made the mice far more anxious.

diverse community of protozoa, fungi, archaea and bacteria aren't just there for a free ride – they seem to get a voting say in what we put down the tube and how we conduct our lives. That they influence our thoughts, emotions and decisions seems to be increasingly clear.

Whether the dysbiosis causes or is caused by these conditions and many others isn't clear, but it's possible that they all have their pathogenic origins in an increased reactivity of the immune system to the microbiome.

This may happen if our diet induces a change in the population of bugs which damages the gut barrier. This barrier is made of tight links between cells, mucus and immune cells, which work together to keep the microbiome on a tight leash. When it's damaged, the gut starts to leak microbes and their waste products into the rest of the body. Lots of things in our diet can change the population of the microbiome and the integrity of the gut wall, including fat, fibre and – not least – emulsifiers.

Two of the most ubiquitous, and thus the most studied, emulsifiers are carboxymethylcellulose and polysorbate 80. Polysorbate 80, also known as polyoxyethylene sorbitan mono-oleate or E433, is an entirely synthetic emulsifier. It's found in lots of kosher pickles, ice cream, aerosols of whipping cream, toothpaste, moisturising cream, shampoo and hair dye. Carboxymethylcellulose – also known as cellulose gum or E466 to you and me – was invented during World War I. It's a polymer made from alkalised plant sugars with a chemical process that uses chloroacetic acid. You'll find it in lots of thick and gloopy UPF products – it stops them separating. Things like Tesco Brownie Flavour Milk, Costa Caramel Latte and Müller's cookie dough flavour milkshake. It's also found in a roll-on deodorant brand called Rexona, eye drops, and even a brand of micro-enema called Norgalax. You can buy it online in big bags if you are into molecular gastronomy or diarrhoea.

So, I'll add a new thought: if you're wondering whether something might be UPF, it's probably a good rule of thumb that, if any of the ingredients can also be found in your deodorant or your enema, then it probably is.

In 2015, a team from the USA and Israel published an elegant series of experiments on carboxymethylcellulose and polysorbate 80 in the prestigious journal *Nature*.[24] (That is not to say that *Nature* papers are never wrong, but this was the first of a growing number that have all shown the same thing.) The researchers tested polysorbate 80 and CMC in mice at concentrations lower than we all eat very regularly.[*]

Over just 12 weeks, the changes were dramatic. The mucus barrier was badly damaged. In healthy mice, gut bacteria are suspended in a layer of mucus away from the cells lining the gut, but in the emulsifier-treated mice, the bacteria were practically touching these cells. Ultimately, the gut started to leak so much that bacterial components could be detected in the mice's bloodstreams. The types of bugs in the microbiome were affected, too, with reduced levels of Bacteroidales – bacteria typically associated with health – and increased levels of bacteria that break down mucus and cause inflammation. Bacteria like *Helicobacter pylori*, which is known to cause cancer and ulcers in humans, began to flourish. Overall, there was a reduction in diversity of the microbiome, which is one of the defining characteristics of health.

Under the microscope the mouse guts were so inflamed that it looked as if they were developing colitis. This inflammation spread through the bodies of the mice, and they started eating more food and gaining weight. As the emulsifiers interrupted their ability to manage glucose, some moved towards type 2 diet-related diabetes.

To check that these effects were mediated through the microbiome, the team repeated the experiments on sterile mice (born

---

[*] They used a concentration of 1 per cent, which is lower than the concentration of the preservatives in many food products. To check the minimum doses, the researchers reduced the concentration down to 0.5 per cent and 0.1 per cent and the effects continued. For polysorbate 80, as little as 0.1 per cent resulted in evidence of low-grade inflammation and increased adiposity.

and raised without any bacteria in their guts) and found none of the effects. Then they transplanted faeces from the emulsifier-treated mice and put it into the colons of the sterile mice, which developed all the same problems. Overall, this study provided robust evidence that, in the case of these two common emulsifiers, the harmful effects are due to damage caused to the microbiome.*

The conclusion to the *Nature* paper proposed that dietary emulsifiers 'may have contributed to the post-mid-twentieth-century increase in incidence of inflammatory bowel disease, metabolic syndrome, and perhaps other chronic inflammatory diseases'.

Overeating may be driven by food additives that alter the microbiome and promote intestinal inflammation. Of course, mice aren't people, but the effect of different components of UPF on the delicate lining of the gut, and the resultant effect on our brains, is becoming increasingly clear.

***

Emulsifiers aren't the only UPF additives that affect our microbiomes, though. Maltodextrins† are synthetic chains of sugar molecules commonly found in UPF. They add texture and shelf life and seem to increase that reward we get from food despite having barely any taste. (Remember they were used in Dana Small's experiments on how we learn to want food.)

At first glance, maltodextrins seem like they would be fairly harmless, but in experiments they seem to cause cellular stress, damage to delicate mucosal linings, intestinal inflammation and reduced immune response to bacteria. They may also be linked to the rise in chronic inflammatory disorders like Crohn's disease and

---

* To translate these results to humans, we'd need to assume that there's an average concentration of at least 0.1 per cent in the human diet which, for some people, perhaps even most people, is very typical.

† Maltodextrin was invented in 1812, and then lost and rediscovered by another industrial chemist called Fred C. Armbruster, whose hobbies included fur trapping, and who operated a part-time pest-control business, Fred's Wildlife Nuisance Control.

type 2 diabetes. Mouse studies have shown that maltodextrins encourage *Salmonella* and *E coli* to start forming slime films and penetrate the body's mucus.[25-28] The evidence shows not that emulsifiers cause inflammation in everyone, but rather that, if you have a genetic risk for inflammatory bowel disease, which may be completely unknown to you, maltodextrin or emulsifiers may expose it.

Then there are all those gums. Xanthan gum is one that we constantly consume. It's an exopolysaccharide: a sugary slime secreted by the bacteria *Xanthomonas campestris*, which forms black rot on vegetables.

The gum is used as a thickener, but it has a remarkable property: when shaken or squirted, it becomes temporarily thinner, so will pour easily. Once at rest again, it thickens and clings. It's used in toothpaste, in drinks for people who have difficulty swallowing and to thicken drilling mud in the oil industry, since it keeps solids suspended in mud (and salad dressing) so that they can be pumped out of an oil well more easily.

I had assumed that xanthan gum was harmless – if disgusting. But a researcher called Matthew Ostrowski in the Department of Microbiology and Immunology at the University of Michigan took a closer look at what xanthan gum does in the body.[29] Ostrowski found that xanthan gum is actually a food for a new bacterial species. From looking at population data, it seems that the gum has driven the colonisation of this bacteria into billions of people. It's completely absent from populations who don't eat it – whom Ostrowski could only find in remote groups of hunter-gatherers. Moreover, if you have this bacterial species, then you may also have another novel species that eats the breakdown products made by the first one. The effects of these bacteria are not understood, but it's clear that xanthan gum creates a food chain in the human gut and, since the bugs it feeds can colonise infants at an early age, it may be having profound effects on immune system development.

Papers about the effect of different additives on the microbiome keep piling up. Trehalose, an additive sugar that was deemed safe in the US in 2000, has been linked to outbreaks of the superbug

Clostridium difficile. Many of the commonly used emulsifiers, including glycerol stearate, sorbitan monostearate, and carrageenans, have been shown to alter overall levels of beneficial bacteria in the gut microbiota when examined in human studies.[30-37]

In light of this, you might expect that food companies wouldn't use these substances.

But if they're so bad, how did they get into our food in the first place?

PART FOUR

But I already paid for this!

15.

Dysregulatory bodies

In June 2017, an Iowa-based company, Corn Oil ONE – then called CoPack Strategies – voluntarily notified the FDA that it intended to market a product called 'COZ corn oil'.[1]

The FDA is the regulator of food additives and drugs in the USA, so it was the right agency to contact. Any medical drug you've ever taken has been licensed by at least one of a small number of allegedly 'stringent' drug regulators like the FDA. Obtaining a drug licence involves submitting volumes of animal and human testing data, as well as giving free access to all research and manufacturing sites to the agency and its experts. That's why it costs so much money to get a drug licence – adequate testing can run into hundreds of millions.*

I assumed that food additives in America would be put through a similar procedure, because they're regulated by the same federal body. I also assumed that, because I was familiar with the reassuring tedium of pharmaceutical regulatory bureaucracy, I'd be able to understand the nuts and bolts of the process. Yet when I went to the FDA website and started reading, I found that I couldn't understand any of the requirements about testing or submission of data at all. I couldn't even understand their definition of an additive. This seemed like a sign that the FDA were taking a complex and detailed approach. But I thought I should ask some experts in food additive regulation to explain it, just in case.

* The reason for all of this oversight and red tape is because, when the pharmaceutical industry wasn't so closely supervised, they proved extremely adept at manipulating data in sophisticated ways to minimise apparent harms and maximise apparent benefits.[2]

Maricel Maffini and Tom Neltner are two of the authors of a twenty-seven-page paper published in 2011 with the title 'Navigating the US food additive regulatory program'.[3] Their names have consistently appeared in prestigious journals atop papers that address (spoiler alert) the significant gaps in the US food regulatory system.[4, 5] I spoke with them separately, but they are very much a dynamic duo. Maffini is a biochemist and physiologist, while Neltner is a chemical engineer and lawyer.

They used the example of COZ corn oil to explain the process of regulating food additives to me.

You might be wondering, as I had, why the company had asked the FDA about something as benign as corn oil. It's a popular cooking oil in America, squeezed from kernels of corn. But this corn oil was made in a novel way.

It was extracted from the corn 'mash' used to produce ethanol biofuel for cars. The mash contains antibiotics and other additives and the 'distillers corn oil' that could be extracted from it had previously only been allowed in livestock feed. The company wanted to process this oil further and feed it to humans to add value to their company's bottom line.

The additional processing and the fact it would now be in human food meant that it should be considered as a new food additive. The company had three options about how to bring it to market.

First, and most rigorously, they could petition the FDA for a full review of the new corn oil and have it formally listed as a food additive. This wouldn't mean quite the same level of scrutiny as for a new medical drug, but it would mean submitting a large volume of data to the FDA. The process might take several years.

The requirements for new ingredients to be formally approved as food additives were laid out in the 1950s when Congress became increasingly concerned about the safety of hundreds of new, industrially produced chemicals that were transforming the way Americans grew, packaged, processed and transported food. A report at the time estimated that more than 700 chemicals were then in use in food, of which only around 400 were known to be safe. The report said: 'Eminent pharmacologists, toxicologists, physiologists and nutritionists expressed the fear that many of the chemicals being added to food today have not been tested sufficiently to establish their non-toxicity and suitability for use in food.'[6]

It could have been written yesterday. The scientists of the 1950s were not so much concerned with things that are immediately toxic, as this can be relatively easily tested for. They were worried about 'substances which may produce noxious effects only after being used for months or years'.

We have fairly good tests for whether molecules cause cancer, birth defects and immediate toxicity, but more subtle long-term harms were – and still are – much harder to assess. Whether an additive causes issues that are detectable only after years of exposure – depression, increased suicidality in teens, weight gain in young adulthood, reduced fertility, inflammatory disease or metabolic disease like type 2 diabetes – is difficult to discern.

In the 1950s, Congress recognised the possible connections between these diseases and food additives, and the challenge of proving them. In particular, they directed the FDA to consider 'the cumulative effect' of these chemicals. 'Cumulative' is an important word here.

Let's take thyroid function as an example. We know that low doses of lots of chemicals that are either added to food or that end up in food from pesticides or packaging can damage the thyroid. Polybrominated-diphenyl-ethers, perchlorate, organophosphate pesticides, per- and polyfluoroalkyl substances (PFAS), bisphenol A, nitrates and ortho-phthalates can all disrupt various aspects of the thyroid hormone system. A low dose of any one of them may be harmless, but what about when they are all present in small doses in foods that are consumed for prolonged periods?

These concerns led to the 1958 Food Additives Amendment, which looked like it would empower the FDA to regulate the hell out of food additives and require extensive testing to ensure they were safe. It sought to protect those who might be vulnerable. That's all of us who eat or have eaten food in the USA, but especially children who are uniquely susceptible to toxic substances in their diet – partly because they are still developing, partly because they are likely to have longer exposures than adults who are first exposed when already halfway through life, and partly because they eat and drink more as a proportion of their size compared with adults.

But – and this is an important 'but' – the amendment allowed an exception to the term 'food additive'. Some substances were to be considered 'generally recognized as safe', or GRAS, a designation that was intended to allow manufacturers of common ingredients, such as vinegar and table salt, to bypass the FDA's lengthy safety-review process when their products were added to processed foods.

Almost immediately, however, this loophole became a way for companies to bypass the FDA entirely. Hundreds of chemicals were immediately added to the GRAS list. Exactly how some got onto the list isn't clear, since lots of the documents are held by the companies that originally made the request, while the documentation and data that were submitted to the regulator have not been published.

Registration of a new additive as GRAS is the second option provided by the FDA and the route that Corn Oil ONE took. If you don't want a lot of innovation-stifling hassle with lots of data requirements, then you can voluntarily apply for a GRAS notification, send the FDA *some* data and (hopefully) they will send back a letter saying that they have no follow-up questions. Phew!

Neltner sent me Corn Oil ONE's eighty-page FDA submission,[7] which claimed that the corn oil was safe based on two unpublished studies and the opinion of four experts convened by the company. I rummaged through and noticed a diagram of the molecular structure of corn oil. This was an odd inclusion for several reasons, but mainly because corn oil doesn't have a molecular structure – it's made of many different molecules. Also, the diagram looked oddly familiar. I dug out a pharmacology textbook. Instead of the structure of an oil, the company had put down the molecular formula of an HIV drug called Lopinavir. Presumably by mistake. But including the wrong molecular structure is a clue that this may not be a company with the sort of thorough, detailed approach that we'd hope when they are determining the safety of additives in our food.

The FDA were also worried and identified other major deficiencies in the company's GRAS determination. The company for example was using a processing aid made by DuPont called FermaSure XL (chlorine dioxide), which according to a blog by Tom Neltner, and an online presentation by DuPont, they market as GRAS even though the FDA turned down a GRAS application in 2011.[8, 9] *

You might think that the FDA could at this point ask to inspect a site, somewhat like they can with a drug company, but as a practical matter they can't do that if the company takes the third option offered, which is to ask the FDA to stop evaluating the additive. This is what Corn Oil ONE did when the FDA questioned the evidence provided. However, although the company asked the FDA to stop evaluating the oil, that did not mean that they had to abandon their idea of including it in food thanks to a reinterpretation of the original GRAS law by a number of companies.

A backlog of GRAS applications built up in the 1960s, 1970s and 1980s, and so the companies decided to make their own safety decisions, in secret, without telling the FDA. In 1997, the FDA proposed that this interpretation of the amendment was absolutely fine, and in 2016 they finalised the rule, meaning that it's legally above board. [10–12] This is known as self-determination. It sounds so affirming and positive, right? You can simply decide whether you think your product is safe and then put it in food.

Because this is so far from how medical drugs are regulated, I had to get Maffini and Neltner to explain this a few times. If the company that will make money from an ingredient disagrees with the FDA's concerns, and it believes that its product is GRAS, then it can withdraw the FDA application and put the molecule in food anyway.

* The company sent in three GRAS determinations. This issue was from the second one, which generated even more questions from the FDA, and the company asked them to stop evaluating the oil.

It's not known whether COZ corn oil ever made it into food, but there's nothing to stop Corn Oil ONE from marketing COZ as safe so long as the scientists there (the same scientists who confused the molecular structure of corn oil with an HIV drug) believe that it is. According to Neltner, the FDA could go to the facility or company headquarters to investigate, but there is no evidence that it does. The corn oil on your kitchen counter, or listed as an ingredient in your lunch, may well have been produced using a technology that leaves it full of unlicensed additives and antibiotics. But all that will be on the label is 'corn oil'.

You might be wondering if this is just one very extreme example. I wondered the same, and asked Neltner how often companies use this loophole. How many molecules have been self-determined to be GRAS isn't known, because the companies that do this don't have to let the FDA know. Since 2000, there have been only ten applications to the FDA for full approval for a new substance. There have been 766 new food chemicals added to the food supply since then, which means that the other 756 (or 98.7 per cent) have been self-determined by the companies that make them.[13]

Maffini and Neltner went through these applications, and found that only one considered the cumulative effects of additives in a meaningful way. Fewer than a quarter undertook the recommended one-month feeding study in animals and fewer than 7 per cent tested for developmental or reproductive effects.[14] In the context of falling fertility in high-income countries, where additive consumption is highest, this is an astonishing deficit of information.*

---

* At this point, you'll probably have a lot of reasonable questions, like 'Surely, even if a company is self-determining, there's a requirement to do specific tests, though?' I ran this past Neltner: 'There's no requirement that the company does a particular test.' Neltner called this 'assumption-based' toxicology. The company can have its own scientists look at the evidence and decide that the product is GRAS. 'If there are problems later,' Neltner continued, 'you might never be able to show it was due to that particular additive because they're not all on the labels. Think of corn oil – how would you ever know how it was produced?'

Neltner estimates that there is a universe of around 10,000 substances added to food in the USA. But because companies are allowed to self-determine, even the FDA doesn't have a complete list, and around 1,000 of these substances are estimated to have been self-determined secretly.

What Maffini and Neltner told me – that there is no functional regulation of food additives in the USA that can ensure food is safe – seemed so bizarre that I thought they were exaggerating. I called Emily Broad Leib to make sure. She's a professor at Harvard and founding director of the Harvard Law School Food Law and Policy Clinic. She said exactly the same thing: that the whole process is now, essentially, voluntary.

As a law professor, she sees the loophole as 'thwarting the will of Congress', which, of course, had demanded that the FDA regulate products. Broad Leib uses the example of trans fats to illustrate why self-determination is a problem. Trans fats are made when hydrogenation is used to turn liquid plant oils into more useful solid fats. The FDA recognised that these fats were causing hundreds of thousands of heart attacks, and tens of thousands of deaths each year. It still took decades to remove them from the food supply in the USA (despite the first concerns being published in the 1950s!) but in that instance, at least we knew what they were. As Broad Leib pointed out, 'If trans fats had been self-approved* then they would never have been on anyone's radar. No one would have been able to link them to the increase in heart attacks and deaths.'†

***

* Two types of trans fats were approved by FDA, but other uses and variants were self-affirmed as GRAS without review. That is why the agency first had to declare them as not GRAS – because they estimated thousands of people died each year – to effectively force the industry to submit a food additive petition, which the agency denied.

† It's worth considering all this from the point of view of the FDA Office of Food Additive Safety, which is responsible for regulating more than 10,000 chemicals and a multi-billion-dollar industry – at least in theory. The office has just 100

Flavours are a separate problem. The Flavor and Extract Manufacturers Association (FEMA) is a trade organisation with around 120 member companies. It has its own GRAS determination process, independent of the FDA. Companies submit GRAS applications to the organisation's expert panel and FEMA has determined more than 2,600 flavouring substances to be GRAS. The flavour industry is literally regulating itself. This is a problem.

Take the case of isoeugenol, a chemical which can be extracted from cloves, basil and gardenias and is commonly added to drinks, gum and baked goods as a flavour. It's been certified GRAS by FEMA. The US National Toxicology Program undertook a study because it has a similar structure to some other molecules that cause cancer.[15] This study found 'clear' evidence that isoeugenol caused liver cancer in mice – 80 per cent of the male mice treated had liver tumours.

Nonetheless FEMA declared isoeugenol to be GRAS because it was a 'high-dose phenomenon without any relevance for assessing the potential cancer risk of the use of isoeugenol as a food flavor ingredient'. FEMA estimated US daily per-capita intake of isoeugenol flavouring at two thousand times lower than the World Health Organization's estimate (which was still lower than what was studied in the mice, but the mice experiments established a dose-dependent effect).[16]

If as a consumer or as a citizen you are worried about this, your options are limited. You could sue an ingredient company, but

---

full-time technical staff and an annual budget of about $1 billion, which is peanuts in comparison to what they need. They're deluged with GRAS referrals. The result is that, from within the FDA, it feels like a regulatory system – they're looking at data and evidence and they're working hard – yet it all means very little, perhaps nothing, because there's no meaningful independent regulation. When it comes to food chemicals, it might make no difference if the FDA sent everyone home and shut the department down. A more honest system might be for the FDA to do exactly that, and simply say that industry is going to look after itself, and we can all just take our chances with however it decides to self-police. This was, to some extent, the approach of Donald Trump's government.

showing the connection will be hard even if you know an ingredient is present, which you might not. Neltner was bleak: 'It's nearly impossible to imagine a scenario in which a consumer could hold anyone accountable without an immediate, demonstratable injury. And I say that as a lawyer.'

In response to one of Maffini and Neltner's studies showing that most additives lacked data on safe maximum intake and reproductive toxicity, John Endres, chief scientific officer at AIBMR Life Sciences, which helps companies interact with the FDA, argued that they were unable to provide any evidence of harm. 'Where are the bodies?' he asked.[17]

The bodies, of course, may be all around us. Imagine that the cocktail of 10,000 chemicals in US food has adverse effects, but that these effects manifest indirectly over many years – by causing, for example, reduced fertility, weight gain, anxiety, depression or metabolic disease. All these things have risen with our intake of these chemicals, but it's nearly impossible to prove or disprove causation when data are so limited and exposure is so universal.

Although, as Broad Leib pointed out, we're not all exposed to the same degree. Additives exacerbate inequalities. After all, people who don't have a lot of money to put food on the table generally eat the cheapest brands, which tends to mean products from smaller companies that are more likely to be using additives that are self-determined. And additive-laden UPF is the only accessible food for many communities who have the knowledge and desire to eat better but simply lack the money.

'It's a huge example of injustice,' she said, 'especially when you think about who's benefitting from the food system: a small number of very wealthy individuals who profit at the expense of a large number of marginalised individuals – lower-income populations, native communities, people of colour.'

The situation in Europe is somewhat better. The EU uses a precautionary approach, maintains a database and publishes everything. It periodically and proactively reviews additives but there are still a lot of gaps in the testing. It's really hard to test for chronic effects mediated through the microbiome so those tests aren't done. The words 'obesity', 'dysbiosis' and 'microbiome' are pretty much absent from European Food Standards Agency reports.

There is an ethical question here as well. We spend around $2 billion on toxicology studies globally each year and kill around 100 million experimental animals.[18] A single two-generation test for reproductive safety might use over 1,000 animals. I don't think that many of us think that food colouring is a good reason to kill this number of animals, but you don't find the number of animals killed to determine the possible safety of the additives written on the pack.

Furthermore, we are not 70kg rats: we absorb and metabolise substances very differently. There are a number of studies that show that animal testing translates poorly to humans.

I acknowledge that I'm happy to use mouse and rat data to support my own point, but there is a difference: I am trying to reduce risk to life, while the makers of food colouring are trying to sell food colouring. It's fair to say that a problem in a mouse could indicate a possible problem in a human. But an absence of a problem in a mouse doesn't make an additive safe.

It's strangely illogical that we don't do more human testing on additives that we are assured are safe in humans. Either ethics committees are declining these proposals, or they are not being funded. Perhaps volunteers to drink a 1 per cent polysorbate solution for a year are in short supply. Or perhaps the more significant problem would be finding people who are not already doing this as part of their normal diet.

As it is, we have a tiny number of academics and activists doing what should be the job of government and trying to protect the most vulnerable. A lawyer like Emily Broad Leib could be making a lot more money working for the food industry. I asked her if she thought about switching sides: 'I couldn't imagine having a job where I was just making money and making things worse ...' She trailed off, and screwed up her face, as if she'd never even thought of it before. 'It's hard to envision how I could do that. What better way to use a law degree than finding these injustices and trying to correct them?'

I put the same question to Neltner, who said he doesn't spend too much time thinking about how much money it has cost him in terms of lost earnings: 'We're committed to this issue. Maricel and I have been working together as a team for twelve years – we're not letting go. We're like a bulldog. No! We're more like a snapping turtle. They never let go!'

It seems obvious to me that both in Europe and in the USA we should take a much more precautionary approach to the molecules we put in our food. The burden of proof should be on the companies that make and use additives to demonstrate long-term safety. And we need far more independent research on how these molecules affect our health in subtle ways in the long term.

Why is the burden of proof on civil society groups, activists and academics to show that adding thousands of entirely synthetic novel molecules to our diet might be harmful? Surely that's not the right way round. The fact that activists have to spend time and money trying to sort this out is just one of the ways that we pay for UPF many times over – as I was to discover on a trip to Brazil.

16.

UPF destroys traditional diets

In early 2020, I went to Brazil. I was working on a (still ongoing) investigation of the baby formula industry for the *British Medical Journal* and the BBC. Part of the project was to examine the effects of the most ambitious industrial food marketing strategy in history, conducted by Nestlé.

Nestlé is a Swiss multinational and is the largest food processing company in the world. Its 2021 revenue was a little over $95 billion – larger than the GDP of most countries. Nestlé controls over 2,000 brands, ranging from global icons to local favourites, and sells its products in 186 countries. In 2016, the company made over 40 per cent of its sales in emerging markets like Brazil. As Mark Schneider, chief executive of Nestlé, told investors in that year, 'at a time when … growth is more subdued in established economies, I think that a strong emerging market posture is going to be a winning position'.[1]

The majority of Nestlé's products are UPF. But the company also makes pet food (a form of UPF), some medical foods (also UPF) and mineral water, which my wife Dinah insists is the ultimate UPF – it might not have any funky additives, but it takes the cheapest ingredient on earth and markets it aggressively for no other reason than financial gain.

A strong traditional food culture is a challenge that modern food companies have to overcome.

Over the past decade, Brazil has become a focus for Nestlé, driven by saturated markets in Europe and North America as well as a mounting public health backlash. To access Brazil's most vulnerable people, Nestlé pioneered the use of novel marketing techniques, especially 'direct sales'. This involves door-to-door sales teams dressed in corporate uniforms wheeling little carts of puddings, cookies and packaged food into slums where the normal distribution infrastructure is lacking.

Following a *New York Times* report on this practice in 2017,[2] the relevant webpage was taken down. But archived pages* show that Nestlé described what it was doing as providing 'value to society',[3] with a network of 200 micro-distributors and 7,000 saleswomen selling fortified Nestlé products to around 700,000 lower income consumers each month. In Nestlé's view, this meant that 'these areas are not only benefiting from new income, but also from products enriched with vitamin A, iron and zinc – the three major nutritional deficiencies in Brazil'.

Nestlé also had plans for further expansion. According to Felipe Barbosa, a supervisor, 'The essence of our program is to reach the poor. What makes it work is the personal connection between the vendor and the customer.'

This is the delivery end of a system that affects all of Brazil. Farmers are encouraged to abandon subsistence crops in favour of growing the raw materials needed for UPF, such as maize, soy and sugar, and policies that favour the UPF companies are then lobbied for.

Nestlé argues that some of the products taken door-to-door are healthy. But even if we accept at face value the company's own definition of health food, according to the door-to-door sales people, customers were only interested in sweet items: KitKats, or yoghurts containing nearly the maximum daily recommended quantity of sugar in a single serving.

While I was in Brazil, I got curious about a rumour I'd heard. It concerned a spectacular marketing effort reportedly announced by Nestlé back in 2010. I managed to find an old press release describing the initiative.[4]

---

* The Wayback Machine is an incredible resource – I make a monthly donation. It trawls through the internet and saves web pages on a regular basis, so that even if companies delete stuff it remains accessible.

Nestlé Até Você a Bordo (Nestlé Takes You Onboard) was a huge floating supermarket staffed by eleven people, which would leave from Belém, the city I was working in, and travel hundreds of miles upriver, serving 800,000 people in remote Amazon communities. According to the press release, 'Nestlé aims at developing another trading channel which offers access to nutrition, health and wellness to the remote communities in the north region.'

On the day that press release was issued, Nestlé's website claimed: 'Our core aim is to enhance the quality of consumers' lives every day, everywhere by offering tastier and healthier food and beverage choices and encouraging a healthy lifestyle.'

***

Founded in 1616, Belém is the second largest city in northern Brazil, and was the final part that Portugal grabbed from the French. It sits on a bay just off the vast Amazon Delta – an accidental location. It was intended to be on the main channel of the Amazon to check on trading excursions. But according to local legend, such is the vastness of the river at that point that it was built in the wrong place. It sits on a minor river – 'minor' in this context being a relative word: the Pará has the appearance of a large brown sea from either bank.

Belém is home to the Ver-o-peso, one of the largest open-air markets in the world.* Carlos Monteiro had recommended that I see this last outpost of the traditional Brazilian diet. It stands at the water's edge, a square kilometre of market stands, covered by a decaying canvas meringue of tents. There are greasy purple açai berries, cupuaçu fruit, little pupunha fruit, dried shrimp, salt fish, manioc roots, tree nuts still in their shells – all products of the Amazon. Across the water is a green rim of what appears to be wilderness.

---

* In the seventeenth century, during the colonial era, taxes on everything extracted from the rainforest were collected here for the Portuguese Crown at the 'Casa do Haver-o-peso' – 'the house to have the weight'. Over three centuries this contracted to Ver-o-peso.

On a day off, I went in search of Nestlé's floating supermarket in the boat yards on the south shore of the city with a local fixer. We walked down a dirt path between two large warehouses, onto a rickety wooden dock on stilts, and there she was – the *Terra Grande*. It was more of a barge than a boat: two storeys at the stern, with the bridge looking over the 'supermarket', a white building with a corrugated roof. A recently repainted deck ran around the whole thing.

It looked like we could just get aboard. Why not? We climbed and waded across logs and broken docks and half-sunk boats, and pushed a little abandoned rowboat over towards the *Terra Grande*. Almost immediately, sirens went off and dogs began barking furiously. Laughing in terror, we jumped back into the rowboat and scrambled back towards the dock. A little adventure, but an unsettling one. Who was guarding the boat? Why was it alarmed and surrounded by dogs? I still don't have answers to these questions.

The next day, I took a boat upstream towards some of the places where the floating supermarket had first brought its products more than a decade earlier. We pulled away from Belém mid-morning in blazing sun, the river ochre, the trees on the bank luminous green. Over a couple of hours, we crossed the bay and made our way between tree-covered islands, before entering the main channel of the Pará.

Immediately we were surrounded by ocean-going container ships and tanker ships. These are some of the biggest ships of their kind in the world, so large that it's hard to describe them in relative terms without breaking them into parts. The bridges at the back are the size of cathedrals, eight stories high with turrets and steeples covered in aerials and masts. The ship bodies were like rusty windowless skyscrapers fallen horizontal. There were twenty or more of these ships being loaded from huge conveyor arms coming out from the Ponta da Montanha grain terminal, in the town of Barcarena, one of the main ports where Amazonian soybeans are exported.

This is an important location for worldwide UPF. In February 2022, Archer-Daniels-Midland, an American multinational food processing and commodities trading corporation, set a record at Barcarena for the largest soybean shipment in history: 84,802 tonnes in a single vessel.[5] That's fifty Olympic swimming pools full of soybeans,[6] all loaded into the *MV Harvest Frost*, which is 237 metres long and forty metres wide, then sent to Rotterdam in the Netherlands.

Brazil is the world's top soy exporter, most of which is used for animal feed in China, Europe and the USA. In the UK, much of our chicken is fed on Brazilian soy. The vast scale of soy farming means that it's cheap. Therefore, it is a great base for making UPF. Estimates suggest that more than 60 per cent of all processed food in the UK contains soy,[7] everything from breakfast cereals and cereal bars to biscuits, cheese spreads, confectionery, cakes, puddings, gravies, noodles, pastries, soups, condiments and much more. The only time you'll see a whole soybean is in the form of edamame beans (soy pods picked before they fully ripen and then boiled in their shells). Edamame have a relatively high sugar and free amino acid content, which gives them a sweet umami flavour.

Unless you're eating edamame or tofu, any soy you consume is ultra-processed through multiple physical and chemical stages: crushed, separated and refined into its different parts, it can appear on food labels as soy flour, hydrolysed vegetable protein, soy protein isolate, protein concentrate, textured vegetable protein, vegetable oil (simple, fully, or partially hydrogenated), plant sterols, or the emulsifier lecithin. Its many guises hint at its value to manufacturers.

Much of the soy from Barcarena comes from farms hundreds of miles south in the state of Mato Grosso.[8] You'll have seen pictures of deforestation in Mato Grosso, even if you don't recognise the name: virgin rainforest on one half of the frame and then a ruler-straight line where the soy fields start. In a statement about Archer-Daniels-Midland's record-breaking soy haul, the company's South America logistics director, Vitor Vinuesa, said enthusiastically, 'This is definitely something we will do again more often.'

As we crossed the Pará, storm clouds built and closed in until the river and sky seemed welded together. The gloom condensed over the far bank, and by the time we arrived in Muaná the rain was so heavy that the air was more liquid than gas. Sheets of water soaked everything. It had taken us five hours to get here, the town that is the sixth stop on the Nestlé supermarket boat's three-week route.

As we landed, it was hard not to think about the development and exploitation that the river had brought to the communities who live on its banks. Muaná is a pretty shambles of huts, palm trees, radio masts and brick buildings. It is home to a few thousand people and the hub for around 40,000 people in the wider Muaná municipality. I interviewed children and local officials, two of whom stood out to me for their descriptions of the problems Nestlé had started.

Paula Costa Ferreira is the head teacher at the local school, and has that bustle and authority common to all great teachers. She remembered the Nestlé boat very well: 'It would come every week; it was like a mall in the city. It was new, and it stayed open late. The young people would go and meet up there. The first thing that happened was that it brought the prices down under the price of the local market.'

In the complex web of claims about proposed economic benefit, this was not an effect that was discussed by Nestlé in press releases or comments to the media. Nestlé did provide employment to a few people, but not to anyone local to Muaná. In the meantime, the low prices made life harder for local traders of whole foods. The shop on the boat went from being a luxury to an essential service.

Costa Ferreira went on to tell me about several local children with type 2 (diet-related) diabetes. I thought the translator had got this wrong, because the presence of *any* children with type 2 diabetes in such a small community would have been astounding. There should have been zero cases. And there *were* zero cases there just a short while ago. This is something that child obesity statistics conceal. The proportion of children who meet the definition of obesity has increased by hundreds of per cent in many places, but the rate of increase in the most severely affected places is essentially infinite. I have not found any evidence that there were children with diet-related diabetes in these parts of Brazil until enterprises like the Nestlé boat.

I went to a small supermarket in the town, Fruteira Pomar, which had huge quantities of traditional foods – rice, beans, yams, papayas, tomatoes, onions – but an array of UPF too. The shopkeeper said he hadn't heard of Nestlé products until the boat came. Now he feels obliged to stock the products because customers began to demand them. Whether or not that was the intention, things have worked out well for Nestlé: the tiniest shops in town now stock Nestlé products, along with other UPF from other manufacturers, from floor to ceiling.

Church NGOs have started to try to manage the public health crisis. Lizete Novaes from the Catholic NGO Pastoral da Criança took me to a village on the outskirts of Muaná that comprised a long row of small wooden houses on stilts in a swamp forest. From a public health perspective, it was a catastrophe. The paths were duckboards running a couple of metres above mud, into which the houses' long-drop toilets emptied directly. There was little running water. The people who lived there worked mainly for a palm hearts company, Novaes told me enigmatically. 'They live here as they have nowhere else to go.'

She took me to see a boy called Leo, who lived with his mum in a tiny house divided into three tinier rooms. Leo was twelve and had severe learning difficulties. His BMI was around 45, which would put him in the heaviest 1 per cent of children his age in the UK.

We walked unsteadily over the boards to the local shop with Leo, who was cheerful and smiling. It took about two minutes to get there. In the heat, it was easy to see the benefit of selling UPF for the shop – no refrigeration required. Many of the products in the shop were made by Nestlé. Leo's mum said that she finds it impossible to stop him coming to the shop: 'Sometimes I tell him not to eat, but he tricks me and comes to the shop anyway. He eats vegetables, but he doesn't like them. I don't know why – he just likes junk food.'

Leo rummaged around the shop and made a pile of things on the counter: chocolate biscuits, strawberry biscuits, powdered milk, crisps. I paid for them all.

Colonists, missionaries, armies: all have used development as a justification for violence in this part of the world. 'Big Food' coming to a place like Muaná also commits violence here, as it does around the world in terms of the damage wrought on bodies and on the environment. At home in London, the violence seems, to me, to be less front of mind – perhaps because it's been so normal for such a long time. In Brazil, it was possible to see the workings, the change taking place. It was the living reality of what Monteiro had seen in his data – the moment when the Nestlé boat first pulled up. As Novaes said, 'The new products that came on the boat were very tasty, and then everyone just started to have these kinds of meals.'

Everyone, from the shopkeepers and Leo's mum to the teachers and the people working for the NGOs, agrees: it all started with the boat. And almost everyone we met – Costa Ferreira, Novaes, Leo's mum and Leo – was living with obesity.

***

The companies that make UPF either displace traditional diets, as they are doing in Brazil, or absorb them and recreate them with new ingredients. I started to notice this early on in my diet.

The day after Emily Broad Leib, the food law professor at Harvard, told me about the inequality that UPF generates, I sat down to try to enjoy some KFC Hot Wings. This was one of the meals I had been most looking forward to on my UPF diet. They were a childhood favourite. Xand and I would get the bus home from school on Wednesdays after sport. We encouraged mum to believe that training frequently over-ran so that we could get home late without any questions being asked. And so, every week, we'd go via KFC.

Even at the time, we knew that those Hot Wings were a special product. The batter casing was a bone-dry crust, almost a shell. Fracturing it released a burst of juices from the moist and tender chicken inside. They were just spicy enough to make me breathless. They were as desirable as any drug and, crucially, they were totally forbidden. I've no idea how we never got caught coming home covered in grease, unable to eat our dinner.

Hot Wings remained a favourite snack throughout my early adult life, but at some point in my late thirties, the combination of a wife and a growing belly reduced my consumption to zero. It didn't feel like my decision so much as something imposed on me by public health messaging, being a doctor and a children's television presenter, environmental concerns and my wife hating that I ate them.

But now I was off the hook. I *had* to eat Hot Wings. It was scientific research. So, I sat down with some one night, finally able to enjoy them fully. They were exactly as I remembered, possibly even better: spicier, with crunchier batter and even more moist and tender chicken. Yet my interpretation of the sensory information was entirely different. The Hot Wings had, like so many other products, become very unpleasant.

The UK ingredients for Hot Wings aren't available online, but I managed to find the Canadian ones as I ate. They included MSG, modified corn starch, partially hydrogenated soybean oil and something called dimethylpolysiloxane.

Dimethylpolysiloxane, or food additive E900, was first evaluated by the Food Standards Agency in 1969. It's used as an antifoaming agent in the frying oil to ensure worker safety.[9] It's also used as a flea treatment, hair conditioner and condom lubricant. Extensive experiments in rats show that hardly any is absorbed when eaten and it passes out unchanged in the faeces. Dimethylpolysiloxane may very well be safe. Or it may be subtly harmful over a long period through some mechanism yet to be discovered. Either way, it occurs nowhere in nature. Whatever it does or doesn't do to the body, we've never encountered it previously, and evolution has had no time to accommodate it.

More troubling to me than the dimethylpolysiloxane were the graphics on the packaging, which as a teenager I'd never thought about. I was eating KFC a few months after the murder of George Floyd by a Minneapolis police officer, Derek Chauvin. The US and British history of enslavement was being discussed everywhere, and someone who looked like a Confederate colonel appeared to be on my chicken box.[10-12]

I remembered a piece in the *Guardian* that had just reinvigorated the conversation about race and fried chicken in the UK: 'I've always loved fried chicken. But the racism surrounding it shamed me'.[13] It was written by Melissa Thompson, a chef, journalist and food historian. Her latest book, *Motherland*, charts the history of Jamaican food.

In that *Guardian* piece, Thompson interweaves her own experiences of racism with the history of fried chicken:

> Historically, chickens held special importance for enslaved black Americans, being the only livestock they were allowed to keep. Black domestic workers would cook fried chicken for their masters and, later, their employers. And then, after emancipation, women known as 'waiter carriers' would hawk trays of fried chicken and biscuits to travellers through open windows as their trains stopped in stations.
>
> But while these black cooks and homemakers effectively invented what would become known as southern food, their contribution was erased. The white folk took the credit for its creation, while Black people were mocked and parodied merely as greedy consumers. It's one of the most outrageous examples of cultural theft.

I got in touch with Thompson and asked her about the KFC packaging. She emphasised that cooking from the American South – southern food, soul food – was established by Black cooks in domestic settings: 'KFC is a company based on Black ingenuity, and yet it does not allude to or celebrate Blackness.'

There's a history of 'The Colonel' on the KFC website. Born in 1890, he left home at thirteen to seek his fortune and, in 1930, took over a service station to serve weary travellers the same fried chicken he ate growing up. It's not clear who cooked it for him as a child – perhaps his mother, perhaps a domestic servant. Either way, he probably wasn't the true originator of the meal I had in front of me: it's hard to believe that the original recipe contained partially hydrogenated vegetable oil, modified corn starch, spice extracts or MSG.

Thompson also talked about the wider relationship between fast-food chains selling UPF and the Black community in the UK. We looked at some adverts together. In July 2021, McDonald's put out a short video on Twitter that showed six Black boys in a park eating and having a fantastic time. I wasn't sure how to respond. It felt inclusive, but problematic at the same time. 'Fast food advertising in this country is definitely inclusive,' Thompson said, 'and you really want to be able to celebrate that. But the very reason it's inclusive is that it's trying to market food that isn't healthy to people who are already marginalised. In that sense, it's predatory.'

Sophisticated marketing campaigns target minority groups so that racial identity is inextricably linked to brands. Critique of these brands then becomes critique of culture, of parenting, of apparent choice. Food that was once a proud part of a cultural identity has been taken over by transnational corporations and is now inextricably associated with poor health. But traditional homemade fried chicken will interact with human appetite in a very different way from the ultra-processed fried chicken available up and down the high street all over the UK.

***

This trend is global. There are KFC outlets in almost every country on earth, with more than 850 in sub-Saharan Africa alone, including Angola, Tanzania, Nigeria, Uganda, Kenya, Ghana and beyond. Public health officials argue that food like KFC is increasing the prevalence of obesity in Ghana, which has risen from less than 2 per cent in 1980 to 13.6 per cent.[14] Charles Agyemang, a Ghanaian professor at the University of Amsterdam, told the *New York Times* that eating local foods in some parts of Ghana is frowned upon: 'People see the European type as civilized.'

Ashok Mohinani, whose company owns all the KFC franchises in Ghana, told the paper that 'We want this to evolve into the idea of getting it to be a daily brand.' When asked whether it was unhealthy for people to eat fried chicken this often, a KFC spokeswoman gave this response: 'At KFC, we're proud of our world famous, freshly in-store prepared fried chicken and believe it can be enjoyed as a part of a balanced diet and healthy lifestyle.' In an interview on CNN, Greg Creed, the former chief executive of YUM! (KFC's parent company), took the argument further, claiming that it's 'so much safer to eat at a KFC in Ghana, than it is to eat, obviously, you know, pretty much anywhere else'.

Ghana is not alone in seeing a massive rise in body weight. By 2017, more people around the world had obesity than were underweight. And while the absolute numbers of people with obesity in the USA, Australia and the UK are shocking, the rate of increase in obesity in other countries is far higher. Between 1980 and 2015, rates of obesity in the USA and the UK little more than doubled. In China, the rates went up by 800 per cent. In Mali, they increased by 1,550 per cent.*

It's clear from the evidence in Brazil and other countries that increasing western fast food (almost all of which is UPF, of course)

---

* This growth in body weight has reflected sales of UPF. Data collected by the market research firm Euromonitor shows that fizzy drinks sales have doubled in Latin America since 2000, such that it has overtaken the USA as a market. Worldwide, fast-food sales grew by 30 per cent between 2011 and 2016. In 2016, Domino's Pizza opened 1,281 stores, one every seven hours, almost all of which were outside the USA.[15] India now has nearly 1,500 Domino's locations.[16]

increases the risks of diabetes, heart disease and death.[17] And in low-income and middle-income countries, health-care infrastructure is far less able to cope with the growing need for drugs to manage diabetes or high blood pressure. This may be especially true in remote or rural regions like the Amazon. But this seems to be of little concern to the UPF companies – developing countries are an important source of revenue and growth, after all. All over the world, traditional diets are being displaced by UPF as part of a global nutritional transition, and the playbook for how to best do this was developed in places like Muaná.

***

When we got back to Belém after visiting Muaná, our fixer managed to track down the manager of Nestlé's supermarket boat, a man named Graciliano Silva Ramo. We walked together out on the dock next to the *Terra Grande* in the gathering gloom on my final evening in the city. He talked about getting the job, how he'd been 'enchanted' when he first saw Nestlé's proposal about the only floating supermarket in the world.

'This river was my home for seven years,' he told me. 'I was so proud of my work and what I did for the project and the population, a needy population who needed a lot of help at the time, especially quality food.

'But,' he went on, 'not all the food we took to the people was nutritious.'

The boat sold hundreds of different products but, according to Ramo (and everyone in the villages), KitKats were the top seller. He said that they had to take a very large stock to serve the population of Ribeirinhos – the riverside people.

He was very upset when Nestlé cancelled the boat service. Ramo had built a life bringing huge excitement to the riverside communities, seeing things that no ordinary urban Brazilian would ever see. He'd never seen the harm, the increasing size of the children, the ones with dental abscesses. But now he felt differently: 'That was the big problem, and it remains the big problem, the poor diet. People ate poorly, they did not eat healthy food. And so they got tooth cavities, and diseases of the stomach.'

By the time he said all this it was nearly dark. The boat was a trojan horse. Its purpose was not to supply food but to create a market. Once you've had ice cream and KitKats you can't go back.

17

The true cost of Pringles

When we were eating Pringles with Andrea, Xand had remembered something as he finished the tube: 'Wasn't there some court case where someone tried to prove Pringles contain so little potato that they are not legally potato crisps? Probably just an urban myth.'

It turns out it wasn't an urban myth at all. If you search through the files of the British and Irish Legal Information Institute (and why wouldn't you?), you'll find the case is entirely real. What lent it the flavour of legend, perhaps, was this detail: it was the manufacturers of Pringles, Procter & Gamble (P&G), who were trying to prove they didn't contain enough potato to be called crisps.

Almost all the bizarre food-based legal cases in the UK that make the news centre around our tax system, internationally regarded as one of the most complex in the world. In the UK, VAT is added to lots of food products, but not to things considered 'essential'.* Tax law in the UK says that 'food' is not subject to VAT, but there is a list of exceptions, which are taxed, and then there are exceptions to the exceptions, which are not taxed.

The result of this is constant squabbling between food manufacturers, who want to squeeze their products into zero-VAT categories and keep the tax money as profit, and His Majesty's Revenue and Customs, who want the extra tax. The most memorable recent case

---

* One of the criticisms of VAT is that poor people spend a far higher proportion of their income on it than rich people and so, to counteract this, certain essential goods are made VAT exempt (or, more properly, given a zero rate, which is the same thing but with a slight legal wrinkle that only tax lawyers understand). VAT is payable on all luxury goods.

was around whether a product called a McVitie's Jaffa Cake was a cake or a biscuit.

The cake/biscuit part of the law may be best summarised like this: VAT is payable on confectionery, with the exception of cakes and biscuits, which are staples, with the exception of chocolate-covered biscuits, which are luxuries, with the exception of chocolate-covered gingerbread men assuming they have no more than a couple of chocolate dots for eyes, which are staples. Gingerbread men with chocolate buttons or belts, however, are, in the eyes of the law, a luxury. Also, when the chocolate on a biscuit is in a sandwich layer between two biscuit halves as in a bourbon, VAT is not payable. It's the same for basket-shaped chocolate biscuits.

None of the tax lawyers I spoke with could explain why chocolate-covered cakes are not a luxury but, for tax purposes, they are not.

This means two things. First, that biscuit company lawyers have strong opinions about gingerbread men's eye colour and state of undress. Second, if a Jaffa Cake were, in fact, a chocolate-covered biscuit, it would be subject to VAT, but if it were a chocolate-covered cake it would be exempt. In the end, McVitie's were spared the tax.

In the Pringles case, the relevant bit of law is that the tax is payable on potato crisps but not on most other snacks. At the time this was written in 1969, the government's intention was to tax food that was not purchased primarily for the purpose of nutrition: potato crisps and nuts were the only real savoury snacks at the time. But by the start of the Pringles case in 2004 many of Pringles' competitors (like Doritos) had no potato content and thus were untaxed.

P&G were set on having their product categorised as something other than 'potato crisps' so that they wouldn't be subject to VAT. Their angle was to work a loophole in the law: if a product requires further preparation, it will avoid the tax – an exception that presumably exists so that sliced potatoes (not a luxury) aren't put in the taxable category. So began a long legal battle.

In 2004, P&G brought out a new product called Pringles Dippers.[1] These had a scoop shape and were slightly thicker to enable the scooping-up of a new range of dips. P&G immediately took their new product to a tax tribunal, claiming that this dipping constituted 'further preparation'. The tribunal agreed, finding in favour of P&G and adding that Pringles Dippers weren't potato crisps, because they lacked both 'similarity and the necessary potato content'. It was this ruling that laid the groundwork for P&G's subsequent cases, which ran from 2007 to 2009.[2-4]

The lawyer employed by P&G was Roderick Cordara KC, who graduated with a first-class law degree from Cambridge, and whose website features endorsements including, appropriately enough, 'hungry to win'. Cordara argued that the combination of the low potato content (around 40 per cent) and the manufacturing process made Pringles more like cake. Cakes are, according to the law, an 'essential' food, and exempt from VAT.

This is how the judgment summarised what Cordara claimed were a Pringle's 'fundamental characteristics'. It's probably one of the most honest accounts of industrial food processing you'll read: 'Unlike a crisp, a Pringle is not made from slicing and frying a potato. Instead, it is produced from a dough, like a cake or biscuit. The dough is pushed into a standardised metal shape and then passed through the cooking process on a conveyor belt ... allowing for uniformity of shape, colour and texture.'

There are further details in the judgment: 'the unique feature of regular Pringles was that the manufacturing process causes oil to go into the spaces throughout the texture of the product replacing the water content removed during the frying. This gives the "mouth-melt" feel when it is eaten. By contrast with potato crisps where most of the fat stays on the surface.'

P&G took the case through two appeals. The 2008 judgment found that regular Pringles should be exempt from VAT – a huge win for the company. But HMRC appealed the decision in 2009, and the presiding judge, Lord Justice Jacob, decided that this was not a question 'calling for or justifying over-elaborate, almost mind-numbing legal analysis'.

Nonetheless the judgment runs to fifteen pages and shows why both sides put in so much effort. It opens in a Shakespearean tone: 'Are Pringles "similar to potato crisps and made from the potato?" That is the question. Upon [this decision] hangs the question of rather a lot of money – as much as £100m of tax for the past and about £20m a year for the future.'

P&G claimed that the product should have a sufficient content of potato to give it a quality of 'potatoness'. But Jacob could not imagine that the government, when it made the law, intended to require something to have this quality: 'It is an Aristotelian question: does the product have an "essence of potato".'

After quoting from legal texts dating back to 1921, Jacob proposed that whether Pringles were made from potato would be better answered by a child than by a food scientist or a culinary pedant: 'I think that most children, if asked whether jellies with raspberries in them were "made from" jelly, would have the good sense to say "Yes", despite the raspberries.'

After years of legal wrangling, P&G lost the final appeal. Pringles, the court ruled, *are* made of potato. VAT still applies to them. The question of whether dipping a crisp into some sauce constituted 'further preparation' was resolved in 2005 in United Biscuits *vs* HMRC concerning McCoy's Dips, when a tribunal held that it obviously did not in any normal sense of the English language. In a scathing judgment, it was said that 'the purchaser of [United Biscuit's] product is required to do no more than open a packet of crisps and a pot of dip. He may, or may not, dip the crisps into the pot. The process of conveying crisp to mouth, whether or not it pauses at the pot, is, in our view, commonly and correctly described as eating; it is not preparation.'

Pringle Dippers, meanwhile, are no longer available. Yet I can't help but wonder if the legal strategy was so sophisticated and so long-range that the company launched that entire range of products for the sole reason of creating the legal precedent used in their various cases. Certainly, the £3.5 million marketing spend on Pringle

Dippers would be very quickly recouped if they had managed to hack off that VAT. And, while it certainly costs HMRC less to fight these cases than to concede them, it's remarkable that they have to fight them at all.

Type the name of any of the dozen or so companies that make most of our UPF into the legal database and you'll find hundreds of these cases, each more entertaining than the last. And HMRC (who represent you and me) often lose: Doritos, Twiglets, Deltas, Skips, Cheeselets, Mignon Morceaux, Ripplins and Wheat Crunchies have all been zero-rated.

It feels like you and I are now essentially subsidising these snacks. And we don't make the money back by getting products more cheaply – if you look at pricing across the range of snacks, it doesn't reflect whether they are taxed or not. When a company doesn't pay the VAT, they are in a way privatising a public good.* Even if you don't eat these snacks, you seem to pay for them twice: you pay the subsidy when they are untaxed, and you pay for the lawyers that HMRC have to employ to beat QCs like Cordara.

These lawsuits are going on the whole time, an arms race with ever more expensive lawyers and arguments of increasing complexity.

Kellogg's recently sued the UK government, disputing the legality of new legislation that would mean lots of Kellogg's products couldn't be promoted or put on the most prominent shelves in supermarkets. The company's argument was that, because we usually have cereal with milk, its cereals' sugar content should be judged with milk, which would obviously, by weight, reduce it very significantly.[5, 6] They lost, but it cost everyone a lot of money. Chris Silcock, managing director of Kellogg's UK, said that they were disappointed with the result and that companies might 'charge higher prices'.

Maybe you'll end up paying more for cereal to cover the Kellogg's lawyers and a little more tax to cover the HMRC lawyers.

---

* For me, the whole episode sits uncomfortably alongside the online claim of P&G's leadership team that it 'always strives to use their knowledge and experience to improve consumers' lives'.

I see the avoidance of tax as part of ultra-processing, as defined by the NOVA system and Monteiro. The legal teams involved in decreasing the tax obligations to increase the profit are a necessary stage in the processing of the food. All food companies have them. And it's not always only about tax. There are a number of other externalised costs of UPF, which link to Monteiro's original definition that the purpose of ultra-processing is to create highly profitable products. I want to focus on the three most significant: environmental destruction (including climate change and land use), antibiotic resistance and plastic pollution.

First: the climate.

Humans have had significant effects on the earth's climate for a long time, but our current food system, driven by demand for UPF, is destroying ecological capital far faster than it regenerates.*

---

* In the 'New World', 1492 marks the beginning of the 'Columbian exchange', a strange euphemism that implies trade and mutual benefit, rather than what actually happened – the start of a period known as the Great Dying, but which would be better described as the Great Killing. Historians of pre-Columbian American history describe a cycle of murder, violence and slavery, catalysed by Columbus and continued by later Europeans to exploit the continent's resources. The arrival of Europeans catalysed waves of epidemic diseases: measles, smallpox, bubonic plague and respiratory viruses like influenza.[7–9] Scientists of various stripes have collaborated to work out a rough estimate of the population shortly after 1492. Colleagues at UCL have estimated the total population of the Americas in 1500 to be around 60 million. There were thriving societies – as many as 20 million people were living in the Amazon where they had complex agricultural systems, farming sweet potato, rice, cassava, peanuts, chilli peppers and maize. Archaeological evidence shows stone-built hill terraces, drainage systems and raised fields, as well as extensive landscape modification using fire, clearing of non-useful plants and seed dispersal. Just 100 years after Columbus's arrival, the population had been reduced to 6 million. The reduction of the population by 90 per cent in a century meant that agricultural land returned to forest. Trees grew again on 56 million hectares of land, removing 7.4 billion tonnes of carbon dioxide from the atmosphere. The team at UCL suggested that this reforestation led to the 'little ice age', seen in depictions of winter scenes in many seventeenth century paintings.[10, 11] The same thing may have happened in Australia. Early human populations burned forests presumably to promote

255

The impact of the current food system is not sustainable for the next few decades – let alone the next few millennia. The environmental cost is so immense that, even if we stopped all fossil-fuel emissions, emissions from the global food system alone will take us well beyond the fatal 1.5°C rise in temperature by 2100.[12] And, while there will always be an environmental impact from farming and processing food for 8 billion people, UPF is a particular driver of carbon emissions and environmental destruction.

If dietary trends continue, per-capita greenhouse-gas emissions from empty calories (calories without significant additional nutritional value) are estimated to nearly double by 2050. In Australia, for example, UPF consumption is already estimated to contribute more than a third of the total diet-related environmental effects.[*]

I went to meet Rob Percival, head of food policy for the Soil Association, to understand the environmental effects of UPF. He speaks like a policy expert with a philosophy degree (which he is and has), while his long hair, goatee and oversized knitwear have a distinct surfer vibe. We met in a pub in east London for a vegan curry. I wanted to understand how much environmental damage is from UPF specifically as compared to simply producing food in general.

'The important question,' he said, 'is not "What is the carbon footprint of a particular product?" but "Which foods would we find

---

grasslands for hunting, and perhaps, as happened in north Africa in the former wetlands that are now the Sahara, this affected the timing of the summer monsoon. These are contentious discussions and rightly so, but it seems that even ancient societies could have had significant effects on global weather, climate and geography. This shouldn't undermine commitments to incorporate Indigenous knowledge into food and environmental policies. Indigenous knowledge has practical value, and Indigenous people have rights to land use. These were and are communities that have lived on the land sustainably for millennia. This doesn't mean zero impact, but rather that they didn't eat into the fundamental ecological capital of the system in under a century.

[*] Specifically, 35 per cent of water use, 39 per cent of energy use, 33 per cent of carbon dioxide equivalents, and 35 per cent of land use.[13]

in a food system that helped to resolve the climate and nature crises?"'

According to Percival, there are obvious environmental questions posed by UPF, but the issue runs much deeper. The prevalence of UPF in our diet is symptomatic of a sickly food system: 'At the moment, the global food system is fundamentally oriented towards producing as much food as possible.'

Given that there are lots of us, and many people are going hungry, this seems eminently sensible. But, as Percival explained, it has led to perverse outcomes. In pursuit of making this quantity of food, agribusinesses have invested in a handful of high-yield crops and products,* typically grown or produced on land that should be tropical forest, using agrochemical inputs – fertilisers, pesticides, herbicides, and lots and lots of fossil fuel of course. Supported by government subsidies, this approach has led to a global glut of commodity crop production, and declining food diversity.

For these commodity crops to be profitable, they need to be turned into something, and there are two options (or three, if you count biofuel): 'You can force the crops through a factory-farmed animal to produce meat, or process them into an aggressively marketed UPF.'

Growing specific foods for specific communities is a hassle. It's much more profitable to grow a small number of things with maximum efficiency, then colour, flavour and market them as diverse foods. As we've seen, everything from chicken nuggets to ice cream can be made from the same base liquids and powders.

'Factory farming and UPFs are two sides of the same industrial food coin,' Percival said. 'And then, of course, lots (though not all) of that factory farmed meat is subsequently turned into UPF.'

The result of this is that, of the thousands of different strains of plants and breeds of animals that have been cultivated since the

---

* Including palm oil, soya protein and soybean oil, sugar, wheat, maize, meat, milk and eggs.

birth of agriculture, just twelve plants and five animals now make up 75 per cent of all the food eaten or thrown away on earth.[14-17]

And while sugar often gets the blame for health effects, a significant part of the calorific load of UPF is from refined vegetable oils. Vegetable oils have gone from being a very small source of calories to the dominant fuel in the global diet. Palm is the oil we now eat most, and is increasingly well known for its environmental impact.

Since 1970, more than half of all the virgin rainforest in Indonesia has been destroyed for oil palm.[18, 19] Between 2015 and 2018, 130,000 hectares was cleared to grow palm in Indonesia.[20] That's an area roughly the size of Greater London. Even if you flew over it in a jetliner, it would stretch from horizon to horizon in all directions. You literally can't see it all without going to space. It was achieved with chainsaws and slash-and-burn techniques – the soil on the forest floor is flammable peat. The scale of carbon released by this is hard to comprehend. On several single days, the fires in 2015 emitted more carbon dioxide than the entire United States economy.[21]

Around three-quarters of the palm oil produced is used in UPF. The rest is used in soap, shaving foam, toothpaste, lipstick and myriad other household products.[22] In my view, if a product contains palm oil it *is* UPF and the same argument could be made for all RBD (remember that's refined, bleached and deodorised) oils. This shows how corrupted our food system has become, because these highly processed oils still count as simple kitchen ingredients or NOVA group 2. There is a separate discussion about their effect on human health that I won't go into here.

Even if you don't accept this, it's hard to find a product with palm oil in it that isn't UPF. While virgin palm oil is used in home cooking in many countries, it is a long way from the highly modified substance that is used to make something like Nutella chocolate spread.

A large-scale boycott would mean replacing the oils in UPF with something else, and this allows the companies to make an efficiency argument. They claim that palm oil plantations are the most efficient form of calorie production because extracting the same amount of oil from coconut palms, for example, would take ten times more land, meaning we'd need to cut down ten times as much rainforest.

Of course, this argument is misguided in several ways. For instance, we can grow other fat sources, like sunflowers, in temperate non-tropical climates. This will take more land but will have far less impact on carbon emissions. Land in temperate climates stores far less carbon than, for example, a Borneo peat swamp, and it has already been farmed for centuries, sometimes millennia, so it is a much less significant contributor to climate change than cutting down virgin tropical forest to grow palm.

The other claim frequently made by industry is that there is such a thing as sustainable palm oil. But nothing about the way we produce UPF is sustainable. The word 'sustainable' has no formal meaning with any independent body. Sustainability criteria are largely set by industry and, in general, the designation just means that a farm growing it can't clear new forest. But if it cleared the forest the year before applying for the designation, that's fine.

And why are we eating palm oil from Indonesia at all? Lots of UPF isn't strictly necessary, so growing its raw ingredients like this is mostly a waste of land. None of the UPF snacks and discretionary products are necessary for human diet, meaning that many of the environmental impacts could be avoided.

Furthermore, the current food system is not efficient, as discussed by a team of food engineers from Wageningen University in a 2016 paper.[23] The authors think about this problem in two nifty ways. First, they point out that there is far less energy in our food than it takes to make it. Neolithic people would not survive if they had to do this level of processing themselves by hand. Mechanisation brings an illusion of energy efficiency, but in fact it's just cost efficiency made possible with enormous amounts of cheap fossil fuel. Oil is cheap for the same reason that UPF is cheap: because, according to the International Monetary Fund and lots of other people, we all subsidise it by paying around $6 trillion (yes trillion) worth of external costs, like increases in healthcare costs due to air pollution and the costs of a changing climate.[24]

The second inefficiency they report is that plants produce a huge amount of potentially nutritious protein, but we eat hardly any of it. Instead, we feed it to animals.[25] Until fairly recently, animals were a way of turning very low-quality plant protein (grass, leaves, food waste and forage) into high-quality edible protein. But the demands of intensive farming, which require that animals are reared quickly, mean that animals are now fed fairly nutritious plants which humans could eat.

It is well known that meat is less carbon efficient than plants as a source of food. Producing 100g of protein from beef emits at least 25kg of carbon dioxide, on average. Chicken produces far less, at 4–5kg of carbon dioxide per 100g, but we eat vastly more chicken than beef. Per 100g, tofu produces 1.6kg carbon dioxide, beans 0.65kg and peas 0.36kg. Some nuts are carbon negative even after transport, because tree nuts are replacing crops and taking carbon from the air.[26]

There are ways of farming beef and chicken that may even help to sequester carbon, and many agroecological systems that farm without chemical inputs and in which grazing and browsing animals help to build soil health and natural capital in a way that supports the local and global ecosystem. But it's doubtful that these methods can produce enough meat to match our current and growing appetite.* If we keep eating more meat, it will require the destruction of more tropical forest, which in turn will drive pandemic disease and climate change.

Because most of what we eat is UPF, most of the meat we eat is *in* UPF. UPF meat (reformulated nuggets, burgers and so on) accounts for 7 per cent of average UK diet, whereas fresh or minimally processed meat accounts for only 5 per cent.[29]

And the nature of UPF means that the manufacturing process typically cannot allow for concern for the environment or high

---

* At present around 80 per cent of the world's farmland is used to graze animals or to produce crops to feed to animals. The combined weight of animals bred for food is now ten times the combined weight of all wild mammals and birds put together.[27, 28]

standards of animal care. It encourages excess consumption of food and necessarily diminishes our knowledge about its origins. If you buy fresh beef or chicken, it will often say on the pack 'grass-fed' or 'corn-fed'. People often want to know which farm it came from. But very few people ask about what the chicken in their prepacked UPF sandwich was fed on, although this is, it turns out, an important question to ask.

Take a soybean, one of the oldest cultivated plants in the world. Traditionally soy has not been widely used as a food crop because it tastes lousy and is hard to digest. You can ferment it and extract good protein in the form of tofu (or harvest it early for edamame), but it's never been a significant source of calories for most people until recently.

But at around 42 per cent protein, soy is very efficient for feeding animals in bulk if it's processed intensively using lots and lots of fossil fuel. The pods are first shaken, to remove stems and dirt, dehydrated in enormous heaters, mechanically dehulled, then crushed by giant rollers into particles, before being rehydrated and rolled into flakes. Oil is extracted using a flammable solvent, hexane, and the flakes can be fed to animals or they can be further heated, cooled, finely ground, dissolved at one pH and then precipitated at another to make 'protein isolate', which can then be added to any UPF for bulk, mouth-feel or to allow the product to be marketed as high in protein. Soy is a good example of the co-dependence of factory farming and UPF industries. Roughly 75 per cent of soy is for animal feed, but the soy oil market is also highly lucrative – soy oil ends up in all sorts of UPFs.[30]

This is *not* an efficient way of making food from a plant (compared with, say, eating the plant), but it is cheap, so cheap that much of the protein in soy is fed to chickens (as well as pigs and dairy cows), which are then used to make UPF.[31]

Chicken is the most popular meat. Around 1 billion chickens are farmed each year in the UK (fifteen for every adult and child – double the global average), and 95 per cent of them are fast-growing breeds that are intensively reared indoors. Almost none are wandering around farmyards. And with bird flu meaning that flocks have to be kept indoors, 'free range' may be a thing of the past.

The best way of making money from a chicken is to spend as little time caring for it as possible. If you keep a chicken as a pet, it will live for around six years. Yet birth-to-slaughter time for 95 per cent of the chicken we eat is just six weeks – less than 2 per cent of their natural lifespan. Free-range chickens live for around eight weeks, and free-range organic chickens for around twelve weeks (that's why it's more expensive). On a purely commercial front, battery farming has proved successful: the cost of chicken, is nearly three times cheaper today than in the 1960s in real terms.[32]

These chickens are fed on a high-protein diet of some fishmeal and a lot of soya.

Each year, 3 million tonnes of soya are imported into the UK, and most of it has caused environmental destruction that is already affecting the global climate.[33–35]

So dominant is soy as industrial animal feed that the average person in the UK or Europe consumes approximately 61kg of soy per year, largely in the form of animal products such as chicken, pork, salmon, cheese, milk and eggs.[36] Only 20–30 per cent of imported soy is 'certified sustainable' (and we have already discussed how little that means). So, if you live in the UK, there is a tennis court of land producing soy in the tropics just for you, and most of it comes from places like Brazil and Argentina where ecosystems that affect global climate are being destroyed.*

On the present course, global meat production is set to almost double in the next 30 years, and we're going to need an area the size of Europe to produce the soy and maize to feed the animals on.

---

* Since the 1960s, half the Cerrado has been lost to soy production and cattle grazing. The UK's overseas 'soy footprint' is an area the size of Wales – 1.7 million hectares of former rainforest that is no longer a home for armadillos, anteaters, jaguars or the humans who lived there for millennia.[37] On a per-person level, this scale of impact also holds true for the USA (which has a population approximately five times larger than the UK) and most western economies.

It's not just habitat destruction. Pesticide use on soy in the Americas is associated with birth defects and higher cancer rates among local populations. In Argentina, since 1990, soy production has quadrupled while herbicide use has gone up eleven-fold. In these areas, miscarriages and birth defects have increased. In Argentina overall, around 20 per cent of deaths are caused by cancer, but in these areas the rate is over 30 per cent.[38–40]

If those effects feel remote, then the effects on global climate shouldn't. The food security that many of us enjoy is the product of a system of production that has kept costs low by destroying wild land and not paying for the costs of atmospheric carbon. These approaches will, ironically, create huge food insecurity. This is happening already around the globe, but nowhere more directly than in the areas of the Amazon that have been deforested to grow soy.

Inland rain requires trees. Rain clouds on their own cannot travel more than 400km from the sea, so rain in the centre of a continent – the very rain that creates the central forest of the Amazon for example – requires continuous forest to the coast. Around half the rain that falls on the Amazon comes from its trees. As every school geography student knows, water evaporates from the sea, then falls as rain on coastal forest. Those trees 'breathe out' water vapour, which creates new clouds that travel further inland in so-called 'flying rivers'.

Crucially, this is how water reaches the soy and corn plantations in central and western Brazil. Once you destroy the forest you get less rain. A 2019 study showed that the rainy season in the state of Mato Grosso had become a month shorter in a decade,[41, 42] and many of the major soy farms in Brazil are now suffering from the very drought that they have caused.

Diverting rivers is not going to be possible, because the river water comes from rain.[43] Hotter temperatures and droughts mean the southeastern Amazon has become a source of carbon dioxide rather than a carbon sink, and by some estimates the Amazon now produces more carbon than it stores.[44, 45]

So, the single greatest threat to Brazilian agribusiness is … Brazilian agribusiness.

Why don't we care about this? Partly because none of this apocalyptic information is mentioned on food packaging. It may be simply that it's hard to wonder about every ingredient on a list of thirty. Packaging and processing create a distance between the consumer and the environment.*

We trust that the manufacturer will have done a good job sourcing their chicken. That's the power of a brand. But if you think that spending more on a fancier brand will mean that more care is taken over the type of chicken in your UPF, then you'd be mistaken.

In spring 2022, *Salmonella* was detected at Cranswick's food-processing plant in Hull during a 'routine internal inspection'. Cranswick bills itself as a producer of 160 tonnes a day of gourmet cooked chicken for sandwiches and meals. *Salmonella* bills itself as a bacterial genus that causes diarrhoea, fever and stomach cramps and kills around fifty people each year in the UK.

Over 100 brands were recalled from the more budget end of the spectrum. But there were also recalls from higher-end places that charge more. The entire spectrum of UK food retail was represented by the recalls: Aldi, Tesco, Starbucks, Amazon, Waitrose, Sainsbury's, Jamie Oliver Deli by Shell, Co-op, M&S, Leon and Pret.

If you're a company making a chicken sandwich, you'd be nuts to spend more than the bare minimum on the chicken. Chicken is chicken. Almost no one thinks about the meat in their UPF, how it is treated or how it affects the planet.

Processing itself is very energy intensive. For UPF, there may be many stages of heating, grinding, chopping and recombining with transport between each one. There are arguments around whether mass-production batch cooking is efficient. It's true that a million people boiling one potato each at home on their hob is less efficient than a factory boiling a million at once. But it's not more efficient when the factory has ground them, dehydrated them, packaged

---

* This lack of connection may be reflected in how much we throw away. The UK is fairly typical, throwing away about 25 per cent of all food.[46]

them and then everyone adds boiling water at home anyway to rehydrate them.

Many UPF products contain ingredients from four or five continents. Your lasagne or ice cream may have palm oil from Asia, cocoa from Africa, soy from South America, wheat from the USA, flavouring from Europe and so on. Many of these ingredients will be shipped more than once – from a farm in South America to a processing plant in Europe, then to a secondary processing and packaging plant in another part of Europe, then to consumers, who might be back in South America right next to the farm.

Remember the soy barges being filled at Barcarena destined for Europe? It's almost certain that some of that soy ended up back in Muaná. That's hardly an argument for efficiency.

We could at least imagine a system arranged around agroecological farming and the consumption of a diverse range of fresh and minimally processed whole foods.[47] Such a system would promote biodiversity and has the capacity to produce enough healthy food for a growing population on a lower land footprint than today with massive climate benefits. We would need to eat significantly less meat, but the modelling is clear that it is possible.[48–53] With this new, organic farming system, fresh and minimally processed whole foods would be more abundant and possibly cheaper. But such a system wouldn't favour the monocultures required for UPF that do so much damage. By fixing the agricultural system so that it becomes sustainable, the production costs of whole foods should fall (without the requirement for fossil-fuel-based agrochemical inputs) – and those of UPF would rise. UPF requires the current destructive way of farming and is the only possible output of this system. With agroecological approaches, we could increase food quality and diversity while reducing all those external costs of ill health and climate change. It may be a fantasy to assume it would fix all problems, and it would almost certainly present new challenges, but they would be nothing compared with the consequences of not changing the food system.

Another existential threat to human life caused by UPF but not mentioned on the packaging is antibiotic resistance.

Suzi Shingler nearly single-handedly runs the Alliance to Save our Antibiotics, an NGO trying to make sure that when you get a urinary tract infection or a skin infection you don't die because it's impossible to treat with existing antibiotics. Treating even minor infections in UK hospitals (my day job) is increasingly difficult because there is so much resistance to antibiotics.*

This is because antibiotics have become a routine part of animal care, and the microbes in the animals' guts become resistant to them. We have been worrying about family doctors 'overprescribing', or giving antibiotics for viral infections (when they're needed only for bacterial infections) for a long time. But this accounts for a trivially small amount of antibiotic use. The place we use the most is on industrial farms, typically to compensate for chronic failings in animal welfare.

There is no 'biosecure' way of rearing animals that keeps the resistant bacteria from their faeces away from us. In the southern USA, intensive pork farms drain faecal waste into 'hog lagoons'. These are frequently aerosolised by tornadoes or overflow into water supply following storms. Flies† carry microbes in and out of farms, and the microbes are found on our meat.

The widespread use of antibiotics on farms means that we could return to an era in which there are no effective antibiotics. If your

---

* The genes that confer resistance to antibiotics are everywhere. You can find them in bacteria in deep caves isolated from the rest of the world for thousands, or even millions of years. The genes exist because microorganisms are in constant conflict with each other. Antibiotics are chemicals that microorganisms use to kill other microorganisms. In the arms race way of these things, both sides in the conflict have evolved defences, which give rise to antibiotic resistance.

† Scientists have looked at resistance genes on bacteria on the feet of flies leaving industrial chicken farms, at which there might be 250,000 birds on one site. The flies can freely move in and out of the buildings carrying resistant bugs. They bring all those resistant bacteria into our lungs, onto vegetable crops and into drinking water.

kid breaks their arm on a trampoline and needs a bone screw, that will become nearly impossible. You won't be able to have chemotherapy for the cancer caused by the UPF you've been eating because chemotherapy frequently needs antibiotics as it suppresses the immune system.[54–56] A simple urinary tract infection could spread to your kidneys and cause permanent damage. And this is already happening. Public Health England reported over 60,000 antibiotic-resistant severe infections in 2018.

As a result, in the UK and Europe we have brought in a number of policies limiting antibiotic use. This sounds good, but, although most UK supermarkets have good policies in place to limit antibiotic use, those policies typically only apply to own-brand, UK-sourced produce. So, if you buy a piece of chicken or beef in a UK supermarket, it will probably have had very limited exposure to medically important antibiotics. But when it comes to imported meat and processed meat in UPF, it's a different story with far more lax regulations. At the time of writing, only M&S and Iceland apply their antibiotic policies to all their suppliers. So, while customers demand – and to some extent get – one set of standards for whole food, UPF is again a very large exception.

The third external cost that I want to touch on is how UPF harms the environment through production and use of plastic. In 2020, Coca-Cola, PepsiCo and Nestlé were named the world's top plastic polluters for the third year in a row in Break Free From Plastic's annual audit, undertaken by 15,000 volunteers around the world.[57] Coca-Cola bottles were the most frequently found plastic discarded on beaches, rivers, parks and other litter sites in fifty-one of fifty-five nations surveyed. Last year it was the most frequently littered bottle in thirty-seven of fifty-one countries surveyed.[58, 59]

A 2020 report by Tearfund found that these three companies and Unilever continue to sell billions of products in single-use bottles, sachets and packets in developing countries, 'and they do this despite knowing that waste isn't properly managed in these contexts; their packaging therefore becomes pollution; and such pollution causes serious harm to the environment and people's health'.

Tearfund looked at a sample of six countries (China, India, the Philippines, Brazil, Mexico and Nigeria) and determined that Coke creates 200,000 tonnes of plastic waste – or about 8 billion bottles – which is burned or dumped each year in those countries alone – enough to cover thirty-three football pitches every day. Each year, globally, Coca-Cola produces 3 million tonnes of plastic waste, and we know that almost none of this is recycled.[60] A staggering 91 per cent of all the plastic waste ever produced has not been recycled and has either been burned, put into landfill or is simply in the environment.[61]

In statements, all the companies affirm their commitments to sustainability and the environment.

What's so odd is that, if you look at the corporate websites, you might believe that these companies are not food companies at all but rather charities committed to improving the environment. This is on the homepage, in July 2022, of Coca-Cola: 'Creating a world without waste: The interconnected global challenges of packaging waste and climate change have made this a focus for our business, and we are taking a hard look at the packaging we use and how we can drive change.'

PART FIVE

What the hell am I supposed to do then?

18

UPF is designed to be overconsumed

So, here we are. This is the science behind how UPF affects the human body:

- The destruction of the food matrix by physical, chemical and thermal processing means that UPF is, in general, soft. This means you eat it fast, which means you eat far more calories per minute and don't feel full until long after you've finished. It also potentially reduces facial bone size and bone density, leading to dental problems.
- UPF typically has a very high calorie density because it's dry, and high in fat and sugar and low in fibre, so you get more calories per mouthful.
- It displaces diverse whole foods from the diet, especially among low-income groups. And UPF itself is often micro-nutrient-deficient, which may also contribute to excess consumption.
- The mismatch between the taste signals from the mouth and the nutrition content in some UPF alters metabolism and appetite in ways that we are only beginning to understand, but that seem to drive excess consumption.
- UPF is addictive, meaning that for some people binges are unavoidable.
- The emulsifiers, preservatives, modified starches and other additives damage the microbiome, which could allow inflammatory bacteria to flourish and cause the gut to leak.
- The convenience, price and marketing of UPF urge us to eat constantly and without thought, which leads to more

snacking, less chewing, faster eating, increased consumption and tooth decay.

- The additives and physical processing mean that UPF affects our satiety system directly. Other additives may affect brain and endocrine function, and plastics from the packaging might affect fertility.
- The production methods used to make UPF require expensive subsidy and drive environmental destruction, carbon emissions and plastic pollution, which harm us all.

These scientific arguments are important, and they allow those with an interest in public health to make the case that UPF is a problem and needs consideration. But I worry that these arguments are unlikely to bring about real change, because the response from industry is to do yet more processing.

They do this already: if emulsifiers damage the microbiome, let's add some probiotics. If the food's too soft, add more gum. If it's too dense in energy, add artificial sweeteners. Their solution to ultra-processing is hyper-processing, also known as reformulation.

This is a very useful strategy for industry because it delays the discussion about warnings on UPF packets. But reformulation won't work for two reasons.

First, many of the ultra-processed products that are currently causing diet-related disease globally have already been reformulated. We've been reformulating UPF for over four decades. Forty years ago, the replacement of fat with sugar coincided with the sharpest increase in obesity. Twenty years ago, the rise of the anti-carb movement had no impact on rising rates of obesity. Artificial sweeteners are reformulation. All those gums to replace fat – that's reformulation.

Almost everything you eat has been reformulated, but the plans are still getting bigger. The Archer-Daniels-Midland Company (aka ADM; revenues around $85 billion) makes ingredients linked to microbiome damage (emulsifiers, stabilisers and modified starches) but they also make enzymes, prebiotics, probiotics, postbiotics as well as selling personalised microbiome services. ADM predict the market for supplements to improve the health of our microbiomes will reach $9.1 billion by 2026. Why would any company remove the emulsifiers when you could add a probiotic powder *and* an emulsifier?

But the main reason that I don't think we can reformulate UPF to make it better for us is that it is designed to be purchased and consumed in the largest possible quantities. And a food that is consumed less will never sell as well as a food that's consumed more.*

There are plenty of public health experts, paediatricians and nutritionists who think this, but we sit outside the industry. So, I went to hear from people inside the industry.

Many of the academic papers I'd been reading didn't talk about a food-supply chain, but rather a value-supply chain or a food-value chain. And I was starting to see that, while I experience food being supplied to me, there's also a stream of my own money flowing in the opposite direction. It flows through the ingredients companies and the processing corporations, just like those electrons flow through the proteins on the mitochondria. Each layer of processing is there to extract a little extra money from those low-quality often-subsidised crops.

For example, the human market for corn cobs is very small, but you can make more money by turning the corn into high-fructose corn syrup, the base ingredient for most of the flavoured-drink market and an additive to almost every product, from barbeque sauce to frozen apple pie. Corn flows one way along the processing chain, and money flows back the other way. These layers of processing increase the range of possible products that corn can become. They extend shelf life, modify flavour profiles and reformulate to appeal to a far wider range of consumers

---

* There are some who think that, because people with increased body-fat percentages eat more food, it's in the food companies' interests to make us gain weight. But I doubt that anyone in the companies is having that conversation. The focus is on next quarter, not the appetites of the future.

than the odd person eating a cob of corn at dinner. After ultra-processing, the corn can be eaten at any time of the day or night by athletes, children, pregnant people, busy commuters or people in need of a treat.

Milk has less added value than baby food, yoghurt and ice cream. People can only eat so many tomatoes, but turn it into ketchup, or pizza and pasta sauce, and the market is huge.

There's an illusion of food supply, but it's primarily a flow of money, driving ever-increasing complexity of processing.

I wanted to follow this flow of money and attempt to understand the incentives along the way. Were companies making food designed to be consumed to excess? And, importantly, could companies choose to change how they operate?

I started with the last person to receive any money when an item of UPF is sold: a farmer. Eddie Rixon was feeding his cows again when we spoke, on a cold, windy day with red kites wheeling overhead. Being a farmer like Eddie isn't a great way of making money, although he's still one of the lucky ones given that he owns his land. By the time the money gets to Eddie, there's not a lot left. Farmers receive, on average, 27 per cent of consumer expenditure on foods consumed at home and a far lower percentage of food consumed away from home.[1]

Producing beef isn't like making a branded product. If you have a brand, then people buy into it and you can charge much more. Eddie is making a commodity, such that his product is exchangeable for the next person's product. 'The price is determined by the market,' he said. 'If I ask for more money because my costs have gone up the supermarkets can just get beef somewhere else. There's no way to avoid being squeezed.'

Eddie has particular insight because he's worked at every stage in the food chain. Before being a farmer, he was a buyer for Waitrose and worked at Kellogg's as a young sales rep just as they were bringing a new snack to the market: the Nutri-Grain bar. He travelled around selling these new bars to supermarkets in the south of England, and got a bonus if he hit certain targets.

I looked up the ingredients on a Nutri-Grain bar as Eddie loaded sacks with mineral mix into the back of his Land Rover. They contain glucose syrup, glycerol, citric acid, invert sugar syrup, palm oil, dextrose, fructose, methylcellulose (a similar molecule to carboxymethylcellulose, which made rodent guts bleed in those microbiome studies) and soy lecithin. There's also some apple purée, fruit concentrate and flour.

Did Eddie think they were healthy? 'We were told that the bars were healthier compared to other breakfast choices at a convenience store, like a Mars bar for example. That's what we told the people at the supermarkets to persuade them to buy,' he said. 'What I believed is irrelevant.'

So, Eddie sold the bars to the supermarket. And the more bars the supermarket bought, the lower the price – they were incentivised to buy and thus sell more. Once the supermarket bought the bars, they were in the hole for that money, and they had to sell them hard to the customer. Eddie's boss, meanwhile, relied on teams of Eddies to sell as much as possible. Everyone within the simple Nutri-Grain value chain was incentivised by one thing – selling as many bars as they could. No one in the system, from the people who developed the bar, through to the people who sold it, could wonder about selling fewer bars. And would it even matter if they did? Kellogg's is in an arms race with other companies selling similar novel bars with similar health claims, all vying for that real estate in the shops that maximises sales. If Kellogg's decided to take a stand, the space would instantly be filled by another product from another company.

Paul Hart told me the same thing about his time at Unilever in the ice cream department. The project, understandably, was ice cream, not public health. The job of his team was to improve sensory and taste experience, and there was also a relentless pressure to drive down costs. Paul told me about life working alongside some of the major innovators in ice cream. Gary Binley was an expert on nozzles and aeration, constantly inventing new methods to extrude frozen foams in different shapes and layers. 'Ice cream isn't new or proprietary,' Paul explained. 'If you're going to stay competitive, the ice cream arms race requires constant evolution.'

Paul clearly idolised some of these scientists, and I could see why based on Binley's list of nozzle patents.[2] This was the team that produced some of the defining ice creams of my generation, including Viennetta and Twisters. 'A Twister is a particularly complex helical extrusion,' Paul said with admiration. 'And all the team thought about was the products.'* Genius takes many forms.

Paul told me about the tasting panels that they used to evolve their food. There were two types. First, there were expert panels. Paul was on an expert low-fat spread tasting panel for many years. He knew all the spreads and how they behaved. This panel was less about personal preference than objective description – using the human mouth as an assay device for all the different variables. 'You'd make up star diagrams with all the different variables for a product: granularity, saltiness, crunchiness, maltiness, burned notes, viscosity and so on,' he said. From there, the products would then go to consumer panels, where it was more about enjoyment and quantities consumed. All this information would then go back to the lab for the next evolution of the product.

Railing against 'evil' food companies starts to feel less sane when you're seeing things from the perspective of Eddie and Paul.

I followed the money further upriver to Robert Plowman, who works at Citigroup, an American multinational investment bank, where he's the head of consumer products in Europe, the Middle East and Africa. He helps companies fulfil their strategic ambitions by raising capital and buying and selling each other, and is 'particularly focused on the food and ingredients value chain'.

Once you start to understand ultra-processing as being about adding value, then you see that it's not just adding emulsifiers.

---

* According to Paul Hart, a flavour release scientist named Patrick Dunphy woke up one morning wondering if they could adapt margarine technology, whereby water is emulsified in fat, for a moisturising lipstick. 'He came up with LipSpa!' Paul told me. '£8 per pop! Moisturising your lips.'

Lawyers, consultants and bankers like Plowman also extract value from the money we pay for UPF. Plowman talks with such fluency that, in over an hour of discussion, there's not a single 'um'. He dresses like someone without an 'um' too.

I asked him to explain the food industry. 'There isn't really a well-defined food industry in the same way there's an aircraft manufacturing industry, with a small number of large players,' he said. 'The food industry is a vast and complicated ecosystem – with hundreds of thousands of food producers of all sizes. Some parts of the industry, like chocolate, are more consolidated but, in general, there are lots of different players all over the world.'

There are layers to the industry though. Farmers, which means large farming businesses as well as small-holding farmers, sell their crops and animals directly to food producers or – more often – to a primary processing industry. In this layer there are big agriculture companies that you've probably never heard of: the aforementioned ADM, Bunge Limited ($43 billion), Cargill Corporation ($114 billion) and Louis Dreyfus Company BV ($36 billion). These four companies (the ABCDs) from the USA and Europe handle most of the global trade in grain.

Other big players like Olam International ($50 billion) and Wilmar International Limited ($50 billion) are based in Asia. Some of these are specialists in 'verticals' like wheat, rice, vegetable oils, chocolate, sugar, coffee and meat, while others make food (modified starch, pet food, glucose syrup), trade, purchase and distribute commodities (like palm oil), raise their own livestock, and even have financial services arms. These are the companies that take those seventeen plants and animals and turn them into the pastes, powders and oils used as the base materials for UPF construction.

The next layer up is the universe of value-added ingredient companies, who make additives for texturing, flavourings and so on. They're producing many of the additive substances that go into UPF that enable on-pack claims such as 'low calorie', 'low fat' or 'low sugar' and help food to last longer, taste better and be easier to eat.

From Robert's perspective, what he calls the 'megatrends' that have been driving the food industry for several decades have been demands from consumers for food products that taste good, are convenient and are good value for money. 'On top of that, we want some products that are healthier and some that are indulgent,' he said. 'And, of course, increasingly consumers are concerned about ethical and sustainable sourcing. So the industry is very focused on meeting all of these needs.'

Companies in the next layer up buy materials from the primary processors and the ingredients companies and ultra-process them into UPF. These multinationals, mid-size companies and start-ups then finally sell to the retailers that you know.

Plowman was blunt about the incentives: 'Every company is trying to do the right thing, on the environment and sustainability, but they are also in business to make money. The financial markets and big investors value growth, margins, cashflow and dividends. CEOs of listed companies are judged by the results they deliver and the share price.'

Results like environmental and sustainability goals? 'Investors do increasingly judge companies on environmental, social and governance (ESG), and pay for directors is increasingly linked to ESG goals,' Plowman said. But the market is more focused on the financial results: 'things like sales growth, margin development, and earnings growth. And, by the way, that's no different to any other industry.'

This is, of course, true and it gives food companies two choices. They can premiumise and sell the same number of units for more money, or they can sell more units to more people more often. In the corporate arms race for money, every company is doing all these things simultaneously as fast as they can.

I asked Plowman about whether UPF is formulated to be bought and consumed as much as possible. 'All these companies constantly launch and improve products, and, of course, they hope they will sell more,' he responded. The requirement for corporate growth is met in different ways: population growth, entry into new markets, taking market share from others, 'and, yes, from existing consumers spending more. Many people in the food industry are incentivised by sales targets, as they are in most businesses.'

Plowman thinks that it's very hard for companies to tackle the public health issue on their own. 'It would be very difficult for one company to say: "We're going to take this on,"' he explained. 'No one company is that big. It would cost them too much and won't ultimately make a difference. The rules of the road have to be set by governments. And in the end, business is really good at reacting to that. Remember the sugar tax that was introduced in the UK in 2018 on the soft drinks industry – that has resulted in a massive reduction in sugar consumed in soft drinks.'

Everyone at every level of the food industry I spoke with agreed: regulation must come from outside. And this needn't harm the economy. Many pointed to the most regulated sectors like pharma and tobacco as being some of the most profitable.

Plowman sent me to speak with a management consultant who specialises in food. This person didn't want to be named because these are their personal opinions and they wanted to speak freely. They talked cheerfully in huge chunks of information, all perfectly organised and simple enough for me to grasp.

I asked them if food manufacturers might evolve products that generate excess consumption because they make more money – for example, if a company tries two formulations of a breakfast cereal and finds that people eat 5 per cent more of one of them during testing trials, is that the one that goes to market? 'Well ...' – the consultant hesitated, like a teacher who, having assured the class that there's 'no such thing as a stupid question', is then asked the stupidest question possible – '... if you are a company that sells breakfast cereal, then selling more breakfast cereal is good. Absolutely.'

Next, Plowman got me an audience with Ibrahim Najafi. He's the CEO of the UK's second largest ice cream company, Froneri, a joint venture between Nestlé and a French private equity house called PAI. I was getting close to the headwaters of the river of

money, a long way from the trickle that makes it to Eddie. Najafi
has a PhD in engineering and grew up in Iraq. You won't meet
anyone more passionate about their job. 'My job is to put smiles on
people's faces. We're so lucky: we make ice cream, we sell ice
cream, we eat ice cream, and we get paid for it. You know, we call
it a job.'

It did sound fun, but I wanted to understand his incentives. 'We
have owners,' he said, 'but the other shareholders – even though
they might not be a financial shareholder – are our consumers,
because they really vote with their pockets. They've got to be
happy.' This requirement to satisfy the consumer was underlined
by everyone within the industry. While the public health perspective
is that industry are forcing products on people, within the industry
it feels much more like they are catering to demand.

Najafi told me about his childhood in Iraq, his mum making ice
cream at home: 'She'd use eggs, sugar, real cream, real vanilla.
We're doing the same, but at a larger scale.' This claim is at the core
of the definition of UPF, which would clearly separate Najafi's
mum's ice cream from almost all commercially available ice
cream. I asked him about the products with the greatest number of
additives including emulsifiers, stabilisers and flavouring. Not
unreasonably, Najafi points out that Froneri do make a variety of
products: 'Look at our Kelly's ice cream, and compare it to one
you'd make at home; they're very similar.' I looked up the Kelly's
ingredients. The list started with 'Cornish whole milk, clotted cream,
sugar', but also included emulsifiers and stabilisers. 'We use these
because handling eggs is difficult and expensive and it's really important to hit the right price point.' A recent salmonella scare in the UK
underlined this point.

We discussed the proliferation of UPF. I realise that in a sense ice
cream is something where the public do arguably have a fairly
accurate view of its effects. Najafi was remarkably comfortable
with my thoughts on regulation and labelling, and had progressive
views on public health education, especially for those with low
incomes, and migrant populations. 'We need education, starting at

a younger age, and the government has to take responsibility for that.'

I was very persuaded that Najafi has a sincere concern for his customers and the quality of his products. But is the purpose of Kelly's ice cream fundamentally different to that of his mother's? This is hard to test. They are both sugary treats designed to bring joy. But it seems to me that there is an additional financial purpose, perhaps an obligation, for Kelly's ice cream. Najafi's mum could choose to limit the supply, but, when it comes to selling less, Najafi himself may be as stuck as Eddie Rixon was when he worked for Kellogg's. If he wanted to put the brakes on, Najafi is answerable to his board, which in turn is answerable to the shareholders.

This is the same problem that faces any company that wants to sell less UPF: they are answerable to their owners. Most of the major food corporations are publicly owned – anyone can buy a piece. And this means that a significant chunk of each company is owned by a few very large funds like BlackRock, Vanguard or Fidelity. Between them, these companies have more than $20 trillion under management. I called a senior investor at a big asset manager about transnational food companies. 'These companies are not really in control of their business model,' they told me, and used Danone as an example.

Institutional investors own a significant percentage of Danone. 'If someone at Danone proposes that they should sell less food for environmental or public health reasons,' the investor said, 'they won't get very far compared to the person who figures out a way of selling more food, which in broad terms equates to more money.' They explained that there were ways to sell less food for more money, but at major corporations all those options have been explored. Prices are as high as the market will bear and production efficiency is maxed out. 'You have to sell enormous volumes to huge numbers of people,' they continued. 'That's why low- and middle-income countries are so important because in the USA and the UK, we are pretty much saturated.'

This may seem obvious to many people, but it wasn't to Emmanuel Faber, the former CEO of Danone. Faber was a poster CEO for ESG (i.e. environmental, social and governance) objectives. He was praised by former Bank of England governor Mark Carney during his BBC Reith lecture about companies creating non-monetary value. Faber led a revolution within Danone, making it the first company to legally dump the primacy of shareholders in place of other objectives around protecting the environment, their employees and suppliers. Faber declared that he had 'toppled the statue of Milton Friedman', the late Nobel economist who in 1970 wrote a seminal essay titled 'The social responsibility of business is to increase its profits'.[3] The board of directors disagreed with what Faber was up to, though. A public campaign was launched by Bluebell Capital and Faber lost his job in March 2021.

Other efforts at activist investing that were met with wide public enthusiasm have stalled when it became clear that it would cost the actual investor money. BlackRock has been outspoken about sustainable investing, but has subsequently stepped back from requiring firms to disclose climate proposals.[4, 5] The reason was simple – BlackRock's clients include public and private pension plans, governments, insurance companies, endowments, universities, charities and, in the end, you and me, whether we're individual investors or we have some of our work pension in their funds. BlackRock have a duty to deliver on long-term durable financial performance. Looked at one way, we all demand the growth from food companies that requires they cut down the Amazon – at least those of us with pensions do, because pension funds are predicated on the idea of growth. There are proposals to divest from food companies, but this is unlikely to work. Divestment doesn't usually meaningfully affect share price,[6] because there is always someone willing to buy a share that will pay a dividend. Cutting off the supply of income is the only real way to change corporate behaviour.

I asked the cheerful management consultant about this. 'Over 250 years, the achievement in terms of providing sufficient food is incredible and that has been driven by the profit motive,' he said. 'So, it can create fantastic things.' But he thinks all those external costs are a problem: 'The incentives in the system are straightforwardly to produce and sell more. It's government that should step up to set rules that deliver proper regulation of markets that don't right themselves. Self-regulation is unlikely to have much impact. Businesses are fundamentally commercial organisations. The incentives are to think very hard about the next six and twelve months.'

That means reducing demand for UPF, and that means policies like reducing the promotions of processed and junk food: 'Promotions drive excess consumption, so if your goal is reducing obesity, in my view it's a no brainer to be moving on that stuff.'

Days after we spoke, the UK government rowed back on regulating the promotions that the management consultant was talking about: buy-one-get-one-free deals on products high in fat, salt and sugar.

Everyone I spoke with in the food industry felt trapped between competing forces much more powerful than they were individually. Consumers might say they want healthy stuff, but they still buy UPF. Supermarkets – and, of course, shareholders – dictate what to sell.

The idea that companies exist to make money and only to make money seems so obvious to some people that it doesn't need saying. But there is genuine confusion about it within companies, and from people like Mark Carney, who clearly felt that Danone could make a different set of choices.

In a speech he gave, Ahmet Bozer, former president of the Coca-Cola Corporation, was clear about the purpose of his company. He talked about how to create yet more growth for a brand that would seem to have conquered the world: 'Because of the fact that half of the world's population have not had a Coke in the last 30 days and the fact that there are 600 million teenagers who have not had a Coke in the last week, we believe a sparkling opportunity is there.'

I love the cheery bluntness of this quote. Until everyone is drinking at least one Coke per day, there will be an opportunity for growth – and even then it would turn out that one Coke wasn't enough. Any moral critique of Bozer or Coca-Cola misunderstands the obligations of the company: this is what they must do until they are required by law to do something different.

Realistic solutions will come only from the understanding that no matter what any company says, it has a single purpose – a purpose that will trump all others. All the major companies that make your food have very significant parts of their websites devoted to their social and environmental projects – which are real. They're great for reputation. But none of these projects can get in the way of creating value for shareholders.

This singular purpose makes sense of a lot of the contradictory things that companies do, selling solutions to the problems they cause. For example, in 2006 Nestlé entered the weight management market (or rather the *other* side of the weight management market) by buying weight-loss brand Jenny Craig.[7] * Peter Brabeck-Letmathe, then chairman and CEO of Nestlé, said it was an important step in Nestlé's transformation into 'a nutrition, health and wellness company that sees weight management as a key competence'.†

* Jenny Craig claimed on its website that 'new research published in the scientific journal *Nature* shows that individuals following our most effective plan ever that includes our revolutionary Recharge Bar, can experience amazing weight loss results and lower blood sugar levels.'[8] The research wasn't published in *Nature* – it was published in the *International Journal of Obesity*, which also published some of the Coca-Cola funded findings I mentioned earlier. It is embarrassingly a *Nature* group journal but it's like calling your Skoda a Bentley because they're owned by the same parent company.

† Jenny Craig was sold for an undisclosed sum in 2013, as part of a larger drive to divest underperforming brands.[9]

As part of this, Nestlé produces a range of UPF called Lean Cuisine. Here's the ingredients list for the Lean Cuisine Grilled Chicken and Vegetables: 'cooked rigatoni pasta (water, durum wheat semolina, wheat gluten), water, cooked seasoned chicken (white meat chicken, water, soy protein isolate, modified corn and tapioca starches, corn maltodextrin, salt, sodium phosphate, seasoning), tomatoes in juice (contain citric acid [acidulant], calcium chloride), yellow zucchini, broccoli, carrots, parmesan and romano cheeses (from milk), modified corn starch, onions, cider vinegar, tomato paste, salt, sugar, garlic purée, soy oil, olive oil, brown sugar, yeast extract, basil, oregano, potassium chloride, flavour, spices.'

Personally, I think it's a stretch to believe that a company that profits from cycles of weight gain and weight loss could make a product that got rid of the problem.

As well as weight-loss solutions, Nestlé have been developing an interest in drugs to treat diet-related disease. Nutrition Science Partners Limited is a 50/50 joint venture formed between Nestlé Health Science and the pharmaceutical and healthcare group Chi-Med. Nutrition Science Partners focuses on gastrointestinal health, and may in the future expand into the metabolic disease and brain health areas.[10] In 2011, Nestlé also bought Prometheus Laboratories, which specialises in diagnostics and licensed speciality pharmaceuticals in gastroenterology. Prometheus Laboratories may already be helping to diagnose and treat some of the health problems caused by the food system of which they are a part.

At the time of writing, Nestlé is apparently considering buying Haleon, the consumer health division of the pharmaceutical giant GSK,[11] whose website says: 'Our digestive health products bring reassuring comfort to millions of people worldwide. We have a portfolio of trusted, market leading brands, including Eno and Tums with a strong heritage in treating heartburn, acid indigestion and gastric discomfort.'

Danone, meanwhile, have hundreds of subsidiaries, including at least two which seem to be pharmaceutical companies.[12] *

It's not hard to imagine that within companies it feels like these projects – asthma inhalers, community farming and so on – are doing good, even while other parts of the same entity may be contributing to disease and environmental destruction. Perhaps Nestlé thought it was doing good when it went up the Amazon. In a *New York Times* piece from 2017, Sean Westcott, then head of food research and development at Nestlé, is quoted as saying obesity was an unexpected side effect of making cheap food widely available: 'We didn't expect what the impact would be.'

It is surprising though, that a company that styles itself as an organisation with deep nutritional expertise couldn't anticipate that, for example, floating a boat full of UPF to remote communities without a public health infrastructure might result in obesity or tooth decay.

There are whole sections of Nestlé devoted to selling products in the poorest places on earth. For example, there is a division called Nestlé Central and West Africa Region, which sells products in Angola, Benin, Burkina Faso, Cameroon, Cabo Verde, Central African Republic, Chad, Congo, Côte d'Ivoire, Democratic Republic of the Congo, Equatorial Guinea, Gabon, Gambia, Ghana, Guinea Bissau, Guinea, Liberia, Mali, Mauritania, Niger, Nigeria, São Tomé and Príncipe, Senegal, Sierra Leone and Togo.

All the major food companies sell products in these regions and are expanding growth. It is a source of constant amazement to public health doctors that you can buy a cold Coke almost anywhere on earth but keeping a vaccine cool enough to get it from a factory to a child is a huge problem.

---

* My personal favourite example of a company causing a problem to which they also sell a solution is Philip Morris, the largest tobacco company in the world. In July 2021, Philip Morris agreed to buy Vectura Group for £1.1 billion[13] – a company that, at the time, made most of its £200m revenue from a portfolio of products to treat smoking-related diseases.

The companies that make our food don't have a choice about the food they make and the way they make it. Many of us don't have a choice about whether we buy it. But there are two groups who can make slightly different choices to create a better situation: governments and the medical profession – including doctors, nurses, public health scientists, nutritionists and everyone else who has signed up to have a single purpose: to care for people.

In these people, we find some solutions in the next chapter.

19.

What we could ask governments to do

Carlos Monteiro told me a story about his time at medical school in the mid-1970s. His wife was also a medical student, and they went together to classes on infant feeding. She was pregnant with their first daughter, so the information perhaps seemed more memorable to them than it did to me when I had similar classes twenty years later. Monteiro even remembered the name of the lecturer. 'He was called Oswaldo Ballarin.'

As well as Carlos's wife, there were several other students and young doctors in the department who were pregnant, and every month they were all sent a package of supplies: diapers and formula milk. When his daughter was born, they breastfed her briefly but then switched to the formula they'd been given. Monteiro told me this was normal: 'Even in the remote valleys where I was studying malnutrition the women would register for formula from feeding centres.'

A few years later he went to New York to study. He met a British couple Derrick and Patrice Jelliffe, paediatricians who were studying infant malnutrition. In a series of papers, they had meticulously documented aggressive marketing practices by the infant formula industry in low-income settings, with a particular focus on Nestlé. Sales representatives with no certification or training were dressed up as 'mothercraft nurses'. They advised impressionable new mothers about the benefits of formula and promoted it in such a way that has since been linked to thousands of avoidable deaths.[1]

Nestlé and some other formula companies were causing a quadruple jeopardy.

First, even formula made with clean water is associated with an increased risk of fatal infection,[2-5] probably because of effects on the infant microbiome. Second, Nestlé was marketing the formula in communities where the possibility of producing an uncontaminated feed was almost zero.[6] In these low-income settings, parents would typically have only one bottle and no way of cleaning it, would have to use river or well water contaminated with sewage and had low literacy rates, which meant they had great difficulty in making up the feeds correctly.

Third, while initial samples were given at low price, or even for free, once the mother had stopped lactating the price went up, creating poverty further and endangering the child and its siblings. In east Africa, for example, to feed an infant properly would take more than a third of a labourer's salary.

Finally, it seemed that to save money mothers diluted the formula so the infants, often already suffering with diarrhoeal disease, were then undernourished: 'Under these circumstances, almost homeopathic quantities of milk are administered with large quantities of bacteria, the result is starvation and diarrhoea, too often leading to death.'[7, 8]

The Jelliffes catalogued instances of formula companies marketing breastfeeding as being 'backwards and insufficient', and in 1972 coined the phrase 'commerciogenic malnutrition' – malnutrition caused by companies.[9] Modern obesity is also a commerciogenic disease.

Reports in the press followed. The cover of the August issue of *New Internationalist* magazine in 1973 showed a photograph of the grave of a Zambian baby. A feeding bottle and an empty tin of milk powder have been placed on the grave by the mother.[10, 11]

By 1977, Nestlé, the largest manufacturer, was the target of a global boycott by NGOs. This inspired Senator Ted Kennedy, chair of the Senate subcommittee on health, to demand that representatives of the major formula milk companies testify in front of congress.

Monteiro followed these hearings with the Jelliffes. One of the first to testify was the chairman of Nestlé's operations in Brazil, Dr

Oswaldo Ballarin. The same doctor who had taught Monteiro and his wife. 'The packages of formula we received were from Nestlé,' Monteiro said. 'They had the names and details of all the student doctors and residents through Ballarin.'

The hearings were disastrous for Nestlé. Ballarin argued that while it would be a poor decision to market products in regions with low literacy levels and without reliable access to sanitary water, it was beyond Nestlé's responsibility to cope with these issues or the deaths that ensued. Of the boycott, he said it was an attack on the free world's economic system. Kennedy pointed out that Ballarin had misunderstood what a free market means. A boycott is of course an important and recognised tool of any free-market system.

The scandal led to a policy document known as The Code. It was written by activists and the World Health Assembly, and it laid out guidelines about the marketing of infant formula.

It was a clever approach. Policies like taxing or banning formula would have been very harmful. Infant formula is UPF, but it is unique among UPFs in the sense that it is an essential food (although some other types of UPF can become essential in contexts where they are the only affordable and available source of calories). People have a right to use it, and should have the freedom to use it. This means that formula must be cheap, high quality and widely available. People also have a right to accurate information about the benefits and harms of different ways of feeding a child, which includes a right not to be exposed to misleading claims.

Nestlé rehabilitated their reputation to the extent that George Clooney felt he could risk his by advertising Nespresso. But dangerous marketing of the type that the Jelliffes described in the early 1970s is still going on.

The marketing budget of the formula industry is almost incomprehensibly large at around $3–5 billion dollars per year – comparable to the entire annual operating budget of the World Health Organization. This spend by industry means that the market for infant formula and follow-on milk is growing eight times faster than the global population. In 1998 the market was worth less than

$15 billion. It is now worth well over $55 billion.[12] The result is that more than 60 per cent of infants under six months old in low-income settings are formula-fed.[13] This has catastrophic effects on the rates of pneumonia and diarrhoea – the two biggest infectious killers of children worldwide.

A report in *The Lancet* estimated that more than 800,000 child deaths could be prevented in low-income and middle-income countries if breastfeeding were nearly universal.[14] That's around 15 per cent of all infant deaths in these countries. In China, India, Indonesia, Mexico and Nigeria, use of formula has been associated with more than 236,000 child deaths a year.[15, 16] Limiting the marketing of formula would be the single most effective intervention for the prevention of deaths in children under five years of age.[17]

One of the most concerning statistics is that the market isn't just increasing because more children are being formula-fed. This increase in sales is because each child is drinking more. In 2008, a child drank on average 5.5kg per year, but now they are drinking almost 8kg, an increase of more than 40 per cent.[18] This is due either to marketing or to new ingredients which make formula hyper-palatable.

A team at Cambridge found that many parents were feeding their babies much more formula than needed. Milk, of course, solves all problems – crying, teething, and so on – and so the babies were consuming hundreds of calories more per day than recommended by the World Health Organization. These babies were being taken to the GP due to symptoms such as crying, fussing and vomiting, and then being diagnosed with allergy or reflux before being prescribed expensive specialist formulas. But, when parents reduced the amount of formula they were offering to recommended levels, these symptoms resolved for many babies.[19–22]

No one throws away powdered formula, so having a very palatable one that is consumed quickly is big business. The result is that formula-fed babies gain weight much more quickly than breastfed babies. I know as a parent how satisfying this can feel, but it's not healthy.

There is other more subtle marketing. Bob Boyle is a paediatric allergy consultant at Imperial College London. He studies allergies in children and has a side-line in investigating claims made on packets. According to the UK Food Standards Agency,[23] The Japanese Society of Allergology,[24] the Australasian Guideline,[25] and The American Academy of Paediatrics,[26] there is no evidence that specialist formulas prevent allergy, and yet Danone Nutricia used one of Boyle's studies to claim that their prebiotic supplemented formula was 'clinically proven' to reduce eczema by over 50 per cent in babies with a family history of allergy, despite the fact his study found the opposite.

These claims are harmful because they encourage the use of expensive formulas in those who don't need them.

I did an investigation of the formula industry in 2018,[27] which exposed the marketing of a diagnosis of cow's milk allergy even in infants who were exclusively breastfed. The symptoms to diagnose the allergy were so broad that it was essentially impossible to avoid diagnosing every child (rash, irritability, diarrhoea, colic and so on), and mothers who were breastfeeding were encouraged to exclude dairy. This adds a barrier to an already difficult task and makes it harder for women who want to breastfeed to do so.

The study also revealed the extent to which the medical profession had been captured by industry. The formula industry fund the basic research, they fund the authors of national feeding guidelines, they fund the professional associations (until recently including the Royal College of Paediatrics and Child Health) and they fund the charities and websites that provide information to patients. When I interviewed the then president of the Royal College of Paediatrics and Child Health, she was about to take a position on Nestlé's scientific board.

This is a huge problem. If a family decides freely and with the best information to use formula, then it's a good choice in a country like the UK. But in the UK the influence of industry over every aspect of infant feeding means that for women who want to breastfeed, there are barriers and a lack of support. For several generations, the UK has had some of the lowest breastfeeding rates in the world. Amy Brown is a professor of public health in Swansea. She explained that if none of a woman's sisters or mother or doctors or midwives or community nurses breastfed themselves, this creates an environment where it's really hard – doubly so when all the education they have has been sponsored by the formula industry.

But how a baby is fed has wider implications than health outcomes. Brown explained that breastfeeding can be important to women for many reasons that are not fixed by giving a bottle, such as protecting their own health, religion or preferred way of caring for their baby. 'When they cannot, this may increase risk of postnatal depression, which is much lower in women who do manage to breastfeed.' Women who stop breastfeeding before they want to have far higher rates of postnatal depression than women who feed their children in the way they want to, and when speaking with Brown they use the language of trauma and bereavement.[28]

The current environment in the UK is stigmatising for all mothers and the marketing harms everyone, especially those trying mixed or formula feeding who may feel that they need to spend money on more expensive products with no efficacy for the problems they claim to solve.

You may have noticed that this has not been a book celebrating the wonders of real food, and similarly this is not a chapter about the benefits of one way of feeding a child.* I am a formula baby, like

---

* Here's a footnote about the best independent evidence around feeding, but if you're out of that (frequently rather grim) stage of childrearing then just skip it. There are a lot of high-quality independent studies comparing never, partially and exclusively breastfed infants. Formula in every country is associated with significantly increased risks of all-cause mortality, diarrhoea and pneumonia mortality,[29] obesity and type 2 diabetes,[30] otitis media,[31] malocclusion,[32] asthma[33] and sudden infant death syndrome.[34] Non-breastfed children also demonstrate significantly lower IQ scores even after accounting for maternal IQ.[35] Formula feeding affects maternal health primarily due to foregone protective effects of breastfeeding against ovarian cancer, breast cancer and type 2 diabetes.[36]

most babies born in London in 1978. My mother made the right choice for our family. She had twins and a career, so went back to work quickly and created the financial security that has enabled so much freedom in my own life. So, I don't care how caregivers feed their children other than that they are fed safely. Many Olympic gold medallists and Nobel Laureates are formula babies.

But the discussions that followed the deaths of children around the world in the 1960s and 1970s due to those marketing techniques provide a template for how to think about policies around UPF in general. Infant formula is the most challenging UPF to consider and so a good place to start.

There are two main policy ideas that come out of the story of formula marketing that inform how we should consider the regulation of NOVA class 4 foods.

First, the people who make policy and inform policy should not take money directly or indirectly from the food industry. Second, the best way to increase rights and freedoms is to restrict marketing.

Let's look first at the role of industry in policy making. It's clear that when it comes to influencing infant-feeding policy the infant formula industry has a conflict of interest. There are some overlapping interests (such as making a good product that's safe), but the companies' purpose is to make money from formula, and that is in conflict with the needs of infants around the globe, whether they are breastfed or formula-fed.

Removing this influence is the most important step. It's very easy to come up with a laundry list of policy initiatives that will promote health, but it can't be done in collaboration with industry.

Policymakers, and that includes doctors and scientists, need to see themselves as regulators.

Obesity and all diet-related diseases are commerciogenic – just like the illnesses caused by inappropriate marketing of infant formula around the world. This means those who seek to limit the harms of these companies must have an adversarial relationship with them.

It doesn't mean that the food industry is inherently immoral or that policymakers shouldn't talk to industry. But I think it does mean that no one should take money. This is a long way from being the case in the USA and the UK at the moment.

In the UK, the UPF industry is deeply involved with food policy. This is why none of those 600 policy proposals I mentioned in the introduction have worked.

Helen Crawley underlined this to me. She is a modest but hugely influential figure in nutrition policy who has spent almost forty years encouraging better food standards for vulnerable groups across the UK and fighting conflicts of interest. The charity she set up, First Steps Nutrition Trust, has been encouraging the avoidance of UPF in the diets of pregnant women, infants and young children for many years. 'You may think of policy as being written by politicians,' Crawley explained, 'but the specifics are frequently hammered out by special interest groups – specifically charities and NGOs and professional groups representing health professionals.'

A range of these organisations have the ear of the government, including the British Nutrition Foundation. The British Nutrition Foundation is a 'public-facing charity which exists to give people, educators and organisations access to reliable information on nutrition'. It describes itself as a 'sounding board for policy development'[37] and has held contracts with numerous government departments, focusing on nutrition policy, communications and school food education. Members of it sit on government advisory groups. The British Nutrition Foundation is funded by almost every food company you can think of, including Coca-Cola, Nestlé, Mondelēz, PepsiCo, Mars, Danone, Kerry and Cargill.[38]

A similar situation exists in the USA, where the Academy of Nutrition and Dietetics, which trains dietitians and helps to shape national food policy, was found to have extensive relationships with the food industry. A report in the peer-reviewed journal *Public Health Nutrition* showed that the organisation accepted more than $4 million from food companies and industry associations, including Coca-Cola, PepsiCo, Nestlé, Hershey, Kellogg's and Conagra.[39]

And this was just between 2011 and 2017. In addition, they had significant equity in UPF companies including more than a million dollars of stocks in PepsiCo, Nestlé and J.M. Smucker.[40]

Meanwhile, back across the Atlantic, Diabetes UK lists Boots, Tesco and Abbott as corporate partners.[41] Cancer Research UK is funded by Compass, Roadchef, Slimming World, Tesco and Warburtons.[42] The British Heart Foundation takes money from Tesco.[43] The British Dietetic Association has Abbott, Danone and Quorn as its current strategic partners, with other food companies as supporters.[44]

The Centre for Social Justice wrote a report about obesity policy that talked about physical activity and sport being 'fundamentally important to tackling our obesity crisis' and said that 'the food and drinks industry must work with the government and civil society to end childhood obesity'. It wasn't exactly all wrong, it was just cosy and collaborative – unsurprising perhaps, given that the report was sponsored by Danone and ASDA. One of the authors confided that the sponsors had requested that wording around promotions be diluted.

It is so, *so* normal to work with and take funding from industry, that many of these groups may not be fully aware of how working with companies that make and sell UPF allows for 'healthwashing' of the brand. It's a great opportunity for the company to get publicity for weak promises and delaying tactics as they fight for 'voluntary' measures to challenge what they do. Organisations that take money from, for example, Coca-Cola, and claim to be fighting obesity are simply extensions of the marketing division of Coca-Cola.

In the UK the lines between food activism and the UPF industry are also very blurred.

Jamie Oliver has been one of the UK's leading food activists for nearly twenty years, campaigning for higher-quality school meals, better food education, and more recently to end buy-one-get-one-free promotions on junk food.

He campaigns for halving the number of children who are obese by 2030, and currently is part of a consortium of funders putting money into a charity called Bite Back 2030, which aims to empower young people to challenge inappropriate food marketing and to engage with UK obesity policy.

I've met Jamie Oliver and worked with many of the people at Bite Back 2030. I have no doubt that their intention is to improve child health, and many who have met and worked with Oliver will attest to his commitment to child health.* But I was concerned by what I saw at a Bite Back 2030 youth summit meeting in October 2021.

Oliver was there with a panel of passionate youth activists, many of whom I've got to know and respect. Alongside the youth activists were the managing director of KFC UK at the time, Paula MacKenzie, Alessandra Bellini, chief customer officer at Tesco, the CEO of Deliveroo and many more highfliers from the food industry.

The conversation during the summit was a mix of enthusiastic but vague commitments, with a sense of equality of purpose of all those there. The young people said some powerful stuff, but it felt to me like industry got more out of the event. There was no understanding that the interests of, for example, KFC and those of obesity campaigners are not, and cannot be, aligned. KFC made a persuasive case that it cares, and I am sure it does, but the company is required by its owners to sell lots of UPF. It cannot be a partner in the fight against obesity.

Bite Back 2030 has also launched something called a 'food systems accelerator', which has partnered with KFC, Tesco, Costa Coffee, Danone, Deliveroo, Innocent, Jamie Oliver Group and Compass Group/Chartwells UK. Young campaigners will be paired with each business to help the senior executives to better understand what consumers actually want from their products.

---

* Like Dr Helen Crawley, for example, who worked with Oliver for years and emphasised Oliver's good intentions to me.

James Toop, chief executive of Bite Back 2030, said: 'Every child has the right to access affordable and nutritious food, so I am pleased that these eight organisations are stepping up and committing to leading the change. Collectively, they represent the shopping and eating habits of the nation, so it's incredibly exciting that Bite Back's tenacious young campaigners will be working with them collaboratively to shape future food systems.'

This is a very enthusiastic endorsement of some companies that I would say will not be able to do anything significant for the reasons that Robert Plowman and Eddie Rixon explained.

The youth summit itself was hosted by Tortoise Media, which works closely with corporate partners such as McDonald's and Unilever and has just launched a 'Better Food Index'. It uses data from a range of sources to determine 106 different indicators of how well companies 'walk the walk and talk the talk' in areas like environment, affordability, nutrition and financial sustainability. Tortoise says that the Better Food Index aims to 'hold power to account' and 'shine a light on some of the best and worst practices within the food industry'.

Rather surprisingly to many of us in the infant feeding world, Nestlé ranks first in this index. Unilever is third (and was once first) in the Tortoise 'Responsibility 100 index' which looks at companies that perform best in key sustainability, social and ethical metrics.

It's really hard to square these rankings with some of the allegations against the companies in terms of health and the environment. For example, a 2019 Greenpeace report alleged that out of the thirty producer groups most linked to Indonesian fires, Nestlé has bought from twenty-eight of them and Unilever from at least twenty-seven.[45] For other examples, see the previous eighteen chapters.

Oliver himself is very much a part of the food industry. His company makes UPF (albeit fairly marginal items but UPF nonetheless due to the presence of flavouring) and makes money from UPF producers and retailers, Tesco and Shell, where his deli-range meal deals include drinks like Cherry Coke, Dr Pepper and Fanta and snacks like Walker's Max Kentucky Fried Chicken flavour crisps.

This clear sense that industry can be a partner in reducing childhood obesity and that industry can help to fund the activism without that activism becoming compromised doesn't seem to be challenged anywhere.

No one thinks that Philip Morris should fund the doctors who generate the research around whether smoking harms you. No one thinks that tobacco legislation should be written by charities funded by British American Tobacco. Why should food policy around health be any different?

Removing industry from the table will require a cultural shift before any shift in legislation. It will gradually become shameful for activists to work with the UPF industry as the understanding spreads that the companies are as responsible for diet-related disease as the tobacco industry is for smoking-related disease. Of course, you can't design national food policy without speaking to industry. But you can make sure that none of the people who write and develop the policy take money from the industry they seek to regulate. The relationship cannot be one of partnership.

Aside from getting industry out of the room, there are a few specific policies that are worth considering.

Chile has some of the highest obesity rates in the world, with three-quarters of adults living with overweight or obesity. Officials have been particularly alarmed by childhood obesity rates that are among the world's highest, with over half of six-year-old children overweight or obese.

In 2016, Chile implemented a set of policies that put marketing restrictions and mandatory black octagonal labels on foods and drinks high in energy, sugar, sodium and saturated fat. These foods were also banned in schools and heavily taxed.[46]

These policies banned treats from Kinder Surprise eggs and removed cartoon animals, including Tony the Tiger and Cheetos' Chester Cheetah, from packaging. PepsiCo, the maker of Cheetos, and Kellogg's, producer of Frosted Flakes (known in the UK as

Frosties), have gone to court, arguing that the regulations infringe on their intellectual property, but at the time of writing Tony and Chester are not on the packs.*

It was a masterclass in the technical side of policy making, developed in consultation with the public and then tested and trialled. All the participants in lay group meetings wanted clear labelling.

The labelling has had a huge impact, with decreases in food purchases and, perhaps most significantly, research showing that the regulation made children ask their parents not to buy the products.[48]

This chimes with my own experience of kids – they're smart. Sure, they're vulnerable to marketing, but they're not entirely motivated by the moment. They care about their own health and the health of their parents.

Whether these policies will shift the dial on obesity, or even stand up to continued industry pressure, isn't yet clear, but they do offer a template for approaching the problem. When people are able to make good choices, they do.

When it comes to specifics, personally I don't think the aim of policy should be for people to eat less UPF. That's not the business of politicians. I don't want to be told what to do any more than Xand did.

I sincerely don't have a moral opinion about eating UPF. None of my friends believe this, but it's true. I don't care how you feed yourself or your child. The goal should be that you live in a world where you have real choices and the freedom to make them.

The NOVA classification system is not the perfect way to consider the food that causes diet-related disease and environmental destruction because there is no perfect classification. In my experience, it captures all the specific foods that so many of us struggle to stop eating while, at least for those with resources, expanding the horizon of possible meals.

---

* After the banning of Kinder Surprise, a company executive from Ferrero claimed that the toy was not a promotional gadget but an 'intrinsic part of the treat', while the Italian ambassador to Chile accused a public health minister of waging 'food terrorism'.[47]

Having decided to try an 80 per cent UPF diet to see if it would put him off UPF, this happened to Xand.

***

Xand called from Costa Coffee on the first day of his diet. He was buying a sausage roll. A fancy one: 'I want to know if I can eat it. Is calcium carbonate UPF?'

I now get calls like this the whole time from friends. It's unsurprising really. Lots of modern British high street snack foods have 'clean labels' – like those lasagnes I'd asked Maria Laura da Costa Louzada about. And I told Xand that, no, the calcium carbonate did not make his sausage roll UPF. It doesn't count as a 'funky' ingredient because it's added by law to most white wheat flour. It's chalk.

But he read out the rest of the ingredients anyway: 'pork, wheatflour (inc calcium carbonate, iron, niacin, thiamin), unsalted butter, onions, potatoes, pasteurised egg, salt, white wine vinegar, rapeseed oil, ground spices (black pepper, white pepper, nutmeg), coriander, parsley, sage, dried thyme, yeast, cracked black pepper. It's fine, no?'

I could hear the people behind him getting irritated as he asked me about the pasteurised egg: 'I don't have *that* in my kitchen.' To be fair to Xand, I find myself having these same debates internally all the time. The NOVA classification has forced me to consider the *purpose* of the food the whole time. Was this created in an environment that is indifferent to my health? Is it sitting within a food system that causes climate change and obesity? Did he know the sausage roll's design process? Was this produced using a system that would favour foods that are eaten in greater quantities? Was it soft? Calorie-dense?

I started telling him about softness and calorie density, and he read out the calories. It contained 294 calories per 100g – a little more than a Big Mac, roughly the same as McDonalds fries. Is it soft? There was no measurement on the pack, but he felt that it was.

I would guess that the M&S Best Ever Sausage Roll (sold at Costa) will be a food that subverts the internal system that regulates energy intake. In my opinion, it might do it a bit less than some other sausage rolls with more ingredients. Greggs describes its sausage rolls as 'the nation's favourite': 'This British classic is made from seasoned sausage meat wrapped in layers of crisp, golden puff pastry, as well as a large dollop of TLC. And that's it. No clever twist. No secret ingredient.'

There are around forty ingredients in the Greggs sausage rolls sold in Iceland, including mono- and diacetyl tartaric acid esters of mono- and diglycerides of fatty acids and carboxymethylcellulose.

It's hard to think of the experiment that you could do to put these two products head-to-head. It would take huge numbers of volunteers and the difference might be very slight.

Xand decided to go elsewhere to get a sausage roll that was definitely UPF.

And then, on day three, Xand stopped eating UPF and hasn't looked back.

20.

What to do if you want to stop eating UPF

If you personally want to stop eating UPF, then you could try what Xand and I did: go on an 80 per cent UPF diet for a few days. You don't need to do the full four weeks. Go and seek it out. Grapple with it. You'll find yourself in front of a cottage pie or a lasagne which is on the cusp of the NOVA 4 definition, with maybe just a little spice extract or some dextrose and you'll try to figure out – is this UPF? And you'll understand what Maria Laura da Costa Louzada meant about fantasy foods. You'll bite into some cheap chocolate or some tangy crisps and you'll hear Fernanda Rauber in your ear: 'It's not food. It's an industrially produced edible substance.'

If you recognise in yourself that you might have an addictive relationship, you can go online and search for the Yale Food Addiction Scale test. If you think you are addicted, get some help if you can – whether from a friend or a relative or your doctor.

You may want to take an approach that you will eat some UPF but will steer clear of the problem products. You may recognise vulnerable moments and foods, so that eating a UPF sandwich for lunch with a friend is not going to prompt a binge, whereas eating crisps at home alone while hungry may be more likely to.

You may find it much easier to be abstinent. Xand and I find this the best approach. Our relationship with it was an addiction, and for us abstinence is the only solution. Xand quit UPF and shed around 20kg in a few months. He is entirely abstinent. No exceptions, ever.

And remember that UPF is just a substance through which other problems are realised. There are often reasons why we eat it. These are often the same reasons why so many of us struggle with addiction to other substances. You may have to fix some of those other problems before you can tackle UPF. You may know what they are. Again, get some help.

If you do stop eating UPF, then you'll need to eat something, and it will cost you more in time and money. There are plenty of cookbooks for those on a budget, but there are two authors I particularly recommend: Allegra McEvedy and Jack Monroe. Their recipes are cheap, easy and delicious. Cooking meals will be a hassle, but one that connects you to a long chain of time-hassled humans who survived long enough to make you.

You may not lose loads of weight. I said at the beginning that this was not a weight-loss book. Barry Smith, after we had worked together on the podcast that preceded this book (*Addicted to Food*), quit UPF. His students started calling him paleo Barry, a reflection of how broken our food system is that simply eating normal food makes you some sort of weird diet freak. Anyway, he felt that having left UPF behind he could eat as much cheese, butter and real bread as he liked. But men of mine and Barry's age have been able to put on weight since long before the invention of maltodextrin. He quickly found out that he did need to moderate his cheese intake.

We are ultra-processed people not just because of the food we eat. Many of the other products we buy are engineered to drive excess consumption; our phones and apps, our clothes, our social media, our games and television. Sometimes these can feel like they take much more than they give. The requirement for growth and the harm it does to our bodies and our planet is so much part of the fabric of our world that it's nearly invisible. You may find that abstinence from some of these other products is helpful too.

Finally, make sure that, like Xand, you own what you want to do. And, whatever happens, don't beat yourself up, but do get in touch and let me know how it goes.

Afterword

For five months after the initial publication of *Ultra-Processed People*, stories were in the press nearly every week around the harms and addictive potential of ultra-processed foods (UPFs). The book arrived at a moment of national frustration around obesity and diet-related disease, and the public seemed ready to absorb the science that clearly described the category of foods making all of us sick.

Then, on September 28, 2023, different headlines appeared in all the major national papers. You may have read some of them.

'Is ultra-processed food bad for you?' queried the *Times*. 'Not always, scientists say'.[1]

The *Independent* led with '10 ultra-processed foods that are actually good for you',[2] and there was similar in the *Telegraph*[3] and other papers.

New Scientist magazine ran an article titled 'Ultra-processed food isn't always unhealthy say UK food officials'.[4] It began like this:

> UK officials have dismissed recent concerns that highly processed food, also known as ultra-processed food (UPF), is automatically unhealthy because of the way that it is made or its artificial ingredients.

Friends, colleagues and strangers on social media sent these stories to me – with the implied, or in some cases directly asked, question: are you wrong?

The stories followed a press conference held the previous day where five scientists said that the science around UPF 'cannot show cause and effect' and that some items classed as UPF were foods that should be encouraged, such as wholemeal bread, whole-grain breakfast cereals and yoghurts.

Only the *Guardian* ran a piece that seemed to explain these scientists' rather surprising position. Of the five speakers, four had significant relationships with companies that make UPF, although there is no suggestion that this was concealed and declarations of potential conflicts of interest appear to have been made at the press conference.

Prof Janet Cade, from the University of Leeds, is the chair of the advisory committee of the British Nutrition Foundation (BNF), whose corporate members include McDonald's, British Sugar and Mars. Some of the companies that help fund the foundation include Nestlé, Mondelēz and Coca-Cola.

Then there was Prof Pete Wilde, from the Quadram Institute in Norwich, who has previously received support for his research from Unilever, Mondelēz and Nestlé. Prof Ciarán Forde also spoke. Remember him from chapter 3 where he initially didn't declare financial relationships with Nestlé on a scientific paper (although he did later issue a correction)? And also from chapter 11 where he claimed to have no "conflicts of interest" on another paper despite also declaring that he was on the scientific advisory council for Kerry Group plc (a multi-billion-dollar manufacturer of UPF)? Once again, he did later issue a correction regarding the conflicts. The *Guardian* reported that he has also received research funding from other companies including PepsiCo and General Mills. He told the briefing that giving advice to avoid UPF 'risks demonising foods that are nutritionally beneficial'.

As chair of the government's Scientific Advisory Committee on Nutrition (SACN – more on them in a moment), Prof Ian Young appeared to bring some credibility to the event, although he has previously accepted research funding from Unilever and the Sugar Bureau (an organisation funded by the sugar industry). These relationships weren't reported in the *Guardian*[5, 6] but made headlines a few years previously when it was questioned whether they influenced his role in developing sugar guidelines.[7] He told the *Grocer* that he was "not influenced by these food industry companies" and that there had been "processes in place to ensure transparency and integrity."

The fifth speaker was Prof Robin May, from the Food Standards Agency. He has no recorded conflicts, and I don't know why he decided to share a platform with those who do.

None of the other publications mentioned these conflicts. And even the *Guardian* didn't mention another layer to the story; while May and Young were UK government officials, this wasn't a press conference held by a government agency, it was held by something called the Science Media Centre, or SMC. It's a press office that claims to provide accurate information about science for the public and policymakers through the media. Many, perhaps even most, of the stories you read about science in the press will have quotes taken from the SMC website or will use SMC contributors. It's hard to overstate their influence over the public discourse around science in the UK. They are the go-to resource for every journalist on the science beat.

The SMC claims that it is 'completely independent in both our governance and funding'. You can probably see where I'm headed with this, but let's do it anyway. So, who does fund the SMC? The *British Medical Journal* investigated this in the weeks after the press conference and published a story that quickly became the most read piece on their website: 'Row over ultra-processed foods panel highlights conflicts of interest issue at heart of UK science reporting'. [8] This piece revealed that the SMC is funded by many of the industries it reports on, including by a food industry body, FoodDrinkEurope (whose members include Cargill, Coca-Cola, Danone and Mars), as well as Nestlé and Procter & Gamble (who you will recall makes Pringles). The SMC has also previously received direct funding from Tate & Lyle, Northern Foods, Kraft Foods and Coca-Cola. Tom Whipple, science editor at the *Times*, is quoted in the *BMJ* article as saying, 'I suppose it would be easy to depict it as a be-tentacled Voldemort of science, with us journalists its credulous marionettes,' and that is exactly how I think it is useful to depict it.

When a scientific paper is published, the SMC gathers comments from scientists about the quality of the research and the context it sits in. These comments are posted on the SMC website. At the bottom of each page of responses is a declaration of these commentators' conflicts of interest. Very often none are declared. For example, Gunter Kuhnle, an associate professor of nutrition and food science at the University of Reading, has over the past year featured in several of the SMC's 'expert reactions' on ultra-processed foods. For each of the SMC responses Kuhnle declared no conflicts of interest.[9-12] A little digging (and a freedom of information request made by Dr Stuart Gillespie, a global nutrition policy expert) revealed that Kuhnle has received unrestricted research grants from Mars (yes, the Mars who makes Mars bars) and has recently co-authored papers with Mars employees. The department he works in at the University of Reading has three main industry funders, all of whom make UPF: Mars, PepsiCo and Roquette Frères.* Between 2018 and 2023, Mars gave £262, 832 in research funding to the department.

Kuhnle told the *BMJ* that he follows the Science Media Centre's guidance to provide 'relevant' declarations of interest and has always been open about his conflicts. But it's really hard to square this with what he has actually declared.

Let's be absolutely clear about what constitutes a 'conflict of interest'. When Kuhnle (and others funded by the UPF industry) speak on the SMC website, their primary interest is the evidence around whether UPF harms human health. This evidence is in direct conflict with the primary interest of Mars, which is to make money from a product portfolio that includes many UPF products. If you take money from Mars while commenting on whether UPF affects human health, you have a conflict of interest. It doesn't make everything these scientists say incorrect, but I would urge the press and the public to be sceptical of opinions from chocolate company scientists. The evidence shows they are likely to be biased. And guess what? Kuhnle is sceptical about UPF as a driver of diet-related disease.[10]

---

* Roquette Frères makes ingredients such as protein isolates, modified starches and so on – for exclusive use in UPF.

Kuhnle isn't the only conflicted scientist* on the SMC website who comments on UPF. Over the past two years, up to the time of writing, the SMC has produced responses to sixteen published scientific papers about UPF. Over 70 per cent of the comments are from 'experts' with ongoing or previous financial relationships with companies that make UPF.

So, the press conference alleging that some UPFs were healthy was held by an industry-funded body using industry-funded scientists. This is how the public 'debate' around UPF is orchestrated in the UK. Industry funds the credible-sounding Science Media Centre, which in turn uses industry-funded scientists, often from the credible-sounding British Nutrition Foundation (funded by Coca-Cola, McDonald's and most food companies you can think of), and the credible-sounding University of Reading's Hugh Sinclair Unit of Human Nutrition (funded by Mars and Pepsi).

But some of the scientists who comment on the SMC website (and one who spoke at the SMC press conference) come from the four UK governments' Scientific Advisory Committee on Nutrition, or SACN, which advises the governments on nutrition and related health matters. This is the most alarming source of doubt and confusion around UPF because it sounds utterly credible – yet members of this committee have declared conflicts with the British Nutrition Foundation, the American Society for Nutrition (funded by Mars, Nestlé, Mondelēz), Cargill, the meat industry, the dairy industry, Coca-Cola and Sprite, Tate & Lyle, Sainsbury's, Danone and (terrifyingly in the Subgroup on Maternal and Child Nutrition) Nestlé.

Look, I can fill pages and pages with this stuff – and I love doing it. The influence of industry is so tentacular that it's nearly

---

* After the scandal emerged, Kuhnle updated his conflicts on a piece so that he mentioned that his research was funded by Mars, and he also provided a long list of other interests that are not conflicts including that he is a 'Trustee of a Parent Teacher Association', indicating that neither he nor the SMC have a real understanding of what conflicts are and how they work.[30]

impossible to describe in totality, and you'll get numb long before I finish and start to wonder, 'Yeah, but do conflicts actually matter?'

We have extremely good evidence that they do. There are lots of data showing that industry-funded science is more likely to find results that are beneficial to industry than is independently funded research. I've cited some in chapter 3, but my favourite example is a 2016 review of the evidence that sugar-sweetened beverages are linked to weight gain and obesity.[13] I'll start by saying that there is a general consensus among the experts that they are – even the British Nutrition Foundation, the Scientific Advisory Committee on Nutrition and the Hugh Sinclair Unit of Human Nutrition at Reading agree on this. Of the thirty-four studies in the review that showed a link between sugar-sweetened beverages and obesity and type 2 diabetes, thirty-three – or 97 per cent – were independent (i.e. not funded by the food and beverage industry). By contrast, of the twenty-six studies that suggested there was no link, twenty-five were funded by industry – including Coca-Cola, PepsiCo, Dr Pepper Snapple Group, Tate & Lyle and other companies that make money from sugary drinks. So, 96 per cent of industry-funded studies suggested that drinking soft drinks is fine, meaning that independent studies were thirty-three times more likely to link sugary drinks with harm.

We find similar patterns across all of science. Industry funding creates bias – which we might also call corruption. But in this specific instance related to UPF we have to ask, could they – the SMC, the British Nutrition Foundation, the University of Reading and the Scientific Advisory Committee on Nutrition – actually be correct?

The clever part of what they do is that when it comes to the granular detail, much of what the scientists at the BNF, or quoted in the SMC, say is artfully true.

For example, on their website the BNF acknowledge that while studies of UPF have shown 'consistent associations, it is difficult to untangle the impact of less healthy dietary patterns and lifestyles and they do not provide clear evidence of a causal association between processing per se and health.' This mirrors many similar statements by conflicted scientists (often from the BNF!) on the Science Media Centre website.

And it's true. You can't prove causation with population studies of the type that link UPF to harm or – come to think of it – the studies that linked cigarettes to lung cancer. In fact, we have never proved causation when it comes to cigarettes and cancer. All we've ever shown is that people who smoke seem to get more lung cancer. And the more they smoke, the more cancer they get.*

The tobacco companies have made a lot of hay out of this uncertainty. In 1953, they set up the Tobacco Industry Research Committee – which I see as being equivalent to the British Nutrition Foundation. This issued a statement[14] to the public in 1954 claiming:

1. That medical research of recent years indicates many possible causes of lung cancer.
2. That there is no agreement among the authorities regarding what the cause is.

---

* In response to a published paper linking increased UPF intake to depression,[26] one commentor (a dietician with no published research papers), said: 'Whilst there is a link in this research we do not know for sure that it was UPF's that are the cause. This is very much a case of correlation and not causation.[9]

The thing is that the paper came out of teams from the medical school and the school of public health at Harvard who do understand roughly how epidemiology works. And they don't claim that their paper is proof, rather that it sits in a context of mounting evidence from several populations that increased UPF intake is associated with depression. It's the fourth large study to make the same finding.[31–33]

One of the important tests of epidemiological data is to ask: Is there a plausible mechanism by which UPF might make people depressed? Yes. We have hundreds of other papers we could cite about additives that cause inflammation, and that have effects on the microbiome. And food that is also associated with obesity and many other health problems might plausibly also drive misery and suffering.

Is the jury in that UPF causes depression? No. Is there enough evidence from really excellent independent groups around the world that it's a risk worth taking seriously and sharing with the public? Yes.

3. That there is no proof that cigarette smoking is one of the causes.
4. That statistics purporting to link cigarette smoking with the disease could apply with equal force to any one of many other aspects of modern life. Indeed, the validity of the statistics themselves is questioned by numerous scientists.

You may hear echoes of this statement in the BNF statement above. There is no proof that smoking causes cancer nor is there proof that UPF causes negative health outcomes ... and yet both are extremely likely.

With every new study that comes out, the SMC hosts 'experts' saying the same stuff. A team at the world-renowned Imperial College London published a paper linking ultra-processed food consumption with cancer. [15] It's the most comprehensive study of the associations between ultra-processed food consumption and risk of overall cancer, as well as thirty-four different cancers. It showed that the higher consumption of ultra-processed foods is associated with a greater risk of overall cancer and specifically ovarian and brain cancer, as well as increased risk of overall, ovarian and breast cancer–associated mortality.

Sure enough, a scientist from the British Nutrition Foundation explained that a limitation of this study is that it does 'not provide evidence of a clear causal link between UPFs and cancer, or the risk of other diseases.' [16] True. But does this really paint a useful picture for journalists or the public? After all, this critique invalidates all epidemiology. The team at Imperial College London are aware of the difficulty of causation, being world-class epidemiologists, and so they make adjustments for smoking and for a range of other possible factors, including sociodemographic, physical activity and other aspects of diet.[17–19]

It's important to acknowledge the limitations of scientific evidence, but by offering a critique of papers one by one, the BNF and the SMC privilege a sceptical view of the evidence that suits the industry. They are doing precisely what the tobacco companies did for many decades – doubt is their product. Unless you've worked in a lab or conducted research, you won't generally understand the extent to which every single published paper and study is flawed. This is especially true in nutrition, where we can't generate the gold standard of evidence, namely a randomised trial.*

There is now such a mountain of evidence on the harms of UPF that it's going to become hard for research ethics committees to permit scientists to randomise participants to a high-UPF diet. Instead, we're going to need to lean on lab experiments on animals, a few small clinical trials and big population data where you follow people who eat different amounts of UPF 'in the wild', as it were, and then see what happens to them. The scientists who undertake this work do their best to make sure that people who eat UPF aren't just all heavy smokers and so on.

When you take a step back and look at the whole body of litera-ture, as we did with smoking, it is utterly persuasive. There are now approaching eighty UPF population studies of the type used to link smoking to cancer, and over 2,000 papers in total that provide evi-dence that a dietary pattern high in UPF is harmful. There is new evidence of links between UPF and cancer, cardiometabolic disease, addiction, emulsifiers and, importantly, eating disorders. [15, 17, 20–26] UPF has met the threshold which means that we can say that, as a category of food, it causes a wide range of what are euphemistically

---

* Ideally, we would take a large number of people and randomly assign them to two diets that varied only in terms of whether they were ultra-processed. We'd need to do this many times with many different diets of course, and even then the question would remain: 'But which ultra-processed products are causing the harm?' So really what you'd do is vary only one single element of a diet in each study. To understand bread, you'd need to randomise people to identical diets that differs only with the type of bread they eat: UPF bread versus non-UPF bread. You'd lock everyone up, ideally from birth, in metabolic labs, like Kevin Hall's, for several decades and see what happens. For a truly perfect experiment you'd separate identical twins at birth and follow them to death. The cost would be prohibitive long before the ethics board shut the whole thing down.

called 'negative health outcomes', a category including everything from cancer to death. So, extremely negative.

Arguing about the flaws in each study suits industry because it delays discussion of what needs to be done about the food we all agree is harmful. More on this in a moment, but essentially bad food needs a warning label. We could start with the products we all agree on like for example cola and all other sugary soft drinks. The sugar in these drinks causes tooth decay, weight gain and metabolic disease. The other acids in these drinks also damage teeth and there is some evidence that they also damage your bones. Drink enough and you may end up peeing out your own skeleton. At the moment, my six-year-old can go into any shop and buy a can without anything telling her (or me) about any of these effects.

Why don't we hear scientists from the British Nutrition Foundation speaking at a Science Media Centre press conference about the crisis of obesity and metabolic disease in children and discussing the best way of labelling these products? In my opinion, one reason might be because the British Nutrition Foundation's Healthy Eating Week in 2023 was sponsored by Coca-Cola. And the SMC is sponsored by FoodDrinkEurope, an industry body partly funded by Coke and other companies that make similar products.

If you, as an individual or an institution, don't buy the UPF evidence but you are committed to reducing diet-related disease and showing a real desire to put a warning label on soft drinks, then no sweat. I can do business with you – I am sure we agree on more than we disagree.

But the silence from industry-funded groups about the crisis and what to do about it is cacophonous.

***

Even while funding their intermediaries to sow doubt and confusion, the UPF industry has been very keen to meet me. A major fast-food chain offered to fly me to their board meeting in America, and other big food companies have offered me obscene amounts to speak to their teams even briefly over Zoom.

At first, I was baffled by this. The most important information in this book came from people inside the food companies themselves. They know far more than I do about many aspects of the food system, from their own commercial incentives to the reasons they use particular emulsifiers. What they don't know they can read in the book or hear in an interview. Paying me tens of thousands of pounds for an hour of my time seemed daft. But I was keen to meet them because I was sure I'd learn more from them than they would from me. And I wrestled with whether I could take the money without becoming conflicted.

Eventually, I decided to take £20,000 from one of the less awful companies. I'd take it in such a way that it would never hit my bank account. Rather, my agents would take it and give it to a non-food charity I work with. So, we set a date. And then the contract arrived.

As I read it, I understood why I was being offered all this money. Section 5, paragraph 1, part f.

WARRANTIES, REPRESENTATIONS AND UNDERTAKINGS
The supplier [that's me] warrants, represents and undertakes that it [me] shall not make any statement or otherwise conduct itself in such a manner as shall, or may in the reasonable opinion of this food company, disparage this food company and/or its customers, or its products or services or bring the food company name into disrepute.

For £20,000 they buy my silence. Of course, they don't want my opinions on UPF, public health or anything else. They want me and all my colleagues and collaborators to shut up.

And the terms of the contract were quite broad extending 'throughout the universe in perpetuity'. I wouldn't be able to disparage this company, their products, or their customers even if I moved to Pluto.

I turned down the money. They cancelled the meeting.*

* A couple of the big companies did still want to meet me even if I wouldn't take their money or sign a gagging agreement, so I went along. In both instances the teams were extremely smart and, in so far as you can tell from a two-hour meeting, decent people. We agreed on the evidence and the products they made that harm human health.

And these meetings revealed that it is really important to speak to the industry you want to regulate. I learned lots of specifics about their constraints, and how if, for example, they took the gums out of their coconut milk, they'd get customer complaints from people who think it's gone rancid because it separates in the can.

I asked one company if they could pivot to being a more 'fruit- and veg-based' business? Awkward looks all round. 'The problem is that we make money from our snacks.'

This is understandable. Selling pears, no matter how good, is difficult. They're a hassle to grow year-round, they bruise easily and they rot in days.

Selling a chocolate brownie made of wheat flour, palm oil and chocolate flavouring with a nearly infinite shelf life is obviously better business. It's what I'd do if I were them.

They asked what I do given unlimited power, and one of the things in my overly long reply was that I would stick a whole bunch of black hexagons on many of their preprepared products and I'd take off the cartoon mascots that are central to so many of their brands. We wrapped things up pretty quickly after that.

Speaking to industry is useful, but if you're paid by them, then you are the industry. If you're interested in public health, then you need a regulatory position. They're not your pal; they're not a partner; they can't give you a single solitary penny.

My refusal of the money created a sort of unbridgeable weirdness that is really important if you want to regulate something. It wasn't that we didn't agree on stuff intellectually, it's just that we want totally different things. I want people to have freedom from predatory marketing and access to affordable available food. As individuals, they also want these things. As a business, they want to make lots of money.

It was like a two-hour blind date where in the first five minutes you establish that you quite like each other but that you have totally incompatible agendas; one of you thrives on art galleries and going to the opera ... and the other wants to live in Antarctica. You can remain cordial, but you're not going to be partners. You're solving different problems.

This brings us nicely to the question of what exactly is being done to improve the food system?

In September 2023, I went to New York for the Global Obesity Forum. This is a WHO-affiliated event that takes place the day before the UN General Assembly meets. It is the only global organisation focused exclusively on obesity.

I gave a talk about UPF and the parallels between Big Food and Big Tobacco, and how we must therefore use a similar regulatory approach. It landed okay, but there was an atmosphere of confusion in the room. I had framed my words defensively in the way that I'm used to having to do in the UK when I speak with MPs, journalists, policymakers and a public steeped in industry messaging. I had laboured the evidence, going over in great detail the responses to the counterarguments. The confusion was not that I had said anything wrong, but rather that I thought that anyone might disagree. I was saying stuff that others around the world have been saying for years.

The truth is that the UK has been left behind. Because, globally, the jury is now in on a diet high in UPF. Public health academics from South and Central America whose speeches followed mine stood up and gave presentations about how they were labelling UPF with black hexagons (see chapter 19) and how it was already driving down purchases. I met colleagues from UNICEF and they told me about their policy on companies that manufacture UPF. I'll quote it here in full, as it's the simplest distillation of how all policymakers and regulators should interact with the food industry.

UNICEF will avoid all partnerships with ultraprocessed food and beverage (UPF) industries.

To preserve our thought and action leadership, align with our programming strategies, and maintain our credibility as a trusted advisor for public policy, normative guidance, and programme implementation for children, UNICEF will avoid all forms of financial and non-financial partnerships and collaborations with the UPF industry. This includes individual companies as well as associations, platforms, and front groups representing UPF industries and their interests.[27]

As well as UNICEF, research groups around the world are very convinced by the data, and many foreign governments have given clear unambiguous guidance on UPF. I'll put them below because they have great clarity, and it may help to read them.

Brazil
Avoid UPF. Always prefer natural or minimally processed foods and freshly made dishes and meals. Do not offer UPF to children.

Belgium
Choose as few ultra-processed products as possible. UPF have no real added value in a healthy and environmentally responsible diet.

Canada
Limit highly processed foods and drinks because they are not part of a healthy eating pattern. If you eat highly processed foods, try to:

- Eat them less often
- Eat them in small amounts
- Replace them with healthier options

Ecuador
Avoid the consumption of UPF.

France
Limit sugary drinks, fatty, sweet, salty and ultra-processed foods. Avoid giving ultra-processed products to under-threes. Avoid giving commercial baby foods and ready meals to under-threes.

I especially love this quote from the French guidance:
Pour varier les goûts et les textures, le fait maison a tout bon.
Plus de goûts, plus de textures, plus de miam!

'To vary tastes and textures, homemade has everything good.
More tastes, more textures, more 'yum'!'

Israel
Reduce the consumption of UPF as much as possible. Avoid processed, industrialised and packaged foods as much as possible. There is no need to buy food made especially for children and babies.

Mexico
Avoid ultra-processed foods. Ultra-processed foods promote preference for very sweet or salty flavours, and increase the risk of both obesity and malnutrition.

Peru
Avoid the consumption of UPF.

Uruguay
Base your diet on natural foods and avoid the regular consumption of ultra-processed products with excessive contents of fat, sugar and salt.

In the UK, progress is slow but, I hope, steady. The Science Media Centre is now, at least, partly discredited and journalists are more and more suspicious of anyone linked to the Coke-funded British Nutrition Foundation. In the first part of 2024, the House of Lords is to hold an inquiry into the links between UPF and obesity thanks to extraordinary efforts by Baroness Anne Jenkin, Baroness Rosie Boycott and Lord Bethell of Romford, along with Dr Dolly van Tulleken. (I interviewed her for this book when she was Dr Dolly Theis, and then collaborated with her sister to get her together with my brother, Xand. This book has had many unexpected outcomes, but this has brought the most joy.)

***

What do we need to do in terms of policy?

There are two separate projects. First, we need to regulate the industry that produces UPF in a way that increases choice and freedom. Second, we need to enable people to choose healthy and affordable food if they wish. There are already many powerful and diverse voices engaged in the second project, celebrating and promoting real, affordable food. My interest lies in the first – regulation.

I believe the approach needs to follow the tobacco control template. It's not about banning anything – bans on addictive substances typically do more harm than good. There are two main things that need to be done.

1. **Put warning labels on harmful foods.** If we try to put black octagons on everything that contains an additive not found in a domestic kitchen, we'll get food industry lawyers whining about the fact that some people have xanthan gum in their kitchens, but that doesn't matter. In Argentina and Mexico, the worst-offending foods have up to five black octagon stop signs (one for each of salt, fat, sugar, trans or saturated fats and calories) and two black boxes for caffeine and sweeteners. This warning-label system for packaged foods, which is based on the World Health Organisation nutrient profile classification, has been shown to work well in many South and Central American countries. Crucially it sweeps up over 95 per cent of UPF. I would suggest additional warnings about synthetic emulsifiers, but once you have one black octagon on food and a threshold for the evidence to do it,

adding another is easy. No company wants to go toe-to-toe with government lawyers over the research showing the stuff they want to put in your food makes rats swell up and die. Labels like this have become law in many countries. A can of Coke in Argentina now has two black octagons – for excess sugar and calories – and crucially it doesn't have the green lights for low fat and salt content like in the UK that imply Coke is more healthy than unhealthy. Once you've put black octagons on products, it's easy to tell people which foods to avoid.

2. **End conflicts of interest.** This step is simple but essential and was vital for tobacco control – industry money came to be seen as dirty. If you seek to improve public health in the UK and the US, then you need to have a regulatory relationship with industry. It can be cordial, with open lines of communication, but you're going to need to make the industry do things it doesn't want to do, so it cannot be merely a partnership. You cannot help to solve a problem you profit from creating. Organisations such as the Scientific Advisory Committee on Nutrition should not have anyone on the committee who has a formal relationship with industry. At the moment, there is a specified industry expert on the committee, and six of the other fourteen members have conflicts of interest with companies like Danone, Mars and Nestlé. And neither should charities: whereas the British Nutrition Foundation and Bite Back have financial links to industry, the best food charities don't take any money. The First Steps Nutrition Trust, UNICEF and the Food Foundation are all incredible organisations. Industry-linked scientists should be rigorously excluded from the policy space and public debate. They shouldn't be quoted in articles or appear on the news any more than tobacco-funded scientists would be. Conflicts of interest undermine trust in science, and nutrition professionals and institutions should avoid and

terminate financial relationships, partnerships, and
co-branding with food companies. Instead, they should
advocate for expanded public funding to support research.

Once we've achieved these first two aims, most other things should
follow easily. Warnings about UPF can be added into the national
nutrition guidance. We stop the targeted marketing of UPF (i.e.
anything with an octagon) to children – meaning nothing on
Spotify or YouTube, no cartoon characters, no McDonald's ads on
bus tickets. And we change the food served in institutions like
schools, hospitals and prisons so it is made on-site (not reheated on-
site) by humans. This creates jobs and improves many different
outcomes for those who prepare it and those who consume it.

Education and taxes are low on my list of priorities. No one serious is proposing taxing staple UPFs that everyone relies on. We
should eventually tax the most harmful products – sweets, soft
drinks, crisps, etc. – and we should use that tax to subsidise real
food and make it more easily available. Local government is already
doing great work in this area, but they have the power to ensure
that you can't stand in one spot in Leicester and see nothing but
Greggs and McDonald's, so they should use it. Meanwhile, improved
education would be amazing – check out the work done by TastEd,
a brilliant food charity – but when kids are steeped in marketing
and can't afford different food it feels uncomfortable.

A wicked problem to be solved is how to make real food affordable. Living in poverty forces a harmful diet, so the first step is to
end poverty. This is possible. The cost of poverty cannot and should
not be expressed purely in financial terms. Poverty is a failure of
justice: children should all have the same opportunities in life irrespective of the household they are born into. But even on a purely
economic level, the arguments for ending poverty are overwhelming, and it should be a priority for even the most hawkish,
right-leaning nationalist who wants a strong military and a world-
beating football team. (I'm guessing not many of you have made it
this far in the book, but hi and welcome if you are still here.)

In the UK, poverty is estimated to cost the government around £78 billion per year in increased healthcare, education, policing, criminal justice, and social care costs and lost tax revenues.[28] This is more money than it would cost to end it. So, it's not just morally right to end poverty, it is way more cost-effective to do so than to spend money fixing the lives it shatters.

The next step is to create a market for real food – the system is too complex to manage from the top down. I don't think it's right to tell people what to eat; rather I want to help to create a world where we all have real choice. Warning labels on packets, education and public health campaigns are regulations that don't nanny people – they empower them. When people understand their food and are free from misleading marketing, they will demand real food. Industry will be very capable of responding to this shift in demand. The old food industry giants may not all survive, but we'll see the rise of new companies with different structures and product portfolios.

There are then a whole suite of changes to be made to the agro-economic system that are way beyond the scope of this book. It is already a very managed system of subsidies and incentives. These could be realigned by government to support a food system that produces affordable, healthy, environmentally sustainable food. But until there is a market for these foods, nothing will change. Politicians won't have a mandate to regulate companies.

What do you want to do?

After boiling down and repeating the core messages of this book over hundreds of lectures and interviews in the last months, I have found a few concepts that are especially helpful. If you're struggling and find yourself eating stuff you don't want to eat, then perhaps these concepts might help you eat the way you want to.

You should keep eating UPF while you learn about it. Not forbidding it seems to be a really important part of recovery. But remember this quick-fire list of ways that UPF harms you:

- It's soft and typically calorie dense, so you eat it at a rate that your body can't keep up with when it comes to feeling full.
- Things like protein isolates, refined oils and modified carbohydrates are absorbed so quickly they may not even reach the part of the gut that sends the fullness signal to the brain. They're not things you have evolved to eat.
- Some of the additives are well known to cause harm – be particularly aware of emulsifiers and artificial sweeteners. Emulsifiers can thin the mucus lining of the gut, allowing faecal bacteria to leak into the blood stream and inflaming your whole body. The non-nutritive sweeteners that tell your body sugar is coming but don't supply any calories seem to cause metabolic stress and changes to the microbiome.
- Other additives that affect the microbiome are maltodextrins, modified starches and lots of the gums and thickeners.
- Flavour enhancers (glutamate, guanylate, inosinate and ribonucleotides on ingredient lists) drive excess consumption. Again, they tell your body a lie about the nutritional content of the food you're eating when they're added out of context.

But the most important thing to remember is the purpose of UPF. This is the most important thing about it. It's not any one of the above properties that is the problem. Every product has hundreds of different properties: acidity, viscosity, fatty mouthfeel, the type of emulsifier, the colouring, the texture, the colour of the font on the packet, the type of cartoon animal used in the ad and on and on. Each of these variables is tested on panels of people and optimised to make you eat and buy as much as possible.

Because the purpose of the food you eat is to make money for its industry.

If your food is made by a transnational conglomerate owned by large institutional investors, they will prioritise making money over your health. And the best way for them to make money is to have an addictive product, which is made using the cheapest possible raw materials.

When you're eating UPF ask yourself who made it and what they were trying to achieve.

Is this real food, made to nourish me?

Or:

Is this an industrially produced edible substance made to turn my health into money for someone else?

If you're struggling, just remember: it's not you, it's the food.

FAQs

I get asked a lot of questions. Here are a few answers.

How can I be sure something is UPF?

If you're reading an ingredients list? It's probably UPF. If you don't recognise an ingredient? Probably UPF. There are some exceptions. In general, preservatives in tinned goods don't mean UPF, nor do the things that many countries require to be added to flour. In the UK, it's calcium, iron, thiamine and niacin. Open Food Facts is a pretty useful database.

Is all UPF bad? What about wholemeal bread.

Emulsified UPF wholemeal bread is likely to drive excess consumption and other problems, due to those emulsifiers and the fact it's very soft. It is almost certainly better than non-wholegrain UPF bread. It is probably worse than real bread. And while there is value in understanding which UPFs are driving the most harm, the degree to which 'better' products can be disentangled is arguably limited. We have a food system that mainly produces UPF and it needs fixing. In the context of an entirely ultra-processed diet, whole grain UPF bread is probably less harmful than some other stuff. But you probably eat more of it than the stuff you know is bad; for example, you don't eat chocolate for breakfast.

If you cook at home with xanthan gum, are you making UPF?

No. UPF is industrially produced for profit. This is part of the definition. If you make food because you love someone and you want to nourish them, then you're not ultra-processing. There are perhaps some exceptions to this general rule. A recipe made entirely of UPF is unlikely to be part of a healthy diet. Grating cheese over flavoured nacho chips doesn't constitute food preparation.

Why are UPFs less expensive than fresh foods? Surely all that 'doing things to them' and packaging should make them more costly.

Additives save money. Palm stearin is cheaper than dairy fat. Stabilizers prolong shelf life, saving money. Flavourings are cheaper than fruit.

How do you stop eating chocolate and ice cream?

Keep eating the ice cream. I'm not judging you. But do read chapter 1 again while you eat, and also take a glance at your ingredients list. There are some non-UPF ice creams, but they are hard to find. I've asked for an ice cream maker for my birthday.

Isn't Alpen heathy?

Alpen Muesli contains milk whey powder, which isn't a typical domestic ingredient. To understand whether this drives excess consumption, buy the other ingredients of the cereal (wholegrain wheat, wholegrain rolled oats, raisins, sugar, skimmed milk powder, hazelnuts, almonds and salt) and see if you can make something as irresistible as Alpen. I haven't been able to. Alpen is made by Post Holdings, a multi-billion-dollar packaged food company. They know what they're doing when it comes to formulating a cereal that you eat a lot of. So, not unhealthy, but you'll eat a lot. I used to eat it for pudding!

Isn't making people afraid of certain foods contributing to eating disorders?

I had been anxious that in criticising a category of food I might be at risk of driving eating disorders. But it does seem important to take this risk, especially because there is some evidence that UPFs contribute to eating disorders. I met the Faculty of Eating Disorders Psychiatry at the Royal College of Psychiatrists to discuss this. They and many others in the community of professionals who treat eating disorders are concerned about the role the UPF may play. In early data, it seems like 100 per cent of the foods that people binge on are UPF.[24, 29] Eating food that isn't produced for nourishment seems to alter our relationship with the way we eat. This is most obvious when it comes to addiction.

All the serious people in the discussion are very alive to the risk of demonising a particular type of food. I don't think there is a perfect way to discuss any of this, but I've tried to show my work, and I don't think there is persuasive evidence that the risks of pointing out the harms of UPF outweigh the benefits.

Is UPF really addictive?

The evidence that many UPF products are addictive is very strong and has grown since the book was first published. I expressed this idea cautiously in chapter 10, when I wrote: 'there may be advantages to considering UPF as an addictive substance.' I no longer feel that caution. I feel more and more that addiction is the best lens through which to see UPF, whether you're thinking about your own kids or making government policy.

Many papers have been published about UPF in the last year, but 'Social, clinical, and policy implications of ultra-processed food addiction', published in the *British Medical Journal* in October 2023, must be one of the most important. [23] This paper reports on two systematic reviews, including 281 studies from thirty-six different countries that found the overall prevalence of food addiction using Yale Food Addiction Scale was 14 per cent in adults and 12 per cent in children. This is similar to the rates of addiction to alcohol (14 per cent) and tobacco 18 per cent in adults, but the level of addiction in children is unprecedented. We are historically good at protecting children from addiction.

Is this a conspiracy? The companies deliberately put their food through design processes, which result in addictive products. And they know that their foods are addictive. We have a cereal called Krave, after all. And the fact that it is impossible to stop eating Pringles once the tube is opened is the basis of their very successful marketing campaign. Ashwin Rodrigues is a journalist with *GQ* magazine. We spoke about UPF, and he made an interesting observation: all the cereal mascots seem to have an addicted relationship with the products they are marketing. This in mind, it's hilarious when you go back through the ads on YouTube but also troubling – it's normalising an addicted relationship with food.

If you feel addicted, then abstinence may be useful for you (if you can afford it!). If you don't live with addiction, then cutting back and having UPF as the occasional treat may be easy (though once you start to regard it as a treat it may not live up to expectation).

Is all UPF equally harmful?

Many important questions remain about UPF. Like what are the least harmful products? There is almost certainly a difference between a salad from Pret a Manger, where the only funky ingredient is a little xanthan gum, and Ms Molly's vanilla ice cream from Tesco, where the only non-funky ingredient is sugar.

The xanthan gum in that Pret salad probably won't hurt you, but it does tell you that it was produced in an industrial system that doesn't care much about your health. The salad is 526 calories, a little more than a Big Mac, and you will find yourself finishing the whole lot because that's the way it was designed. When you eat the Ms Molly's, at least you're absolutely clear what you're getting into.

The crucial thing to remember is that the evidence is about the proportion of your diet that comes from UPF. A bowl of Coco Pops isn't toxic. But a diet built around products like Coco Pops seems to be very harmful.

Isn't this a culture war against people who live in poverty and already have enough to deal with?

This is a point made by Prof Janet Cade from the industry-funded British Nutrition Foundation, at the industry-funded Science Media Centre press conference.

People rely on processed foods for a wide number of reasons, so the bottom line would be that if we remove them from our diets, this would require a huge change in the food supply, which is really unachievable for most people, and potentially resulting in further stigmatisation, guilt, etc in those who rely on processed foods, promoting further inequalities in disadvantaged groups.

I agree with almost every word of this. But whereas they land on 'so keep eating UPF' I land on 'we need to have a huge change in the food supply system'. Using this argument to stifle regulation that would improve life for many feels cynical and cruel. What promotes inequalities is forcing disadvantaged groups to eat terrible food. All of us are immersed in misleading predatory marketing.

@RoadsideMum (aka Louisa Britain) is a poverty and disability campaigner and activist who understands far better than me how this food interacts with poverty.

If there's a culture war on here it's not against the working class. I had UPF pizza last night and it cost me much less than the beef stew I'm making tonight. So being anti-UPF isn't saying 'pah, peasants need to lay off the dirty fishfingers', it's saying, 'can someone go and get some proper oversight on those food companies please?'

All the proposed solutions made by activists are about reducing inequality and disadvantage.

It's about making real, actual, proper food, the standard rather than almost-food /industrially produced food-like substances ...

Acknowledgements

I have only one real skill in life, and it is surrounding myself with people who are far more competent than me. This has proved crucial, because I hugely underestimated writing this book and I needed a lot of help from a lot of people to get it done.

This is a list, in no particular order, of people without whom the book would not exist, people without whom the book would be much worse, and people and places that supported and enabled me to write the book.

My mother Kit and my father Anthony. Mum and Dad come first not just because of the logic of biology but because, for my entire life, they have created an environment for me (and my brothers) where everything seems possible. Mum is also the best cook I know and was a professional editor, so she also literally helped to create the book and many of the ideas in it.

I have had three absurdly talented editors who returned comments on the second draft so thorough that they totalled almost 20 per cent of the length of the final book. Helen Conford at Cornerstone Press has soaked up the stress caused by my missed deadlines like a carbon rod in a fission reactor ... so much so that I barely knew there was any stress until much later. She is sometimes brutal, always unpredictable, extremely funny and absolutely the best editor I could have wished for.

Melanie Tortoroli at WW Norton in the US and Rick Meier in Canada at Knopf wrapped their much-needed and brilliant critiques with such warmth and humour that I almost enjoyed trying to fix all the problems. Their enthusiasm for an early draft kept me going.

The team at Cornerstone Press have supported me far beyond expectations. My publicist Etty Eastwood has worked tirelessly to bring the ideas in this book to as many people as possible. Claire

Bush and Charlotte Bush (no relation) did heroics with marketing and publicity respectively. Matt Waterson in sales and Penny Liechti in rights helped my book reach readers. Joanna Taylor supervised the editorial process, and Odhran O'Donoghue copy-edited to a level of detail that was, at times, humiliating but absolutely necessary. Any remaining errors are of course my own.

Zoë Waldie at RCW is the best possible literary agent. She's been a friend, mentor and a guide at every stage, from the big decisions about structure and contracts to the placement of commas. The book would not exist without her or the team at RCW.

Miranda Chadwick was my friend before she started to represent me. The book would not exist without her either. She is the best broadcasting agent bar none, and is the reason I have a career. Jamie Slattery is the yin to her yang and without him no aspect of my life would function. Together they are two of the most important people in my life.

James Browning (or 'Bames' as Sasha would have it) was sent to me by Zoë to assist with the proposal and a year later he feels like one of the family. He's acted as editor/counsellor week to week, helping me to understand the difference between a book and a series of unconnected factual statements.

Alexander Greene has been my pal since before I can remember and has never wavered in his enthusiasm or encouragement for this whole idea. His farm in Italy sells some of the best real food you'll ever eat. Go to https://potentino.com/.

Lizzie Bolton first gave me the papers on UPF to read – she's one of the brains behind many of my BBC documentaries, including *What Are We Feeding Our Kids?*, the programme about UPF that filmed the diet experiment in this book. The book wouldn't exist without her or Dominique Walker (who superbly exec produces most of my documentaries), Jack Bootle (who develops, execs and now commissions them) or Tom McDonald (who looked after me for many years at the BBC). The BBC is unique in having no commercial funding and a brave team of in-house commissioners and lawyers who have boldly supported me broadcasting about commercial determinants of health for many years. We're all lucky it exists.

Helen Crawley is a food policy expert, was one of my expert reviewers and is perhaps my most trusted source on every aspect of food, from the details of scientific nutrition evidence to how policy is created. She's a brilliant person.

Carlos Monteiro and his team gave me huge amounts of time and advice, especially Carlos himself, Fernanda Rauber, Geoffrey Cannon (who spoke for hours and sent me a huge quantity of valuable research), Maria Laura da Costa Louzada, Gyorgy Scrinis and Jean-Claude Moubarac.

Rob Percival and Helen Browning from the Soil Association. Rob feels nearly omniscient about almost every aspect of the problem. Helen provided the first and still the clearest explanation of the economics of commodity foods I've ever been given. It was after speaking with them for the first time that I really 'got it'.

As I started to write, I interviewed Dolly Theis as someone who deeply understands the theory and politics of food and the policies that surround it, and she is now part of my family. She is at the core of many of the ideas throughout this book, especially those in the final chapter about the way forward.

Andrew and Claire Cavey are two of my dearest friends, and I have hassled them about every word in the book. Andrew's intolerance of sloppy argument is infuriating but one of the best things about him.

Giles Yeo is awesome and has influenced me more than he can possibly know. Buy his books – *Gene Eating* and *Why Calories Don't Count* – and read them.

Melissa Thompson told me far more about food and history and culture than I could possibly include. Buy her book *Motherland: A Jamaican Cookbook*.

Aubrey Gordon presents the *Maintenance Phase* podcast, which is required listening for anyone interested in science, health, weight and humanity. She was hugely generous with advice about how to discuss weight without stigma. Her books *What We Don't Talk About When We Talk About Fat* and *'You Just Need to Lose Weight': And 19 Other Myths About Fat People* are essential.

At UCL, Rachel Batterham has been a friend and mentor over many projects. Sam Dicken, Janine Makaronidis and Claudia Gandini Wheeler-Kingshott have contributed more to this book and other projects than they realise.

Bee Wilson wrote the best account of UPF I've ever read in the *Guardian* (handed to me by Lizzie Bolton). I'm lucky to count her as a friend. As well as her thoughtful comments on some ideas, she introduced me to Naomi Alderman, who told me about how to accept criticism and how money works.

Kevin Hall gave me huge amounts of time and kept me within the bounds of the evidence (for the most part!).

Chris Snowdon was very generous with his time and arguments. We agree on a lot, and I am hopeful that one day he'll leave the Institute of Economic Affairs and put his considerable talents towards making the world a better place for everyone.

In Muaná, Brazil – Paula Costa Ferreira, Lizete Novaes from the Catholic Pastoral da Criança, Graciliano Silva Ramo and Leo and his family. Tristan Quinn directed the Brazil portion of the BBC documentary *What Are We Feeding Our Kids?* Alasdair Livingston was the superb DOP and Tom Bell kept everything together.

Paul Hart tracked me down and made sure that I didn't go too far off-piste. He kindly reviewed the text as well as contributing massive technical and ethical expertise. He and Sharon made a lot of the research fun.

Gary Taubes: I may not agree about insulin, but I really enjoyed speaking with him and admired him more at the end of our chat than I did at the beginning.

Barry Smith illuminated a whole new area of philosophy and neuroscience that I had never thought about and that helped me understand how UPF works on the body and brain. He was incredibly generous with a vast number of ideas.

Clare Llewellyn studies twins at UCL and has done some of the most important work describing the relationships between genes and environment. Discussions with her and her research in general are some of the most important concepts in the book.

Anthony Fardet told me about the food matrix and tweaked the way I approach scientific problems.

Suzi Shingler runs the Alliance to Save our Antibiotics, and is helping keep us all alive.

Ben Scheindlin spoke to me at length about Clara Davis, as did Canadian journalist Stephen Strauss, who spent years digging up everything he could find on her. Stephen was unbelievably generous sharing this research as well as lots of other fascinating miscellany on nutrition.

Matt Bosworth offered invaluable and terrifying early legal advice (for free!).

Tom Neltner and Maricel Maffini work at and with the Environmental Defense Fund, trying to hold the FDA to account about food additives. They are truly snapping turtles. Emily Broad Leib at Harvard works on the same issue and, in the best way, I also consider her to be a snapping turtle: she helped me understand that additives don't affect us all equally.

Sarah Finer is a twin, a friend, a doctor and a scientist who has shaped my thoughts over many years and many discussions.

I was lucky to have a great number of tolerant and expert teachers at medical school, but Huw Dorkins and Paul Dennis particularly supported me and shaped my subsequent career more than either of them can imagine.

Sharon Newson: what I didn't say about Sharon in the text is the extent to which she has changed my mind about aspects of obesity and how we discuss weight. I spent a long time pushing her in the wrong direction before she started to push me in the right one. She's a true expert and a great pal.

Eddie Rixon brilliantly explained farming and the food business in snatches of time while *Operation Ouch!* took over his farm.

Tim Cole at UCL took so much time to explain exactly how subtly but surely wrong people who try to claim that childhood obesity is a myth are. A lovely, inspiring man.

David Biller has the banker's omniscience about all things and made me a little less naïve as well as connecting me to industry experts like Robert Plowman, the anonymous management consultant, and Ibrahim Najafi. These contributors had nothing to gain (and plenty to lose) from speaking with me, and were incredibly generous with their time and knowledge.

Patti Rundall understands the arms race among food companies better than anyone and she is a huge force protecting children around the world from predatory marketing and a constant inspiration. Her influence is on every page of this book.

I'm really proud to work alongside the whole team at UNICEF UK, both professionally and as a supporter – especially Katherine Shats, Grainne Moloney, Claire Quarrell and Jessica Gray.

Experts and colleagues at the World Health Organization have helped with much of the academic work that preceded this book, and I am very proud to work alongside them, including Nigel Rollins, Tony Waterston, Larry Grummer-Strawn, Nina Chad and Anna Gruending.

Victoria Kent and Sarah Halpin refined many ideas about UPF and cooked me lots of non-UPF. Vic explained investment and money in a way that even I could understand.

The team at the National Food Strategy has fed me well many times and shaped much of the discussion in the book. Tamsin Cooper and Henry (and Jemima) Dimbleby really taught me how to approach this subject. That's why you will see their plan referenced so often in these pages.

Jo Rowntree, Philly Beaumont, Richard Berry and Hester Cant made the podcast *Addicted to Food*, which preceded this book. They're all amazing and made me think harder about food than I ever have before.

Thanks also to Marion Nestle, Phil Baker, Nicole Avena, Sadaf Farooqi, Andrea Sella, Mélissa Mialon, Bob Boyle, Gordon Hamilton and his whole family and Susan Jebb (over many documentaries together, Susan has been incredibly helpful).

The scientists, activists and clinicians who take big pay cuts to spend their lives reducing inequality and making the world a better, nicer place for everyone that lives in it, including for me and my children. It's always easier to take the money from Coke.

Everyone at the Hospital for Tropical Diseases (but especially Sarah Logan, Phil Gothard and Mike Brown) has helped to find a way of making my professional life work. I'm lucky to work at a world-class hospital, UCLH, surrounded by people who support and challenge me as well as giving me the flexibility to have a career that sits alongside my clinical work.

The people I work with each week are a source of continuous inspiration, brilliant people in every respect. Anna Checkley, Anna Last and Nicky Longley get a special shout-out.

The comms team at UCLH are unsurprisingly central to much of the overlap between my clinical, academic and broadcasting work, especially Rachel Maybank, Sharon Spiteri and Michaela Keating.

Being an NHS doctor is a privilege and the people I learn the most from are my patients, who have taught me that what we eat is much more about our environment than our desires. The NHS is one of the last bulwarks against the commercial forces that are now the leading cause of early death on our planet. If we privatise healthcare and allow it to operate with the same set of incentives as the food and tobacco companies, we will lose something that can never be rebuilt. This is a real and urgent risk.

I'm grateful to UCL for giving me an academic home and huge freedom to go with it. Greg Towers and Richard Milne coaxed a PhD out of me, and their way of investigating the world influences everything I do. They both read early drafts and were very helpful.

The *British Medical Journal* (in particular: Rebecca Coombes, Fi Godlee, Kamran Abbasi, Jennifer Richardson and Peter Doshi) has supported my academic work over many years. More than that, it has responded to its own publications by refusing formula industry sponsorship. I am always impossibly proud to publish in its pages.

Julian Marks from Barfoots was incredibly generous with his time and knowledge and perfectly explained all things fruit and veg. My friend Nick Seddon helped me understand at least some of the inner workings of government and policy.

Thanks to the whole Sheldrake family but especially Merlin for explaining how to write a book: 'It's like a party – everyone has to know where the toilets are and everyone needs a drink.' April Smith and Jackie Dalton hold the whole show together for us at home. Elke Maier sent me invaluable research about coal butter. Adam Rutherford, Hannah Fry, Mark Schatzker, Gin Drinkers of Oak Room, Dr Ronx, Amy Brown, Henry and Nicola Byam-Cook, Margaret McCartney, Ralph Woodling (who told me about electrons and chemistry), Max Hardy, Nick Macan, Rupert Winckler, Ed vdBurg, Bruce Parry, James Blount, Hen Peace, Stuart Gillespie, Caroline and Imogen Barter (Caroline is responsible for so much that is good in my life, including Imogen), the SBs, Layal Liverpool, Eszter Vamos, Dev Sharma, Christina Adane, Jamie Oliver, Nicki Whiteman, Vicki Cooper, Monika Ghosh, The SBWAG, Zeba Lowe and Dan Brocklebank (another old pal who understands money and is good at explaining it). Rosie Haines (who owns the Scolt Head pub and Sweet Thursday pizzeria, which are my best and only sources of non-UPF fast food), Andreas Wesemann (who told me about economics and abused me for lazy thinking). Alasdair Cant fixed my relationship with my brother and made me understand that demanding change is not the best way to achieve it. The *Operation Ouch!* team are like family and have tolerated weeks of useful UPF discussion.

I live with my amazing mother-in-law, Christine, who is a constant inspiration to me, Dinah and my daughters. I rest my computer on her PhD thesis, so I am literally basing this book on her work (and she has a huge influence over my general behaviour in the best way).

My brothers and sisters-in-law (Ryan, Chid, Martha and Leah) are the very best and I'm impossibly lucky to have them as family.

Acknowledgements

My brothers, Xand and J (Bratty), are my best friends, and I don't do anything without discussing it at tedious length with both of them. Their opinion counts for more than anyone else's, apart from (in this case) Helen Conford's. Xand, my twin, shaped the central thesis over a decade of physical fights and screaming arguments, which in the end he has won. J is the glue that binds me and Xand together.

My perfect nephew Julian probably doesn't realise how much he makes me and Xand think about lots of stuff in these pages.

My two daughters are the only people in these acknowledgements who have taken no interest whatsoever in this book. They are both avid consumers of UPF and, aside from being unsurprisingly willing participants in many eating trials, their contribution has been exclusively negative.

Finally, my wife Dinah, who is responsible for everything good in my life. She hates this sort of thing, but she's the best person I've ever met.

Notes

Introduction

1 Jacobs FMJ, Greenberg D, Nguyen N, et al. An evolutionary arms race between KRAB zinc-finger genes *ZNF91/93* and *SVA/L1* retrotransposons. *Nature* 2014; 516: 242–45.

2 Villarreal L. *Viruses and the Evolution of Life*. London: ASM Press, 2005.

3 Hauge HS. Anomalies on Alaskan wolf skulls. 1985. Available from: http://www.adfg.alaska.gov/static/home/library/pdfs/wildlife/research_pdfs/anomalies_alaskan_wolf_skulls.pdf.

4 Mech LD, Nelson ME. Evidence of prey-caused mortality in three wolves. *The American Midland Naturalist* 1990; 123: 207–08.

5 Rauber F, Chang K, Vamos EP, et al. Ultra-processed food consumption and risk of obesity: a prospective cohort study of UK Biobank. *European Journal of Nutrition* 2020; 60: 2169–80.

6 Chang K, Khandpur N, Neri D, et al. Association between childhood consumption of ultraprocessed food and adiposity trajectories in the Avon Longitudinal Study of Parents and Children birth cohort. *JAMA Pediatrics* 2021; 175: e211573.

7 Baraldi LG, Martinez Steele E, Canella DS, et al. Consumption of ultra-processed foods and associated sociodemographic factors in the USA between 2007 and 2012: evidence from a nationally representative cross-sectional study. *BMJ Open* 2018; 8: e020574.

8 Rodgers A, Woodward A, Swinburn B, Dietz WH. Prevalence trends tell us what did not precipitate the US obesity epidemic. *Lancet Public Health*. 2018 Apr; 3(4):e162–3.

9 Theis DRZ, White M. Is obesity policy in England fit for purpose? Analysis of government strategies and policies, 1992–2020. *The Milbank Quarterly* 2021; 99: 126–70.

10 Cole T. Personal communication. 2022.

11 NCD Risk Factor Collaboration. Height and body-mass index trajectories of school-aged children and adolescents from 1985 to 2019 in 200 countries and territories: a pooled analysis of 2181 population-based studies with 65 million participants. *Lancet* 2020; 396: 1511–24.

12 National Food Strategy. National food strategy (independent review): the plan. 2021. Available from: https://assets.publishing.service.gov.uk/government/uploads/system/uploads/attachment_data/file/1025825/national-food-strategy-the-plan.pdf.

13 UK Government. Obesity statistics. 2022. Available from: https://researchbriefings.files.parliament.uk/documents/SN03336/SN03336.pdf.

14 Hiscock R, Bauld L, Amos A, Platt S. Smoking and socioeconomic status in England: the rise of the never smoker and the disadvantaged smoker. *Journal of Public Health* 2012; 34: 390–96.

1. Why is there bacterial slime in my ice cream? The invention of UPF

1 Avison Z. Why UK consumers spend 8% of their money on food. 2020. Available from: https://ahdb.org.uk/news/consumer-insight-why-uk-consumers-spend-8-of-their-money-on-food.

2 Office for National Statistics. Living costs and food survey. 2017. Available from: https://www.ons.gov.uk/peoplepopulationandcommunity/personalandhouseholdfinances/incomeandwealth/methodologies/livingcostsandfoodsurvey.

3 Scott C, Sutherland J, Taylor A. Affordability of the UK's Eatwell Guide. 2018. Available from https://foodfoundation.org.uk/sites/default/files/2021-10/Affordability-of-the-Eatwell-Guide_Final_Web-Version.pdf.

4 BeMiller JN. One hundred years of commercial food carbohydrates in the United States. *Journal of Agricultural and Food Chemistry* 2009; 57: 8125–29.

5 Centre for Industrial Rheology. Hellman's [sic] *vs* Heinz: mayonnaise fat reduction rheology. Available from: https://www.rheologylab.com/articles/food/fat-replacement/.

6 di Lernia S, Gallinaro M. The date and context of neolithic rock art in the Sahara: engravings and ceremonial monuments from Messak Settafet (south-west Libya). *Antiquity* 2010; 84: 954–75.

7 di Lernia S, Gallinaro M, 2010.

8 Dunne J, Evershed RP, Salque M, et al. First dairying in green Saharan Africa in the fifth millennium BC. *Nature* 2012; 486: 390–94.

9 Evershed RP, Davey Smith G, Roffet-Salque M, et al. Dairying, diseases and the evolution of lactase persistence in Europe. *Nature* 2022; 608: 336–45.

10 List GR. Hippolyte Mège (1817–1880). *Inform* 2006; 17: 264.

11 Rupp R. The butter wars: when margarine was pink. 2014. Available from: https://www.nationalgeographic.com/culture/article/the-butter-wars-when-margarine-was-pink.

12 Khosrova E. *Butter: A Rich History*. London: Appetite by Random House, 2016.

13 McGee H. *On Food and Cooking: The Science and Lore of the Kitchen* (revised edition). London: Scribner, 2007.

14 Snodgrass K. Margarine as a butter substitute. *Oil & Fat Industries* 1931; 8: 153.

15 SCRAN. Whale oil uses. 2002. Available from: http://www.scran.ac.uk/packs/exhibitions/learning_materials/webs/40/margarine.htm.

16 Nixon HC. The rise of the American cottonseed oil industry. *Journal of Political Economy* 1930; 38: 73–85.

2. I'd rather have five bowls of Coco Pops: the discovery of UPF

1 Monteiro CA, Cannon G, Lawrence M, et al. Ultra-processed foods, diet quality, and health using the NOVA classification system. Rome: Food and Agriculture Organization of the United Nations, 2019.

2 Ioannidis JPA. Why most published research findings are false. *pLoS Medicine* 2005; 2: e124.

3 Rauber F, da Costa Louzada ML, Steele EM, et al. Ultra-processed food consumption and chronic non-communicable diseases-related dietary nutrient profile in the UK (2008–2014). *Nutrients* 2018; 10: 587.

4 Rauber et al, 2020.

5 Chang et al, 2021.

6 Rauber F, Steele EM, da Costa Louzada ML, et al. Ultra-processed food consumption and indicators of obesity in the United Kingdom population (2008–2016). *pLoS One* 2020; 15: e0232676.

7 Martínez Steele E, Juul F, Neri D, Rauber F, Monteiro CA. Dietary share of ultra-processed foods and metabolic syndrome in the US adult population. *Preventive Medicine* 2019; 125: 40–48.

8 Public Health England. Annex A: The 2018 review of the UK Nutrient Profiling Model. 2018. Available at https://assets.publishing.service.gov.uk/government/uploads/system/uploads/attachment_data/file/694145/Annex__A_the_2018_review_of_the_UK_nutrient_profiling_model.pdf.

9 Levy-Costa RB, Sichieri R, dos Santos Pontes N, et al. Household food availability in Brazil: distribution and trends (1974–2003). *Revista de Saúde Pública* 2005; 39: 530–40.

10 Pollan, M. Unhappy meals. 2007. Available at https://www.nytimes.com/2007/01/28/magazine/28nutritionism.t.html.

11 Rutjes AW, Denton DA, Di Nisio M, et al. Vitamin and mineral supplementation for maintaining cognitive function in cognitively healthy people in mid and late life. *Cochrane Database of Systematic Reviews* 2018; 12: CD011906.

12 Singal M, Banh HL, Allan GM. Daily multivitamins to reduce mortality, cardiovascular disease, and cancer. *Canadian Family Physician* 2013; 59: 847.

13 Officer CE. Antioxidant supplements for prevention of mortality in healthy participants and patients with various diseases. *Cochrane Database of Systematic Reviews* 2012; 3: CD007176.

14 Snowdon C. What is "ultra-processed food"? 2022. Available from: https://velvetgloveironfist.blogspot.com/2022/01/what-is-ultra-processed-food.html.

15 Your Fat Friend. The bizarre and racist history of the BMI. 2019. Available from: https://elemental.medium.com/the-bizarre-and-racist-history-of-the-bmi-7d8dc2aa33bb.

3. Sure, 'ultra-processed food' sounds bad, but is it really a problem?

1 Hall KD, Sacks G, Chandramohan D, et al. Quantification of the effect of energy imbalance on bodyweight. *Lancet* 2011; 378: 826–37.

2 Fothergill E, Guo J, Howard L, et al. Diet versus exercise in 'The Biggest Loser' weight loss competition. *Obesity* 2013; 21: 957–59.

3 Hall KD, Ayuketah A, Brychta R, et al. Ultra-processed diets cause excess calorie intake and weight gain: an inpatient randomized controlled trial of ad libitum food intake. *Cellular Metabolism* 2019; 30: 67–77.

4 Martini D, Godos J, Bonaccio M, et al. Ultra-processed foods and nutritional dietary profile: a meta-analysis of nationally representative samples. *Nutrients* 2021; 13: 3390.

5 October 28. Health inequalities and obesity. 2020. Available from: https://www.rcplondon.ac.uk/news/health-inequalities-and-obesity.

6 Fiolet T, Srour B, Sellem L, et al. Consumption of ultra-processed foods and cancer risk: results from NutriNet-Santé prospective cohort. *British Medical Journal* 2018; 360: k322.

7 Zhong G-C, Gu H-T, Peng Y, et al. Association of ultra-processed food consumption with cardiovascular mortality in the US population: long-term results from a large prospective multicenter study. *International Journal of Behavioral Nutrition and Physical Activity* 2021; 18: 21.

8 Schnabel L, Kesse-Guyot E, Allès B, et al. Association between ultra-processed food consumption and risk of mortality among middle-aged adults in France. *JAMA Internal Medicine* 2019; 179: 490–98.

9 Rico-Campà A, Martínez-González MA, Alvarez-Alvarez I, et al. Association between consumption of ultra-processed foods and all cause mortality: SUN prospective cohort study. *British Medical Journal* 2019; 365: l1949.

10 Kim H, Hu EA, Rebholz CM. Ultra-processed food intake and mortality in the USA: results from the Third National Health and Nutrition Examination Survey (NHANES III, 1988–1994). *Public Health Nutrition* 2019; 22: 1777–85.

11 Bonaccio M, Di Castelnuovo A, Costanzo S, et al. Ultra-processed food consumption is associated with increased risk of all-cause and cardiovascular mortality in the Moli-sani Study. *American Journal of Clinical Nutrition* 2021; 113: 446–55.

12 Chen X, Chu J, Hu W, et al. Associations of ultra-processed food consumption with cardiovascular disease and all-cause mortality: UK Biobank. *European Journal of Public Health* 2022; 32: 779–85.

13 Bonaccio et al, 2021.

14 Kim et al, 2021.

15 Srour B, Fezeu LK, Kesse-Guyot E, et al. Ultra-processed food intake and risk of cardiovascular disease: prospective cohort study (Nutri-Net-Santé). *British Medical Journal* 2019; 365: l1451.

16 Fiolet et al, 2018.

17 Llavero-Valero M, Martín JE-S, Martínez-González MA, et al. Ultra-processed foods and type-2 diabetes risk in the SUN project: a prospective cohort study. *Clinical Nutrition* 2021; 40: 2817–24.

18 Srour B, Fezeu LK, Kesse-Guyot E, et al. Ultraprocessed food consumption and risk of type 2 diabetes among participants of the NutriNet-Santé prospective cohort. *JAMA Internal Medicine* 2020; 180: 283–91.

19 Jardim MZ, Costa BVdL, Pessoa MC, et al. Ultra-processed foods increase noncommunicable chronic disease risk. *Nutrition Research* 2021; 95: 19–34.

20 Silva Meneguelli T, Viana Hinkelmann J, Hermsdorff HHM, et al. Food consumption by degree of processing and cardiometabolic risk: a systematic review. *International Journal of Food Sciences and Nutrition* 2020; 71: 678–92.

21 de Mendonça RD, Lopes ACS, Pimenta AM, et al. Ultra-processed food consumption and the incidence of hypertension in a Mediterranean cohort: the Seguimiento Universidad de Navarra Project. *American Journal of Hypertension* 2017; 30: 358–66.

22 Zhang S, Gan S, Zhang Q, et al. Ultra-processed food consumption and the risk of non-alcoholic fatty liver disease in the Tianjin Chronic Low-Grade Systemic Inflammation and Health Cohort Study. *International Journal of Epidemiology* 2021; 51: 237–49.

23 Narula N, Wong ECL, Dehghan M, et al. Association of ultra-processed food intake with risk of inflammatory bowel disease: prospective cohort study. *British Medical Journal* 2021; 374: n1554.

24 Lo C-H, Khandpur N, Rossato S, et al. Ultra-processed foods and risk of Crohn's disease and ulcerative colitis: a prospective cohort study. *Clinical Gastroenterology and Hepatology* 2022; 20: 1323–37.

25 Gómez-Donoso C, Sánchez-Villegas A, Martínez-González MA, et al. Ultra-processed food consumption and the incidence of depression in

a Mediterranean cohort: the SUN project. *European Journal of Nutrition* 2020; 59:1093–103.

26 Schnabel L, Buscail C, Sabate J-M, et al. Association between ultra-processed food consumption and functional gastrointestinal disorders: results from the French NutriNet-Santé cohort. *American Journal of Gastroenterology* 2018; 113: 1217–28.

27 Zhang S, Gu Y, Rayamajhi S, et al. Ultra-processed food intake is associated with grip strength decline in middle-aged and older adults: a prospective analysis of the TCLSIH study. *European Journal of Nutrition* 2022; 61: 1331–41.

28 Schnabel et al, 2018.

29 Li H, Li S, Yang H, et al. Association of ultraprocessed food consumption with risk of dementia: a prospective cohort study. *Neurology* 2022; 99: e1056–66.

30 Li et al, 2022.

31 Bonaccio et al, 2021.

32 Kim et al, 2019.

33 Chen et al, 2022.

34 Rico-Campà et al, 2019.

35 Romero Ferreiro C, Lora Pablos D, Gómez de la Cámara A. Two dimensions of nutritional value: Nutri-Score and NOVA. *Nutrients* 2021; 13(8).

36 Gibney MJ, Forde CG, Mullally D, Gibney ER. Ultra-processed foods in human health: a critical appraisal. *American Journal of Clinical Nutrition* 2017; 106: 717–24.

37 Tobias DK, Hall KD. Eliminate or reformulate ultra-processed foods? Biological mechanisms matter. *Cell Metabolism* 2021; 33: 2314–15.

38 Corrigendum to *The American Journal of Clinical Nutrition*, Volume 107, Issue 3, March 2018, Pages 482–3. Available from: https://academic.oup.com/ajcn/article/107/3/482/4939379.

39 Jones JM. Food processing: criteria for dietary guidance and public health? *Proceedings of the Nutrition Society* 2019; 78: 4–18.

40 Knorr D, Watzke H. Food processing at a crossroad. *Frontiers in Nutrition* 2019; 6: 85.

41 Sadler CR, Grassby T, Hart K, et al. "Even we are confused": a thematic analysis of professionals' perceptions of processed foods

and challenges for communication. *Frontiers in Nutrition* 2022; 9: 826162.

42 Flacco ME, Manzoli L, Boccia S, et al. Head-to-head randomized trials are mostly industry sponsored and almost always favor the industry sponsor. *Journal of Clinical Epidemiology* 2015; 68: 811–20.

43 Stamatakis E, Weiler R, Ioannidis JPA. Undue industry influences that distort healthcare research, strategy, expenditure and practice: a review. European Journal of Clinical Investigation 2013; 43: 469–75.

44 Ioannidis JPA. Evidence-based medicine has been hijacked: a report to David Sackett. *Journal of Clinical Epidemiology* 2016; 73: 82–86.

45 Fabbri A, Lai A, Grundy Q, Bero LA. The influence of industry sponsorship on the research agenda: a scoping review. *American Journal of Public Health* 2018; 108: e9–16.

46 Lundh A, Lexchin J, Mintzes B, et al. Industry sponsorship and research outcome. *Cochrane Database of Systematic Reviews* 2017; 2: MR000033.

47 Rasmussen K, Bero L, Redberg R, et al. Collaboration between academics and industry in clinical trials: cross sectional study of publications and survey of lead academic authors. *British Medical Journal* 2018; 363: 3654.

4. *(I can't believe it's not) coal butter: the ultimate UPF*

1 Engelberg S, Gordon MR. Germans accused of helping Libya build nerve gas plant. 1989. Available from: https://www.nytimes.com/1989/01/01/world/germans-accused-of-helping-libya-build-nerve-gas-plant.html.

2 Second Wiki. Arthur Imhausen. 2007 [cited 2022 Mar 21]. Available from: https://second.wiki/wiki/arthur_imhausen.

3 Maier E. Coal – in liquid form. 2016. Available from: https://www.mpg.de/10856815/S004_Flashback_078–079.pdf.

4 Imhausen A. Die Fettsäure-Synthese und ihre Bedeutung für die Sicherung der deutschen Fettversorgung. *Kolloid-Zeitschrift* 1943; 103: 105–08.

5 Imhausen A, 1943.

6 Barona JL. *From Hunger to Malnutrition: The Political Economy of Scientific Knowledge in Europe, 1918–1960*. Pieterlen, Switzerland: Peter Lang AG, 2012.

7 Evonik. Arthur Imhausen, chemist and entrepreneur. 2020. Available from: https://history.evonik.com/en/personalities/imhausen-arthur.

8 Maier, 2016.

9 Dockrell M. Clearing up some myths around e-cigarettes. 2018. Available from: https://ukhsa.blog.gov.uk/2018/02/20/clearing-up-some-myths-around-e-cigarettes/.

10 Kopper C. Helmut Maier, Chemiker im 'Dritten Reich'. Die Deutsche Chemische Gesellschaft und der Verein Deutscher Chemiker im NS-Herrschaftsapparat. Im Auftrag der Gesellschaft Deutscher Chemiker. Weinheim, Wiley-VCH 2015. *Historische Zeitschrift* 2017; 305: 269–70.

11 Von Cornberg JNMSF. Willkür in der Willkür: Befreiungen von den antisemitischen Nürnberger Gesetzen. *Vierteljahrshefte für Zeitgeschichte* 1998; 46: 143–87.

12 Von Cornberg, 1998.

13 Stolberg-Wernigerode O. *Neue Deutsche Biographie*. Berlin: Duncker & Humblot, 1974.

14 Emessen TR. *Aus Görings Schreibtisch ein Dokumentenfund*. Dortmund: Historisches Kabinett, Allgemeiner Deutscher Verlag, 1947.

15 Breitman R. *The Architect of Genocide: Himmler and the Final Solution*. New York: Alfred A Knopf, 1991.

16 Imhausen A, 1943.

17 Proctor R. *The Nazi War on Cancer*. Princeton: Princeton University Press, 2000.

18 British Intelligence Objectives Sub-Committee. Available from: http://www.fischer-tropsch.org/primary_documents/gvt_reports/BIOS/biostoc.htm.

19 Floessner O. *Synthetische Fette Beitraege zur Ernaehrungsphysiologie*. Leipzig: Barth, 1948.

20 British Intelligence Objectives Sub-Committee. Synthetic Fatty Acids and Detergents. Available from: http://www.fischer-tropsch.org/primary_documents/gvt_reports/BIOS/bios_1722htm/bios_1722_htm_sec14.htm.

21 Kraut H. The physiological value of synthetic fats. *British Journal of Nutrition* 1949; 3: 355–58.

22 *The Eagle Valley Enterprise.* Butter is made by Germans from coal. 1946. Available from: https://www.coloradohistoricnewspapers. org/?a=d&d=EVE19460906-01.2.29&e=-------en-20--1--img-txIN%7ct xCO%7ctxTA--------o------.

23 Thompson J. Butter from coal: The Grafic Laboratory of Popular Science. *Chicago Daily Tribune* 1946; C2.

24 Historische Kommission für Westfalen. Ingenieure im Ruhrgebiet Rheinisch-Westfälische Wirtschaftsbiographien Volume 17. Aschendorff; 2019.

25 Evonik, 2020.

26 Andrews EL. The business world; IG Farben: a lingering relic of the Nazi years. 1999. Available from: https://www.nytimes.com/1999/ 05/02/business/the-business-world-ig-farben-a-lingering-relic-of-the-nazi-years.html.

27 Marek M. Norbert Wollheim gegen IG Farben. 2012. Available from: https://www.dw.com/de/norbert-wollheim-gegen-ig-farben/a-16373141.

28 Johnson JA. Corporate morality in the Third Reich. 2009. Available from: https://www.sciencehistory.org/distillations/corporate-morality-in-the-third-reich.

29 Andrews, 1999.

30 Marek, 2012.

31 Johnson, 2009.

32 Staunton D. Holocaust survivors protest at IG Farben meeting. 1999. Available from: https://www.irishtimes.com/news/holocaust-survivors-protest-at-ig-farben-meeting-1.218051.

33 *Der Spiegel.* IG-Farben-Insolvenz: Ehemalige Zwangsarbeiter gehen leer aus. 2003. Available from: https://www.spiegel.de/wirtschaft/i-g-farben-insolvenz-ehemalige-zwangsarbeiter-gehen-leer-aus-a-273365.html.

34 Charles J. Former Zyklon-B maker goes bust. 2003. Available from: http://news.bbc.co.uk/1/hi/business/3257403.stm.

35 *Der Spiegel*, 2003.

36 *Der Spiegel.* Die Schweizer Konten waren alle abgeräumt. 1993. Available from: https://www-spiegel-de.translate.goog/politik/die-schweizer-konten-waren-alle-abgeraeumt-a-e59c3df1-0002–0001-0000–000009286542.

37 *Der Spiegel*. Zwanzig Minuten Kohlenklau. 1947. Available from: https://www.spiegel.de/politik/zwanzig-minuten-kohlenklau-a-9896e990-0002–0001-0000–000041123785?context=issue.

38 Daepp MIG, Hamilton MJ, et al. The mortality of companies. *Journal of the Royal Society Interface* 2015; 12: 20150120.

39 Strotz LC, Simões M, Girard MG, et al. Getting somewhere with the Red Queen: chasing a biologically modern definition of the hypothesis. *Biology Letters* 2018; 14: 20170734.

40 Van Valen L. Extinction of taxa and Van Valen's law (reply). *Nature* 1975; 257: 515–16.

41 Van Valen L. A new evolutionary law. *Evolutionary Theory* 1973; 1: 1–30.

42 Van Valen L. The Red Queen. *American Naturalist* 1977; 111: 809–10.

43 Kraut, 1949.

5. The three ages of eating

1 Bell EA, Boehnke P, Harrison TM, et al. Potentially biogenic carbon preserved in a 4.1-billion-year-old zircon. *Proceedings of the National Academy of Sciences USA* 2015; 112: 14518–21.

2 Bell et al, 2015.

3 Alleon J, Bernard S, Le Guillo C, et al. Chemical nature of the 3.4 Ga Strelley Pool microfossils. *Geochemical Perspectives Letters* 2018; 7: 37–42.

4 Cavalazzi B, Lemelle L, Simionovici A, et al. Cellular remains in a ~3.42-billion-year-old subseafloor hydrothermal environment. *Science Advances* 2021; 7: abf3963.

5 Dodd MS, Papineau D, Grenne T, et al. Evidence for early life in Earth's oldest hydrothermal vent precipitates. *Nature* 2017; 543: 60–64.

6 Gramling C. Hints of oldest fossil life found in Greenland rocks. 2016. Available from: http://www.sciencemag.org/news/2016/08/hints-oldest-fossil-life-found-greenland-rocks.

7 Li W, Beard BL, Johnson CM. Biologically recycled continental iron is a major component in banded iron formations. *Proceedings of the National Academy of Sciences USA* 2015; 112: 8193–98.

8   Haugaard R, Pecoits E, Lalonde S, et al. The Joffre banded iron forma-
    tion, Hamersley Group, Western Australia: assessing the palaeo-
    environment through detailed petrology and chemostratigraphy.
    Precambrian Research 2016; 273: 12–37.

9   Powell H. Fertilizing the ocean with iron. 2022. Available from:
    https://www.whoi.edu/oceanus/feature/fertilizing-the-ocean-with-
    iron/.

10 Retallack GJ. First evidence for locomotion in the Ediacara biota from
    the 565 Ma Mistaken Point Formation, Newfoundland: COMMENT.
    Geology 2010; 38: e223.

11 Chen Z, Zhou C, Meyer M, et al. Trace fossil evidence for Ediacaran
    bilaterian animals with complex behaviors. *Precambrian Research* 2013;
    224: 690–701.

12 Retallack, 2010.

13 Peterson KJ, Cotton JA, Gehling JG, et al. The Ediacaran emergence
    of bilaterians: congruence between the genetic and the geological
    fossil records. *Philosophical Transactions of the Royal Society B* 2008; 363:
    1435–43.

14 Weidenbach K. *Rock Star: The Story of Reg Sprigg – an Outback Legend.*
    Kensington: East Street Publications, 2008.

15 Weidenbach, 2008.

16 Mote T, Villalba JJ, Provenza FD. Foraging sequence influences the
    ability of lambs to consume foods containing tannins and terpenes.
    *Behavioral Education for Human, Animal, Vegetation, and Ecosystem Man-
    agement* 2008; 113: 57–68.

17 Villalba JJ, Provenza FD, Manteca X. Links between ruminants' food
    preference and their welfare. *Animal* 2010; 4: 1240–47.

18 Provenza F. *Nourishment: What Animals Can Teach Us about Rediscovering
    Our Nutritional Wisdom.* Hartford, VT: Chelsea Green Publishing, 2018.

19 Mote et al, 2008.

20 Hoste H, Meza-Ocampos G, Marchand S, et al. Use of agro-industrial
    by-products containing tannins for the integrated control of gastro-
    intestinal nematodes in ruminants. *Parasite* 2022; 29:10.

21 Boback SM, Cox CL, Ott BD, et al. Cooking and grinding reduces the
    cost of meat digestion. *Comparative Biochemistry & Physiology* 2007;
    148: 651–66.

22 Furness JB, Bravo DM. Humans as cucinivores: comparisons with other species. *Journal of Comparative Physiology B* 2015; 185: 825–34.

23 Zink KD, Lieberman DE, Lucas PW. Food material properties and early hominin processing techniques. *Journal of Human Evolution* 2014; 77: 155–66.

24 Stevens CE, Hume ID. *Comparative Physiology of the Vertebrate Digestive System*. Cambridge: Cambridge University Press, 2004.

25 Koebnick C, Strassner C, Hoffmann I, et al. Consequences of a long-term raw food diet on body weight and menstruation: results of a questionnaire survey. *Annals of Nutrition and Metabolism* 1999; 43: 69–79.

26 *Scientific American*. The inventor of saccharin. 1886. Available from: https://web.archive.org/web/20170314015912/https:/books.google.com/books?id=f4I9AQAAIAAJ&pg=PA36#v=onepage&q&f=false.

27 Brown HT, Morris GH. On the non-crystallisable products of the action of diastase upon starch. *Journal of the Chemical Society, Transactions* 1885; 47: 527–70.

28 Mepham B. Food additives: an ethical evaluation. *British Medical Bulletin* 2011; 99: 7–23.

29 Powers G. Infant feeding. Historical background and modern practice. *Journal of the American Medical Association* 1935; 105: 753–61.

30 Scheindlin B. "Take one more bite for me": Clara Davis and the feeding of young children. *Gastronomica* 2005; 5: 65–69.

31 Davis CM. Self-regulation of diet in childhood. *Health Education Journal* 1947; 5: 37–40.

32 Scheindlin, 2005.

6. How our bodies really manage calories

1 Chusyd DE, Nagy TR, Golzarri-Arroyo L, et al. Adiposity, reproductive and metabolic health, and activity levels in zoo Asian elephant (*Elephas maximus*). *Journal of Experimental Biology* 2021; 224: jeb219543.

2 Pontzer H, Brown MH, Raichlen DA, et al. Metabolic acceleration and the evolution of human brain size and life history. *Nature* 2016; 533: 390–92.

3 Pontzer H, Raichlen DA, Wood BM, Mabulla AZP, Racette SB, Marlowe FW. Hunter-gatherer energetics and human obesity. *pLoS One* 2012; 7: e40503.

4 Klimentidis YC, Beasley TM, Lin H-Y, et al. Canaries in the coal mine: a cross-species analysis of the plurality of obesity epidemics. *Proceedings of the Royal Society B* 2011; 278: 1626–32.

5 *ABC News*. Is 'Big Food's' big money influencing the science of nutrition? 2011. Available from: https://abcnews.go.com/US/big-food-money-accused-influencing-science/story?id=13845186.

6 Saul S. Obesity Researcher Quits Over New York Menu Fight. The *New York Times* [Internet]. 2008 Mar 3 [cited 2022 Feb 28]; Available from: https://www.nytimes.com/2008/03/03/business/03cnd-obese.html.

7 McDermott L. Self-representation in upper paleolithic female figurines. *Current Anthropology* 1996; 37: 227–75.

8 Michalopoulos A, Tzelepis G, Geroulanos S. Morbid obesity and hypersomnolence in several members of an ancient royal family. *Thorax* 2003; 58: 281–82.

9 Buchwald H. A brief history of obesity: truths and illusions. 2018. Available from: https://www.clinicaloncology.com/Current-Practice/Article/07–18/A-Brief-History-of-Obesity-Truths-and-Illusions/51221.

10 O'Rahilly S. Harveian Oration 2016: some observations on the causes and consequences of obesity. *Clinical Medicine* 2016; 16: 551–64.

11 Corbyn Z. Could 'young' blood stop us getting old? 2020. Available from: https://amp.theguardian.com/society/2020/feb/02/could-young-blood-stop-us-getting-old-transfusions-experiments-mice-plasma.

12 Kosoff M. Peter Thiel wants to inject himself with young people's blood. 2016. Available from: https://www.vanityfair.com/news/2016/08/peter-thiel-wants-to-inject-himself-with-young-peoples-blood.

13 Hervey GR. The effects of lesions in the hypothalamus in parabiotic rats. *J Physiol.* 1959 Mar 3;145(2):336–52.

14 Paz-Filho G, Mastronardi C, Delibasi T, et al. Congenital leptin deficiency: diagnosis and effects of leptin replacement therapy. *Arquivos Brasileiros de Endocrinologia & Metabologia* 2010; 54: 690–97.

15 Murray EA, Wise SP, Rhodes SEV. What can different brains do with reward? In: Gottfried JA, editor. *Neurobiology of Sensation and Reward.* Boca Raton, FL: CRC Press/Taylor & Francis, 2012.

16 Hall KD, Farooqi IS, Friedman JM, et al. The energy balance model of obesity: beyond calories in, calories out. *American Journal of Clinical Nutrition* 2022; 115: 1243–54.

7. *Why it isn't about sugar ...*

1 Petersen MC, Shulman GI. Mechanisms of insulin action and insulin resistance. *Physiological Reviews* 2018; 98: 2133–223.

2 Liebman, Bonnie/Center for Science in the Public Interest. Big Fat Lies – The Truth About the Atkins Diet. Nutrition Action [Internet]. 2002 Nov; 29. Available from: https://cspinet.org/sites/default/files/attachment/bigfatlies.pdf.

3 Hall KD, Chen KY, Guo J, et al. Energy expenditure and body composition changes after an isocaloric ketogenic diet in overweight and obese men. *American Journal of Clinical Nutrition* 2016; 104: 324–33.

4 Hall KD. A review of the carbohydrate-insulin model of obesity. *European Journal of Clinical Nutrition* 2017; 71: 323–26.

5 Gardner CD, Trepanowski JF, Del Gobbo LC, et al. Effect of low-fat vs low-carbohydrate diet on 12-month weight loss in overweight adults and the association with genotype pattern or insulin secretion: the DIETFITS randomized clinical trial. *Journal of the American Medical Association* 2018; 319: 667–79.

6 Low-fat diet compared to low-carb diet [Internet]. National Institutes of Health (NIH). 2021 [cited 2022 Sep 4]. Available from: https://www.nih.gov/news-events/nih-research-matters/low-fat-diet-compared-low-carb-diet.

7 Hall KD, Guo J, Courville AB, et al. Effect of a plant-based, low-fat diet versus an animal-based, ketogenic diet on ad libitum energy intake. *Nature Medicine* 2021; 27: 344–53.

8 Foster GD, Wyatt HR, Hill JO, et al. A randomized trial of a low-carbohydrate diet for obesity. *New England Journal of Medicine* 2003; 348: 2082–90.

9 Ebbeling CB, Feldman HA, Klein GL, et al. Effects of a low carbohydrate diet on energy expenditure during weight loss maintenance: randomized trial. *British Medical Journal* 2018; 363: k4583.

10 Hall KD, Guo J, Speakman JR. Do low-carbohydrate diets increase energy expenditure? *International Journal of Obesity* 2019; 43: 2350–54.

11 Martin-McGill KJ, Bresnahan R, Levy RG. Ketogenic diets for drug-resistant epilepsy. *Cochrane Database of Systematic Reviews* 2020; 6: CD001903.

12 Mintz SW. *Sweetness and Power: The Place of Sugar in Modern History.* London: Penguin Publishing Group, 1985.

13 Hardy K, Brand-Miller J, Brown KD, et al. The importance of dietary carbohydrate in human evolution. *Quarterly Review of Biology* 2015; 90: 251–68.

14 Soares S, Amaral JS, Oliveira MBPP, Mafra I. A comprehensive review on the main honey authentication issues: production and origin. *Comprehensive Reviews in Food Science and Food Safety* 2017; 16: 1072–100.

15 Sammataro D, Weiss M. Comparison of productivity of colonies of honey bees, *Apis mellifera*, supplemented with sucrose or high fructose corn syrup. *Journal of Insect Science* 2013; 13: 19.

16 Marlowe FW, Berbesque JC, Wood B, et al. Honey, Hadza, hunter-gatherers, and human evolution. *Journal of Human Evolution* 2014; 71: 119–28.

17 Reddy A, Norris DF, Momeni SS, et al. The pH of beverages in the United States. *Journal of the American Dental Association* 2016; 147: 255–63.

18 Public Health England. Child oral health: applying All Our Health. 2022. Available from: https://www.gov.uk/government/publications/child-oral-health-applying-all-our-health/child-oral-health-applying-all-our-health.

19 Public Health England. National Dental Epidemiology Programme for England: oral health survey of five-year-old children 2017. Available from: https://assets.publishing.service.gov.uk/government/uploads/system/uploads/attachment_data/file/768368/NDEP_for_England_OH_Survey_5yr_2017_Report.pdf.

20 Touger-Decker R, van Loveren C. Sugars and dental caries. *American Journal of Clinical Nutrition* 2003; 78: 881S–92S.

21 Towle I, Irish JD, Sabbi KH, et al. Dental caries in wild primates: interproximal cavities on anterior teeth. *American Journal of Primatology* 2022; 84: e23349.

22 Grine FE, Gwinnett AJ, Oaks JH. Early hominid dental pathology: interproximal caries in 1.5 million-year-old *Paranthropus robustus* from Swartkrans. *Archives of Oral Biology* 1990; 35: 381–86.

23 Coppa A, Bondioli L, Cucina A, et al. Palaeontology: early neolithic tradition of dentistry. *Nature* 2006; 440: 755–56.

24 Coppa et al, 2006.

25 Waldron T. Dental disease. In: *Palaeopathology*. Cambridge: Cambridge University Press, 2008: 236–48.

26 Oxilia G, Peresani M, Romandini M, et al. Earliest evidence of dental caries manipulation in the late upper palaeolithic. *Scientific Reports* 2015; 5: 12150.

27 Adler CJ, Dobney K, Weyrich LS, Kaidonis J, Walker AW, Haak W, et al. Sequencing ancient calcified dental plaque shows changes in oral microbiota with dietary shifts of the neolithic and industrial revolutions. *Nature Genetics* 2013; 45: 450–55.

8. ... or about exercise

1 Hill JO, Wyatt HR, Peters JC. The importance of energy balance. *European Endocrinology* 2013; 9: 111–15.

2 Hill JO, Wyatt HR, Peters JC. Energy balance and obesity. *Circulation* 2012; 126: 126–32.

3 Webber J. Energy balance in obesity. *Proceedings of the Nutrition Society* 2003; 62: 539–43.

4 Hill JO. Understanding and addressing the epidemic of obesity: an energy balance perspective. *Endocrine Reviews* 2006; 27: 750–61.

5 Shook RP, Blair SN, Duperly J, et al. What is causing the worldwide rise in body weight? *European Journal of Endocrinology* 2014; 10: 136–44.

6 Hand GA, Blair SN. Energy flux and its role in obesity and metabolic disease. *European Endocrinology* 2014; 10: 131–35.

7   Tudor-Locke C, Craig CL, Brown WJ, et al. How many steps/day are enough? For adults. *International Journal of Behavioral Nutrition and Physical Activity* 2011; 8: 79.

8   Katzmarzyk PT, Barreira TV, Broyles ST, et al. Relationship between lifestyle behaviors and obesity in children ages 9–11: results from a 12-country study. *Obesity* 2015; 23: 1696–702.

9   Griffith R, Lluberas R, Lührmann M. Gluttony and sloth? Calories, labor market activity and the rise of obesity. *Journal of the European Economic Association* 2016; 14: 1253–86.

10 Snowdon C. The fat lie. 2014. Available from: https://papers.ssrn.com/abstract=3903961.

11 Ladabaum U, Mannalithara A, Myer PA, et al. Obesity, abdominal obesity, physical activity, and caloric intake in US adults: 1988 to 2010. *American Journal of Medicine* 2014; 127: 717–27.

12 Church TS, Thomas DM, Tudor-Locke C, et al. Trends over 5 decades in US occupation-related physical activity and their associations with obesity. *pLoS One* 2011; 6: e19657.

13 Hill et al, 2012.

14 Shook et al, 2014.

15 Katzmarzyk et al, 2015.

16 Lindsay C. A century of labour market change: 1900 to 2000. 2003. Available from: http://www.ons.gov.uk/ons/rel/lms/labour-market-trends–discontinued-/volume-111–no–3/a-century-of-labour-market-change–1900-to-2000.pdf.

17 Office for National Statistics. Long-term trends in UK employment: 1861 to 2018. 2019. Available from: https://www.ons.gov.uk/economy/nationalaccounts/uksectoraccounts/compendium/economicreview/april2019/longtermtrendsinukemployment1861to2018.

18 British Heart Foundation. Physical activity statistics 2012. London: British Heart Foundation, 2017.

19 Church et al, 2011.

20 Fox M. Mo Farah – base training (typical week). Available from: https://www.sweatelite.co/mo-farah-base-training-typical-week/.

21 Dennehy C. The surprisingly simple training of the world's fastest marathoner. 2021. Available from: https://www.outsideonline.com/health/running/eliud-kipchoge-marathon-workout-training-principles/.

22 Snowdon, 2014.

23 Department for Environment, Food & Rural Affairs. Family Food 2012. 2013. Available from: https://www.gov.uk/government/statistics/family-food-2012.24.

24 Harper H, Hallsworth M. Counting calories: how under-reporting can explain the apparent fall in calorie intake. 2016. Available from: https://www.bi.team/wp-content/uploads/2016/08/16-07-12-Counting-Calories-Final.pdf.

25 Lennox A, Bluck L, Page P, Pell D, Cole D, Ziauddeen N, et al. Appendix X Misreporting in the National Diet and Nutrition Survey Rolling Programme (NDNS RP): summary of results and their interpretation [Internet]. [cited 2022 Sep 6]. Available from: https://www.food.gov.uk/sites/default/files/media/document/ndns-appendix-x.pdf.

26 Church et al, 2011.

27 Harper H, Hallsworth M. Counting calories: how under-reporting can explain the apparent fall in calorie intake. 2016. Available from: https://www.bi.team/wp-content/uploads/2016/08/16-07-12-Counting-Calories-Final.pdf.

28 Health and Social Care Information Centre. Health Survey for England – 2012. 2013. Available from: https://digital.nhs.uk/data-and-information/publications/statistical/health-survey-for-england/health-survey-for-england-2012.

29 NielsenIQ. The power of snacking. 2018. Available from: https://nielseniq.com/global/en/insights/report/2018/the-power-of-snacking/.

30 Nielsen. Snack attack: what consumers are reaching for around the world. Available from: https://www.nielsen.com/wp-content/uploads/sites/2/2019/04/nielsen-global-snacking-report-september-2014.pdf.

31 Bee C, Meyer B, Sullivan JX. The validity of consumption data: are the Consumer Expenditure Interview and Diary Surveys informative? 2012. Available from: https://EconPapers.repec.org/RePEc:nbr:nberwo:18308.

32 Office for National Statistics. Survey sampling for Family Food. 2015. Available from: https://assets.publishing.service.gov.uk/government/uploads/system/uploads/attachment_data/file/486047/familyfood-method-sampling-17dec15.pdf.

33 Bean C. Independent review of UK economic statistics: final report. 2016. Available from: https://www.gov.uk/government/publications/independent-review-of-uk-economic-statistics-final-report.

34 Barrett G, Levell P, Milligan K. A comparison of micro and macro expenditure measures across countries using differing survey methods. In: Carroll CD, Crossley TF, Sabelhaus J (eds). *Improving the Measurement of Consumer Expenditures*. Chicago, IL: University of Chicago Press, 2015: 263–86.

35 Meyer BD, Mok WKC, Sullivan JX. Household surveys in crisis. *Journal of Economic Perspectives* 2015; 29: 199–226.

36 British Heart Foundation. Portion distortion. 2013. Available from: https://www.bhf.org.uk/what-we-do/news-from-the-bhf/news-archive/2013/october/portion-distortion.

37 Waste and Resources Action Programme. Household food and drink waste in the United Kingdom 2012. 2013. Available from: https://wrap.org.uk/resources/report/household-food-and-drink-waste-united-kingdom-2012.

38 Dray S. Food waste in the UK. 2021. Available from: https://lordslibrary.parliament.uk/food-waste-in-the-uk/.

39 Kantar. Consumer panels. 2022. Available from: https://www.kantarworldpanel.com/id/About-us/consumer-panels.

40 Pontzer et al, 2012.

41 Ebersole KE, Dugas LR, et al. Energy expenditure and adiposity in Nigerian and African-American women. *Obesity* 2008; 16: 2148–54.

42 Pontzer et al, 2016.

43 Pontzer H. Energy constraint as a novel mechanism linking exercise and health. *Physiology* 2018; 33: 384–93.

44 Pontzer H, Yamada Y, Sagayama H, et al. Daily energy expenditure through the human life course. *Science* 2021; 373: 808–12.

45 Kraft TS, Venkataraman VV, Wallace IJ, et al. The energetics of uniquely human subsistence strategies. *Science* 2021; 374: eabf0130.

46 Ferro-Luzzi A, Martino L. Obesity and physical activity. *Ciba Foundation Symposium* 1996; 201: 207–21; discussion 221–7.

47 Luke A, Dugas LR, Ebersole K, et al. Energy expenditure does not predict weight change in either Nigerian or African American women. *American Journal of Clinical Nutrition* 2009; 89: 169–76.

48 Dugas LR, Harders R, Merrill S, et al. Energy expenditure in adults living in developing compared with industrialized countries: a meta-analysis of doubly labeled water studies. *American Journal of Clinical Nutrition* 2011; 93: 427–41.

49 Pontzer H. The crown joules: energetics, ecology, and evolution in humans and other primates. *Evolutionary Anthropology* 2017; 26: 12–24.

50 Pontzer H, Durazo-Arvizu R, Dugas LR, et al. Constrained total energy expenditure and metabolic adaptation to physical activity in adult humans. *Current Biology* 2016; 26: 410–17.

51 Pontzer H, Raichlen DA, Gordon AD, et al. Primate energy expenditure and life history. *Proceedings of the National Academy of Sciences USA* 2014; 111: 1433–37.

52 Bilici S, Saglam F, Beyhan Y, Barut-Uyar B, Dikmen D, Goktas Z, et al. Energy expenditure and nutritional status of coal miners: a cross-sectional study. *Archives of Environmental & Occupational Health* 2016; 71: 293–99.

53 Ellison PT. Energetics and reproductive effort. *American Journal of Human Biology* 2003; 15: 342–51.

54 Ellison PT, Lager C. Moderate recreational running is associated with lowered salivary progesterone profiles in women. *American Journal of Ostetrics and Gynecology* 1986; 154: 1000–03.

55 Pontzer H. Energy constraint as a novel mechanism linking exercise and health. *Physiology* 2018; 33: 384–93.

56 Nabkasorn C, Miyai N, Sootmongkol A, et al. Effects of physical exercise on depression, neuroendocrine stress hormones and physiological fitness in adolescent females with depressive symptoms. *European Journal of Public Health* 2006; 16: 179–84.

57 @TateLyleSugars. 'Come along to the #IEA #ThinkTent for steaming porridge & Lyle's Golden Syrup & to discuss global trade: producers vs. consumers – where does the balance lie?' 2 October 2018. Available from: https://twitter.com/tatelylesugars/status/1047037066952028166.

58 Institute of Economic Affairs. After Brexit, building a global free trade environment. 2016. Available from: https://iea.org.uk/events/exiting-the-eu-reclaiming-trade-sovereignty/.

59 Lee I-M, Shiroma EJ, Lobelo F, Puska P, Blair SN, Katzmarzyk PT, et al. Effect of physical inactivity on major non-communicable diseases

worldwide: an analysis of burden of disease and life expectancy. *Lancet* 2012; 380: 219–29.

60 Church et al, 2011.

61 Hill et al, 2012.

62 Wood B, Ruskin G, Sacks G. How Coca-Cola shaped the international congress on physical activity and public health: an analysis of email exchanges between 2012 and 2014. *International Journal of Environmental Research and Public Health* 2020; 17: 8996.

63 Serôdio PM, McKee M, Stuckler D. Coca-Cola – a model of transparency in research partnerships? A network analysis of Coca-Cola's research funding (2008–2016). *Public Health Nutrition* 2018; 21: 1594–607.

64 O'Connor A. Coca-Cola funds scientists who shift blame for obesity away from bad diets. 2015. Available from: https://well.blogs.nytimes.com/2015/08/09/coca-cola-funds-scientists-who-shift-blame-for-obesity-away-from-bad-diets/.

65 Wood et al, 2020.

66 O'Connor et al, 2015.

67 Serôdio et al, 2018.

68 Serôdio et al, 2018.

69 Coca-Cola. Transparency Research Report. 2022. Available from: https://www.coca-colacompany.com/content/dam/journey/us/en/policies/pdf/research-and-studies/transparency-research-report.pdf.

70 Botkin JR. Should failure to disclose significant financial conflicts of interest be considered research misconduct? *Journal of the American Medical Association* 2018; 320: 2307–08.

71 Anderson TS, Dave S, Good CB, et al. Academic medical center leadership on pharmaceutical company boards of directors. *Journal of the American Medical Association* 2014; 311: 1353–55.

72 Coca-Cola. Exercise is the best medicine. 2009. Available from: https://investors.coca-colacompany.com/news-events/press-releases/detail/392/exercise-is-the-best-medicine.

73 Flacco ME, Manzoli L, Boccia S, et al. Head-to-head randomized trials are mostly industry sponsored and almost always favor the industry sponsor. *Journal of Clinical Epidemiology* 2015; 68: 811–20.

74 Stamatakis E, Weiler R, Ioannidis JPA. Undue industry influences that distort healthcare research, strategy, expenditure and practice: a review. *European Journal of Clinical Investigation* 2013; 43: 469–75.

75 Ioannidis JPA. Evidence-based medicine has been hijacked: a report to David Sackett. *Journal of Clinical Epidemiology* 2016; 73: 82–86.

76 Fabbri A, Lai A, Grundy Q, Bero LA. The influence of industry sponsorship on the research agenda: a scoping review. *American Journal of Public Health* 2018; 108: e9–16.

77 Lundh et al, 2017.

78 Rasmussen K, Bero L, Redberg R, et al. Collaboration between academics and industry in clinical trials: cross sectional study of publications and survey of lead academic authors. *British Medical Journal* 2018; 363: 3654.

79 Bes-Rastrollo M, Schulze MB, Ruiz-Canela M, et al. Financial conflicts of interest and reporting bias regarding the association between sugar-sweetened beverages and weight gain: a systematic review of systematic reviews. *PLoS Medicine* 2013; 10: e1001578.

80 Serôdio et al, 2018.

81 Serôdio et al, 2018. 'Three hundred and eighty-nine articles, published in 169 different journals, and authored by 907 researchers, cite funding from The Coca-Cola Company. But Coca-Cola's transparency lists are far from complete. After incorporating the results from a survey, our search identified up to 471 authors corresponding to 128 articles whose names do not appear on Coca-Cola's lists, but whose articles acknowledge funding from the company.'

82 Leme ACB, Ferrari G, Fisberg RM, et al. Co-occurrence and clustering of sedentary behaviors, diet, sugar-sweetened beverages, and alcohol intake among adolescents and adults: the Latin American Nutrition and Health Study (ELANS). *Nutrients* 2021; 13: 1809.

9. ... or about willpower

1 @matthewsyed. 'Here I say that some obese people could lose weight with willpower – more exercise, less food. I explicitly exclude those with thyroid & other conditions. That this has caused offence

underlines my point: we've seen a collapse in individual responsibility'. 14 February 2021. Available from: https://twitter.com/matthewsyed/status/1360913923340394499.

2 Cooksey-Stowers K, Schwartz MB, Brownell KD. Food swamps predict obesity rates better than food deserts in the United States. *International Journal of Environmental Research and Public Health* 2017; 14: 1366.

3 National Food Strategy, 2021.

4 National Food Strategy, 2021.

5 Folkvord F, Anschütz DJ, Wiers RW, et al. The role of attentional bias in the effect of food advertising on actual food intake among children. *Appetite* 2015; 84: 251–58.

6 Harris JL, Speers SE, Schwartz MB, et al. US food company branded advergames on the internet: children's exposure and effects on snack consumption. *Journal of Children and Media* 2012; 6: 51–68.

7 Folkvord F, Anschütz DJ, Buijzen M, et al. The effect of playing advergames that promote energy-dense snacks or fruit on actual food intake among children. *American Journal of Clinical Nutrition* 2013; 97: 239–45.

8 Harris JL, Bargh JA, Brownell KD. Priming effects of television food advertising on eating behavior. *Health Psychology* 2009; 28: 404–13.

9 Boyland E, McGale L, Maden M, et al. Association of food and non-alcoholic beverage marketing with children and adolescents' eating behaviors and health: a systematic review and meta-analysis. *JAMA Pediatrics* 2022; 176: e221037.

10 Laraia BA, Leak TM, Tester JM, et al. Biobehavioral factors that shape nutrition in low-income populations: a narrative review. *American Journal of Preventive Medicine* 2017; 52: S118–26.

11 Adam TC, Epel ES. Stress, eating and the reward system. *Physiology & Behavior* 2007; 9: 449–58.

12 Schrempft S, van Jaarsveld CHM, Fisher A, et al. Variation in the heritability of child body mass index by obesogenic home environment. *JAMA Pediatrics* 2018; 172: 1153–60.

13 Schrempft S et al, 2018.

14 Baraldi LG, Martinez Steele E, Canella DS, et al. Consumption of ultra-processed foods and associated sociodemographic factors in the USA between 2007 and 2012: evidence from a nationally representative cross-sectional study. *BMJ Open* 2018; 8: e020574.

15 Leung CW, Fulay AP, Parnarouskis L, et al. Food insecurity and ultra-processed food consumption: the modifying role of participation in the Supplemental Nutrition Assistance Program (SNAP). *American Journal of Clinical Nutrition* 2022; 116: 197–205.

16 Marchese L, Livingstone KM, Woods JL, et al. Ultra-processed food consumption, socio-demographics and diet quality in Australian adults. *Public Health Nutrition* 2022; 25: 94–104.

17 Mischel W, Shoda Y, Rodriguez MI. Delay of gratification in children. *Science* 1989; 244: 933–38.

18 Mischel W, Ebbesen EB, Zeiss AR. Cognitive and attentional mechanisms in delay of gratification. *Journal of Personality and Social Psychology* 1972; 21: 204–18.

19 Watts TW, Duncan GJ, Quan H. Revisiting the marshmallow test: a conceptual replication investigating links between early delay of gratification and later outcomes. *Psychological Science* 2018; 29: 1159–77.

20 Watts et al, 2018.

21 Falk A, Kosse F, Pinger P. Re-revisiting the marshmallow test: a direct comparison of studies by Shoda, Mischel, and Peake (1990) and Watts, Duncan, and Quan (2018). *Psychological Science* 2020; 31: 100–04.

22 Evans GW, English K. The environment of poverty: multiple stressor exposure, psychophysiological stress, and socioemotional adjustment. *Child Development* 2002; 73: 1238–48.

23 Sturge-Apple ML, Suor JH, Davies PT, et al. Vagal tone and children's delay of gratification: differential sensitivity in resource-poor and resource-rich environments. *Psychological Science* 2016; 27: 885–93.

24 Kidd C, Palmeri H, Aslin RN. Rational snacking: young children's decision-making on the marshmallow task is moderated by beliefs about environmental reliability. *Cognition* 2013; 126: 109–14.

25 Raver CC, Jones SM, Li-Grining C, et al. CSRP's impact on low-income preschoolers' preacademic skills: self-regulation as a mediating mechanism. *Child Development* 2011; 82: 362–78.

26 *The Economist*. Desire delayed: Walter Mischel on the test that became his life's work. 2014. Available from: https://www.economist.com/books-and-arts/2014/10/11/desire-delayed.

27 Gill D. New study disavows marshmallow test's predictive powers. 2021. https://anderson-review.ucla.edu/new-study-disavows-marshmallow-tests-predictive-powers/.

10. *How UPF hacks our brains*

1   Library of Congress. Who "invented" the TV dinner? 2019. Available from: https://www.loc.gov/everyday-mysteries/food-and-nutrition/item/who-invented-the-tv-dinner/.

2   Lynch, B. Understanding opportunities in the chilled ready meals category in the UK. 2021. Available from: https://www.bordbia.ie/industry/news/food-alerts/2020/understanding-opportunities-in-the-chilled-ready-meals-category-in-the-uk/.

3   Frings D, Albery IP, Moss AC, et al. Comparison of Allen Carr's Easyway programme with a specialist behavioural and pharmacological smoking cessation support service: a randomized controlled trial. *Addiction* 2020; 115: 977–85.

4   Carr A, Dicey J. *Allen Carr's Easy Way to Quit Smoking Without Willpower – Includes Quit Vaping: The Best-selling Quit Smoking Method Updated for the 2020s.* London: Arcturus, 2020.

5   Keogan S, Li S, Clancy L. Allen Carr's Easyway to Stop Smoking – a randomised clinical trial. *Tobacco Control* 2019; 28: 414–19.

6   World Health Organization. Allen Carr's Easyway. 2021. Available from: https://www.who.int/campaigns/world-no-tobacco-day/2021/quitting-toolkit/allen-carr-s-easyway.

7   Fletcher PC, Kenny PJ. Food addiction: a valid concept? *Neuropsychopharmacology* 2018; 43: 2506–13.

8   Fletcher & Kenny, 2018.

9   Polk SE, Schulte EM, Furman CR, et al. Wanting and liking: separable components in problematic eating behavior? *Appetite* 2017; 115: 45–53.

10 Morales I, Berridge KC. "Liking" and "wanting" in eating and food reward: brain mechanisms and clinical implications. *Physiology & Behavior* 2020; 227: 113152.

11 Ellin A. I was powerless over Diet Coke. 2021. Available from: https://www.nytimes.com/2021/08/11/well/eat/diet-coke-addiction.html.

12 Fletcher & Kenny, 2018.

13 Hebebrand J, Albayrak Ö, Adan R, et al. "Eating addiction", rather than "food addiction", better captures addictive-like eating behavior. *Neuroscience & Biobehavioral Reviews*; 47: 295–306.

14 Polk et al, 2017.

15 Gearhardt AN, Schulte EM. Is food addictive? A review of the science. *Annual Review of Nutrition* 2021; 41: 387–410.

16 Schulte EM, Sonneville KR, Gearhardt AN. Subjective experiences of highly processed food consumption in individuals with food addiction. *Psychology of Addictive Behaviors* 2019; 33: 144–53.

17 Schulte EM, Avena NM, Gearhardt AN. Which foods may be addictive? The roles of processing, fat content, and glycemic load. *PLoS One* 2015; 10: e0117959.

18 Allison S, Timmerman GM. Anatomy of a binge: food environment and characteristics of nonpurge binge episodes. *Eating Behaviors* 2007; 8: 31–38.

19 Tanofsky-Kraff M, McDuffie JR, et al. Laboratory assessment of the food intake of children and adolescents with loss of control eating. *American Journal of Clinical Nutrition* 2009; 89: 738–45.

20 Grant BF, Goldstein RB, Saha TD, et al. Epidemiology of DSM-5 alcohol use disorder: results from the national epidemiologic survey on alcohol and related conditions III. *JAMA Psychiatry* 2015; 72: 757–66.

21 Martin CB, Herrick KA, Sarafrazi N, Ogden CL. Attempts to lose weight among adults in the United States, 2013–2016. *National Center for Health Statistics Data Brief* 2018; 313: 1–8.

22 Grant et al, 2015.

23 Lopez-Quintero C, de los Cobos JP, Hasin DS, et al. Probability and predictors of transition from first use to dependence on nicotine, alcohol, cannabis, and cocaine: results of the National Epidemiologic Survey on Alcohol and Related Conditions (NESARC). *Drug and Alcohol Dependence* 2011; 115: 120–30.

24 Volkow ND, Wang G-J, Fowler JS, et al. Overlapping neuronal circuits in addiction and obesity: evidence of systems pathology. *Philosophical Transactions of the Royal Society B* 2008; 363: 3191–200.

25 Volkow ND, Wang GJ, Fowler JS, et al. Food and drug reward: over-lapping circuits in human obesity and addiction. *Current Topics in Behavioral Neurosciences* 2012; 11: 1–24.

26 Afshin A, Sur PJ, Fay KA, et al. Health effects of dietary risks in 195 countries, 1990–2017: a systematic analysis for the Global Burden of Disease Study 2017. *Lancet* 2019; 393: 1958–72.

11. *UPF is pre-chewed*

1 Haber GB, Heaton KW, Murphy D, Burroughs LF. Depletion and dis-ruption of dietary fibre. Effects on satiety, plasma-glucose, and serum-insulin. *Lancet* 1977; 2: 679–82.

2 Ungoed-Thomas J. An honest crust? Craft bakeries rise up against 'sourfaux' bread. 2022. Available from: https://amp.theguardian.com/food/2022/apr/23/fake-bake-uk-government-steps-in-over-sourfaux-threat-to-craft-bakers.

3 Dodson TB, Susarla SM. Impacted wisdom teeth. *BMJ Clinical Evidence* 2014; 2014: 1302.

4 Corruccini RS. *How Anthropology Informs the Orthodontic Diagnosis of Malocclusion's Causes*. London: Edwin Mellen Press, 1999.

5 Lieberman, D. *The Story of the Human Body: Evolution, Health and Disease*. London: Penguin Books, 2011.

6 Corruccini RS. Australian aboriginal tooth succession, interproximal attrition, and Begg's theory. *American Journal of Orthodontics and Dentofacial Orthopedics* 1990; 97: 349–57.

7 Corruccini RS. An epidemiologic transition in dental occlusion in world populations. *American Journal of Orthodontics* 1984; 86: 419–26.

8 Lieberman DE, Krovitz GE, Yates FW, et al. Effects of food process-ing on masticatory strain and craniofacial growth in a retrognathic face. *Journal of Human Evolution* 2004; 46: 655–77.

9 BBC News. *Mary Rose* skeletons studied by Swansea sports scientists. 2012. Available from: https://www.bbc.co.uk/news/uk-wales-17309665.

10 Ingervall B, Bitsanis E. A pilot study of the effect of masticatory muscle training on facial growth in long-face children. *European Journal of Orthodontics* 1987 Feb; 9(1):15–23.

11 *Business Insider.* There's a very simple reason why McDonald's hamburgers don't rot. 2017. Available from: https://www.businessinsider.com/why-mcdonalds-hamburgers-do-not-rot-2016-2?r=US&IR=T.

12 Rolls BJ. The relationship between dietary energy density and energy intake. *Physiology & Behavior* 2009; 97: 609–15.

13 Bell EA, Castellanos VH, Pelkman CL, et al. Energy density of foods affects energy intake in normal-weight women. *American Journal of Clinical Nutrition* 1998; 67: 412–20.

14 Rolls BJ, Cunningham PM, Diktas HE. Properties of ultraprocessed foods that can drive excess intake. *Nutrition Today* 2020; 55: 109.

15 Bell et al, 1998.

16 Rolls et al, 2020.

17 Ohkuma T, Hirakawa Y, Nakamura U, et al. Association between eating rate and obesity: a systematic review and meta-analysis. *International Journal of Obesity* 2015; 39: 1589–96.

18 de Graaf C. Texture and satiation: the role of oro-sensory exposure time. *Physiology & Behavior* 2012; 107: 496–501.

19 Wee MSM, Goh AT, Stieger M, et al. Correlation of instrumental texture properties from textural profile analysis (TPA) with eating behaviours and macronutrient composition for a wide range of solid foods. *Food & Function* 2018; 9: 5301–12.

20 Zhu Y, Hsu WH, Hollis JH. Increasing the number of masticatory cycles is associated with reduced appetite and altered postprandial plasma concentrations of gut hormones, insulin and glucose. *British Journal of Nutrition* 2013; 110: 384–90.

21 Fogel A, Goh AT, Fries LR, et al. A description of an "obesogenic" eating style that promotes higher energy intake and is associated with greater adiposity in 4.5-year-old children: results from the GUSTO cohort. *Physiology & Behavior* 2017; 176: 107–16.

22 Llewellyn CH, van Jaarsveld CHM, Boniface D, et al. Eating rate is a heritable phenotype related to weight in children. *American Journal of Clinical Nutrition* 2008; 88: 1560–66.

23 de Wijk RA, Zijlstra N, Mars M, et al. The effects of food viscosity on bite size, bite effort and food intake. *Physiology & Behavior* 2008; 95: 527–32.

24 Forde CG, Mars M, de Graaf K. Ultra-processing or oral processing? A role for energy density and eating rate in moderating energy intake from processed foods. *Current Developments in Nutrition* 2020; 4: nzaa019.

25 Bell et al, 1998.

26 Gearhardt & Schulte, 2021.

12. UPF smells funny

1 Morrot G, Brochet F, Dubourdieu D. The color of odors. *Brain and Language* 2001; 79: 309–20.

2 Brochet F. Chemical object representation in the field of consciousness. Available from: https://web.archive.org/web/20070928231853if_/http://www.academie-amorim.com/us/laureat_2001/brochet.pdf.

3 Bushdid C, Magnasco MO, Vosshall LB, et al. Humans can discriminate more than 1 trillion olfactory stimuli. *Science* 2014; 343: 1370–72.

4 McGann JP. Poor human olfaction is a 19th-century myth. *Science* 2017; 356: eaam7263.

5 Sclafani A. Oral and postoral determinants of food reward. *Physiology & Behavior* 2004; 81: 773–79.

6 de Araujo IE, Lin T, Veldhuizen MG, et al. Metabolic regulation of brain response to food cues. *Current Biology* 2013; 23: 878–83.

7 Holman EW. Immediate and delayed reinforcers for flavor preferences in rats. *Learning and Motivation* 1975; 6: 91–100.

8 Holman GL. Intragastric reinforcement effect. *Journal of Comparative and Physiological Psychology* 1969; 69: 432–41.

9 Mennella JA, Jagnow CP, Beauchamp GK. Prenatal and postnatal flavor learning by human infants. *Pediatrics* 2001; 107: E88.

10 Barabási A-L, Menichetti G, Loscalzo J. The unmapped chemical complexity of our diet. *Nature Food* 2020; 1: 33–37.

11 Holliday RJ, Helfter J. *A Holistic Vet's Prescription for a Healthy Herd: A Guide to Livestock Nutrition, Free-choice Minerals, and Holistic Cattle Care.* Greeley: Acres USA, 2014.

12 Scrinis G. Reframing malnutrition in all its forms: a critique of the tripartite classification of malnutrition. *Global Food Security* 2020; 26: 100396.

13 Scrinis G. Ultra-processed foods and the corporate capture of nutrition – an essay by Gyorgy Scrinis. *British Medical Journal* 2020; 371: m4601.

14 Elizabeth L, Machado P, Zinocker M, et al. Ultra-processed foods and health outcomes: a narrative review. *Nutrients* 2020; 12: 1955.

15 Reardon T, Tschirley D, Liverpool-Tasie LSO, et al. The processed food revolution in African food systems and the double burden of malnutrition. Global Food Security 2021; 28: 100466.

16 Swinburn BA, Kraak VI, Allender S, Atkins VJ, Baker PI, Bogard JR, et al. The global syndemic of obesity, undernutrition, and climate change: the *Lancet* Commission report. *Lancet* 2019; 393: 791–846.

17 National Food Strategy, 2021.

18 OECDiLibrary. Obesity Among Children. 2019 Available from: https://www.oecd-ilibrary.org/sites/health_glance_eur-2018-26-en/index.html?itemId=/content/component/health_glance_eur-2018-26-en.

19 Enserink M. Did natural selection make the Dutch the tallest people on the planet? 2015. Available from: https://www.science.org/content/article/did-natural-selection-make-dutch-tallest-people-planet.

20 Haines G. Why are the Dutch so tall? 2020. Available from: https://www.bbc.com/travel/article/20200823-why-are-the-dutch-so-tall#:~:text=A%20land%20of%20giants%2C%20the,cm%20and%20163.5cm%20respectively.

21 García OP, Long KZ, Rosado JL. Impact of micronutrient deficiencies on obesity. *Nutrition Review* 2009; 67: 559–72.

13. UPF tastes odd

1 Chandrashekar J, Kuhn C, Oka Y, et al. The cells and peripheral representation of sodium taste in mice. *Nature* 2010; 464: 297–301.

2 Breslin PAS. An evolutionary perspective on food and human taste. *Current Biology* 2013; 23: R409–18.

3 Keast RSJ, Breslin PAS. An overview of binary taste–taste interactions. *Food Quality and Preference* 2003; 14: 111–24.

4 Henquin J-C. Do pancreatic β cells "taste" nutrients to secrete insulin? *Science Signaling* 2012; 5: e36.

5 Behrens M, Meyerhof W. Gustatory and extragustatory functions of mammalian taste receptors. *Physiology & Behavior* 2011; 105: 4–13.

6 Chandrashekar et al, 2010.

7 Breslin, 2013.

8 Breslin, 2013.

9 Breslin, 2013.

10 Coca-Cola. Does Coca-Cola contain cocaine? 2020. Available from: https://www.coca-cola.co.uk/our-business/faqs/does-coca-cola-contain-cocaine.

11 Tucker KL, Morita K, Qiao N, Hannan MT, Cupples LA, Kiel DP. Colas, but not other carbonated beverages, are associated with low bone mineral density in older women: The Framingham Osteoporosis Study. *American Journal of Clinical Nutrition* 2006; 84: 936–42.

12 Veldhuizen MG, Babbs RK, Patel B, et al. Integration of sweet taste and metabolism determines carbohydrate reward. *Current Biology* 2017; 27: 2476–2485.

13 Lopez O, Jacobs A. In town with little water, Coca-Cola is everywhere. So is diabetes. 2018. Available from: https://www.nytimes.com/2018/07/14/world/americas/mexico-coca-cola-diabetes.html.

14 Imamura F, O'Connor L, Ye Z, et al. Consumption of sugar sweetened beverages, artificially sweetened beverages, and fruit juice and incidence of type 2 diabetes: systematic review, meta-analysis, and estimation of population attributable fraction. *British Medical Journal* 2015; 351: h3576.

15 Fowler SP, Williams K, Resendez RG, et al. Fueling the obesity epidemic? Artificially sweetened beverage use and long-term weight gain. *Obesity* 2008; 16: 1894–900.

16 Fowler SPG. Low-calorie sweetener use and energy balance: results from experimental studies in animals, and large-scale prospective studies in humans. *Physiology & Behavior* 2016; 164: 517–23.

17 Nettleton JA, Lutsey PL, Wang Y, et al. Diet soda intake and risk of incident metabolic syndrome and type 2 diabetes in the

Multi-Ethnic Study of Atherosclerosis (MESA). *Diabetes Care* 2009; 32: 688–94.

18 Gallagher AM, Ashwell M, Halford JCG, et al. Low-calorie sweeteners in the human diet: scientific evidence, recommendations, challenges and future needs. A symposium report from the FENS 2019 conference. *Journal of Nutritional Science* 2021; 10: e7.

19 Tate DF, Turner-McGrievy G, Lyons E, et al. Replacing caloric beverages with water or diet beverages for weight loss in adults: main results of the Choose Healthy Options Consciously Everyday (CHOICE) randomized clinical trial. *American Journal of Clinical Nutrition* 2012; 95: 555–63.

20 Miller PE, Perez V. Low-calorie sweeteners and body weight and composition: a meta-analysis of randomized controlled trials and prospective cohort studies. *American Journal of Clinical Nutrition* 2014; 100: 765–77.

21 Tate et al, 2012.

22 Sylvetsky AC, Figueroa J, Zimmerman T, et al. Consumption of low-calorie sweetened beverages is associated with higher total energy and sugar intake among children, NHANES 2011–2016. *Pediatric Obesity* 2019; 14: e12535.

23 Dalenberg JR, Patel BP, Denis R, et al. Short-term consumption of sucralose with, but not without, carbohydrate impairs neural and metabolic sensitivity to sugar in humans. *Cellular Metabolism* 2020; 31: 493–502.

24 Swithers SE, Sample CH, Davidson TL. Adverse effects of high-intensity sweeteners on energy intake and weight control in male and obesity-prone female rats. *Behavioral Neuroscience* 2013; 127: 262–74.

25 Onaolapo AY, Onaolapo OJ. Food additives, food and the concept of 'food addiction': is stimulation of the brain reward circuit by food sufficient to trigger addiction? *Pathophysiology* 2018; 25: 263–76.

26 Bartolotto C. Does consuming sugar and artificial sweeteners change taste preferences? *Permanente Journal* 2015; 19: 81–84.

27 Rodriguez-Palacios A, Harding A, Menghini P, et al. The artificial sweetener Splenda promotes gut *Proteobacteria*, dysbiosis, and myeloperoxidase reactivity in Crohn's disease-like ileitis. *Inflammatory Bowel Disease* 2018; 24: 1005–20.

28 de-la-Cruz M, Millán-Aldaco D, Soriano-Nava DM, et al. The artificial sweetener Splenda intake promotes changes in expression of

c-Fos and NeuN in hypothalamus and hippocampus of rats. *Brain Research* 2018; 1700: 181–89.

29 Suez J, Korem T, Zeevi D, et al. Artificial sweeteners induce glucose intolerance by altering the gut microbiota. *Nature* 2014; 514: 181–86.

30 HM Treasury. Soft drinks industry levy comes into effect. 2018. Available from: https://www.gov.uk/government/news/soft-drinks-industry-levy-comes-into-effect.

31 Pell D, Mytton O, Penney TL, et al. Changes in soft drinks purchased by British households associated with the UK soft drinks industry levy: controlled interrupted time series analysis. *British Medical Journal* 2021; 372: n254.

32 First Steps Nutrition Trust, 2019.

33 First Steps Nutrition Trust, 2019.

34 Breslin, 2013.

14. *Additive anxiety*

1 Wood Z. Pret a Manger censured over natural sandwich ingredients claim. 2018. Available from: http://www.theguardian.com/business/2018/apr/18/pret-a-manger-censured-over-natural-sandwich-ingredients-claim.

2 Sustain. Pret's progress. 2018. Available from: https://www.sustainweb.org/news/dec18_pret_progress/.

3 Jab Holding Company. Annual report 2020. 2021. Available from: https://www.jabholco.com/documents/2/FY20_JAB_Holding_Company_Sarl_Consolidated_Financial_Statements.pdf.

4 Appelbaum B. Bagels and war crimes. 2019. Available from: https://www.nytimes.com/2019/03/27/opinion/bagels-war-crimes-nazi-reimann.html.

5 Bennhold K. Germany's second-richest family discovers a dark Nazi past. 2019. Available from: https://www.nytimes.com/2019/03/25/world/europe/nazi-laborers-jab-holding.html.

6 Kiewel M. 33 Milliarden Euro reich: die Nazi-Vergangenheit der Calgon-Familie. 2019. Available from: https://www.bild.de/bild-plus/politik/inland/politik-inland/33-milliarden-euro-reich-die-nazi-vergangenheit-der-calgon-familie-60835802,view=conversionToLogin.bild.html.

7 Rising D. Family who owns Krispy Kreme, Panera, Peet's Coffee acknowledges Nazi past. 2019. Available from: https://www.nbcbayarea. com/news/national-international/family-that-owns-krispy-kreme-panera-peets-coffee-acknowledges-nazi-past/159805/.

8 McCann D, Barrett A, Cooper A, et al. Food additives and hyper-active behaviour in 3-year-old and 8/9-year-old children in the community: a randomised, double-blinded, placebo-controlled trial. *Lancet* 2007; 370: 1560–67.

9 Neltner TG, Kulkarni NR, Alger HM, et al. Navigating the US food additive regulatory program. *Comprehensive Reviews in Food Science and Food Safety* 2011; 10: 342–68.

10 Naimi S, Viennois E, Gewirtz AT, et al. Direct impact of commonly used dietary emulsifiers on human gut microbiota. *Microbiome* 2021; 9: 66.

11 Richey Levine A, Picoraro JA, Dorfzaun S, et al. Emulsifiers and intes-tinal health: an introduction. *Journal of Pediatric Gastroenterology and Nutrition* 2022; 74: 314–19.

12 Dupont Nutrition and Biosciences. Panodan DATEM: emulsifier for efficient processing and fat reduction. Available from: https://www. dupontnutritionandbiosciences.com/products/panodan.html.

13 Environmental Protection Agency. Lifetime health advisories and health effects support documents for perfluorooctanoic acid and perfluorooctane sulfonate. 2016. Available from: https://www. regulations.gov/document/EPA-HQ-OW-2014–0138-0037.

14 Rich N. The lawyer who became DuPont's worst nightmare. 2016. Available from: https://www.nytimes.com/2016/01/10/magazine/the-lawyer-who-became-duponts-worst-nightmare.html.

15 Rich, 2016.

16 Morgenson G, Mendell D. How DuPont may avoid paying to clean up a toxic "forever chemical". 2020. Available from: https://www.nbcnews. com/health/cancer/how-dupont-may-avoid-paying-clean-toxic-forever-chemical-n1138766.

17 Morgenson & Mendell, 2020.

18 Sevelsted A, Stokholm J, Bønnelykke K, et al. Cesarean section and chronic immune disorders. *Pediatrics* 2015; 135: e92–98.

19 Nickerson KP, Homer CR, Kessler SP, et al. The dietary polysaccharide maltodextrin promotes *Salmonella* survival and mucosal colonization in mice. *PLoS One* 2014; 9: e101789.

20 Bäckhed F, Fraser CM, Ringel Y, et al. Defining a healthy human gut microbiome: current concepts, future directions, and clinical applications. *Cell Host & Microbe* 2012; 12: 611–22.

21 Dinan TG, Stilling RM, Stanton C, Cryan JF. Collective unconscious: how gut microbes shape human behavior. *Journal of Psychiatric Research* 2015; 63: 1–9.

22 Gilbert JA, Blaser MJ, Caporaso JG, et al. Current understanding of the human microbiome. *Nature Medicine* 2018; 24: 392–400.

23 Holder MK, Peters NV, Whylings J, et al. Dietary emulsifiers consumption alters anxiety-like and social-related behaviors in mice in a sex-dependent manner. *Scientific Reports* 2019; 9: 172.

24 Chassaing B, Koren O, Goodrich JK, et al. Dietary emulsifiers impact the mouse gut microbiota promoting colitis and metabolic syndrome. *Nature* 2015; 519: 92–96.

25 Nickerson et al, 2014.

26 Nickerson KP, McDonald C. Crohn's disease-associated adherent-invasive *Escherichia coli* adhesion is enhanced by exposure to the ubiquitous dietary polysaccharide maltodextrin. *PLoS One* 2012; 7: e52132.

27 Arnold AR, Chassaing B. Maltodextrin, modern stressor of the intestinal environment. *Cellular and Molecular Gastroenterology and Hepatology* 2019; 7: 475–76.

28 Hofman DL, van Buul VJ, Brouns FJPH. Nutrition, health, and regulatory aspects of digestible maltodextrins. *Critical Reviews in Food Science and Nutrition* 2016; 56: 2091–100.

29 Ostrowski MP, La Rosa SL, Kunath BJ, et al. The food additive xanthan gum drives adaptation of the human gut microbiota. *bioRxiv* (preprint) 2021. DOI:10.1101/2021.06.02.446819.

30 Rodriguez-Palacios et al, 2018.

31 Naimi et al, 2021.

32 Nickerson et al, 2014.

33 Chassaing et al, 2015.

34 Nickerson & McDonald, 2012.

35 Arnold & Chassaing, 2019.

36 Nair DVT, Paudel D, Prakash D, et al. Food additive guar gum aggravates colonic inflammation in experimental models of inflammatory bowel disease. *Current Developments in Nutrition* 2021; 5: 1142.

37 Roberts CL, Keita AV, Duncan SH, et al. Translocation of Crohn's disease *Escherichia coli* across M-cells: contrasting effects of soluble plant fibres and emulsifiers. *Gut* 2010; 59: 1331–39.

15. Dysregulatory bodies

1 Maffini M, Neltner T. Broken GRAS: a scary maze of questions a corn oil producer couldn't answer. 2022. Available from: http://blogs.edf.org/health/2022/03/25/broken-gras-a-scary-maze-of-questions-a-corn-oil-producer-couldnt-answer/.

2 Goldacre B. *Bad Pharma: How Medicine is Broken, And How We Can Fix It*. London: HarperCollins, 2012.

3 Neltner TG, Kulkarni NR, Alger HM, Maffini MV, Bongard ED, Fortin ND and Olson ED, Navigating the U.S. Food Additive Regulatory Program. *Comprehensive Reviews in Food Science and Food Safety* 2011; 10: 342–68. https://doi.org/10.1111/j.1541-4337.2011.00166.x.

4 Maffini MV, Neltner TG, Vogel S. We are what we eat: regulatory gaps in the United States that put our health at risk. *PLoS Biology* 2017; 15: e2003578.

5 Neltner TG, Alger HM, O'Reilly JT, et al. Conflicts of interest in approvals of additives to food determined to be generally recognized as safe: out of balance. *JAMA Internal Medicine* 2013; 173: 2032–36.

6 Delaney JJ. Investigation of the use of chemicals in food products. 1951. Available from: https://aseh.org/resources/Documents/Delaney-Investigation..Use%20of%20Chemicals%20in%20Foods-1.3.51.pdf.

7 Corn Oil ONE. FDA GRAS 704 Corn Oil Zero 1st Application. Available from: https://www.fda.gov/media/107554/download.

8 Maffini & Neltner, 2022.

9 Okull D. Stabilized chlorine dioxide in fuel ethanol fermentation: efficacy, mechanisms and residuals. 2019. Available from: https://distillersgrains.org/wp-content/uploads/2019/05/5-Okull-Stabilized-Chlorine-Dioxide-Fuel-Ethanol-Fermentation.pdf.

10 Maffini & Neltner, 2022.

11 Neltner et al, 2011.

12 Maffini et al, 2017.

13 Backhaus O, Benesh M. EWG analysis: Almost all new food chemicals greenlighted by industry, not the FDA. 2022. Available from: https://www.ewg.org/news-insights/news/2022/04/ewg-analysis-almost-all-new-food-chemicals-greenlighted-industry-not-fda.

14 Neltner TG, Alger HM, Leonard JE, et al. Data gaps in toxicity testing of chemicals allowed in food in the United States. *Reproductive Toxicology* 2013; 42: 85–94.

15 US National Toxicology Program. NTP technical report on the toxicology and carcinogenesis studies of isoeugenol (CAS no. 97–54-1) in F344/N rats and B6C3F1 mice. 2010. Available from: https://ntp.niehs.nih.gov/ntp/htdocs/lt_rpts/tr551.pdf?utm_source=direct&utm_medium=prod&utm_campaign=ntpgolinks&utm_term=tr551.

16 Nicole W. Secret ingredients: who knows what's in your food? *Environmental Health Perspectives* 2013; 121: A126–33.

17 Watson E. Where are the dead bodies? Toxicology experts hit back at latest attack on food additive safety system. 2013. Available from: https://www.beveragedaily.com/Article/2013/08/15/Where-are-the-dead-bodies-Toxicology-experts-hit-back-at-latest-attack-on-food-additive-safety-system.

18 Hartung T. Toxicology for the twenty-first century. *Nature* 2009; 460: 208–12.

16. *UPF destroys traditional diets*

1 Nestlé. 2016 full year results conference call transcript. 2017. Available from: https://www.nestle.com/sites/default/files/asset-library/documents/investors/transcripts/2016-full-year-results-investor-call-transcript.pdf.

2 Jacobs A, Richtel M. How big business got Brazil hooked on junk food. 2017. Available from: https://www.nytimes.com/interactive/2017/09/16/health/brazil-obesity-nestle.html.

3 Nestlé. Door-to-door sales of fortified products. 2015. Available from: https://web.archive.org/web/20150923094209/https://www.nestle.com/csv/case-studies/allcasestudies/door-to-doorsalesoffortifiedproducts,brazil.

4 Nestlé. Nestlé launches first floating supermarket in the Brazilian north region. 2010. Available from: https://www.nestle.com/sites/default/files/asset-library/documents/media/press-release/2010-february/nestl%C3%A9%20brazil%20press%20release%20-%20a%20bordo.pdf.

5 Figueiredo N. ADM sets record for single soybean shipment from northern Brazil. 2022. Available from: https://www.reuters.com/business/energy/adm-sets-record-single-soybean-shipment-northern-brazil-2022-02-22/.

6 Weight to Volume conversions for select substances and materials [Internet]. [cited 2022 May 8]. Available from: https://www.aqua-calc.com/calculate/weight-to-volume.

7 Lawrence F. Should we worry about soya in our food? 2006. Available from: http://www.theguardian.com/news/2006/jul/25/food.foodanddrink.

8 *Dry Cargo International.* Barcarena now handling export soya. 2015. Available from: https://www.drycargomag.com/barcarena-now-handling-export-soya.

9 EFSA Panel on Food Additives and Flavourings. Re-evaluation of dimethyl polysiloxane (E 900) as a food additive. *EFSA Journal* 2020; 18: e06107.

10 Hall AB, Huff C, Kuriwaki S. Wealth, slaveownership, and fighting for the Confederacy: an empirical study of the American Civil War. *American Political Science Review* 2019; 113: 658–73.

11 Eskridge L. After 150 years, we still ask: why 'this cruel war'? 2011. Available from: https://web.archive.org/web/20110201183505/http://www.cantondailyledger.com/topstories/x1868081570/After-150-years-we-still-ask-Why-this-cruel-war.

12 Gallagher G. Remembering the Civil War. 2011. Available from: https://www.c-span.org/video/?298125-1/remembering-civil-war.

13 Thompson M. I've always loved fried chicken. But the racism surrounding it shamed me. The Guardian [Internet]. 2020 Oct 13 [cited 2022

May 9]; Available from: http://www.theguardian.com/food/2020/.
oct/13/ive-always-loved-fried-chicken-but-the-racism-surround
ing-it-shamed-me.

14 Searcey D, Richtel M. Obesity was rising as Ghana embraced fast food. Then came KFC. 2017. Available from: https://www.nytimes.com/2017/10/02/health/ghana-kfc-obesity.html.

15 Domino's Pizza. Annual report 2016. 2016. Available from: https://ir.dominos.com/static-files/315497fc-5e31-42f9-8beb-f182d9282f21.

16 Statista. Number of Domino's Pizza outlets in India from 2006 to 2021. 2022. Available from: https://www.statista.com/statistics/277347/number-of-dominos-pizza-stores-india/.

17 Odegaard AO, Koh WP, Yuan J-M, et al. Western-style fast food intake and cardiometabolic risk in an Eastern country. *Circulation* 2012; 126: 182–88.

17. *The true cost of Pringles*

1 Monckton Chambers. Regular Pringles – once you pop (open VATA 1994, Schedule 8, Group 1, Excepted Item 5), the fun doesn't stop! 2007. Available from: https://www.monckton.com/wp-content/uploads/2008/11/ProcterGamblePringlesAug07AM.pdf.

2 Monckton Chambers, 2007.

3 British and Irish Legal Information Institute Tribunal. Procter & Gamble (UK) v Revenue & Customs [2007] UKVAT V20205. 2007. Available from: https://www.bailii.org/cgi-bin/format.cgi?doc=/uk/cases/UKVAT/2007/V20205.html.

4 British and Irish Legal Information Institute Tribunal. Revenue & Customs v Procter & Gamble UK EWCA Civ 407. 2009. Available from: https://www.bailii.org/cgi-bin/format.cgi?doc=/ew/cases/EWCA/Civ/2009/407.html&query=(18381).

5 Hansen J. Kellogg's is taking the government to court over putting milk in cereal. 2022. Available from: https://london.eater.com/23044506/kelloggs-breakfast-cereal-milk-suing-government-coco-pops-frosties.

6 Sweney M. Kellogg's to challenge new UK rules for high-sugar cereals in court. 2022. Available from: https://amp.theguardian.com/business/2022/apr/27/kelloggs-court-challenge-new-uk-rules-high-sugar-cereals.

7 Cook SF, Borah W. *Essays in Population History: Mexico and California*. Berkeley, CA: University of California Press, 1979.

8 Denevan WM, Lovell WG. *The Native Population of the Americas in 1492*. Madison, WI: University of Wisconsin Press, 1992.

9 Nunn N, Qian N. The Columbian Exchange: a history of disease, food, and ideas. *Journal of Economic Perspectives* 2010; 24: 163–88.

10 Marshall M, Climate crisis: what lessons can we learn from the last great cooling-off period? 2022. Available from: theguardian.com/environment/2022/may/09/climate-crisis-lessons-to-learn-from-the-little-ice-age-cooling.

11 Koch A, Brierley C, Maslin MM, et al. Earth system impacts of the European arrival and Great Dying in the Americas after 1492. *Quaternary Science Reviews* 2019; 207: 13–36.

12 Clark MA, Domingo MGG, Colgan K, et al. Global food system emissions could preclude achieving the 1.5° and 2°C climate change targets. *Science* 2020; 370: 705–08.

13 Anastasioua K, Baker P, Hadjikakou M. A conceptual framework for understanding the environmental impacts of ultra-processed foods and implications for sustainable food systems. *Journal of Cleaner Production* 2022; 368: 133155.

14 Soil Association. Ultra-processed planet: the impact of ultra-processed diets on climate, nature and health (and what to do about it). 2021. Available from: https://www.soilassociation.org/media/23032/ultra-processed-planet-final.pdf.

15 National Food Strategy, 2021.

16 Fardet A, Rock E. Perspective: reductionist nutrition research has meaning only within the framework of holistic and ethical thinking. *Advances in Nutrition* 2018; 9: 655–70.

17 International Food Policy Research Institute. Women: The key to food security. 1995. Available from: https://www.ifpri.org/publication/women-key-food-security.

18 Wilson B. The irreplaceable. 2022. Available from: https://www.lrb.co.uk/the-paper/v44/n12/bee-wilson/the-irreplaceable.

19 Edwards RB, Naylor RL, Higgins MM, et al. Causes of Indonesia's forest fires. *World Development* 2020; 127: 104717.

20 Greenpeace International. The final countdown. 2018. Available from: https://www.greenpeace.org/international/publication/18455/the-final-countdown-forests-indonesia-palm-oil/.

21 Edwards et al, 2020.

22 Pearce F. UK animal feed helping to destroy Asian rainforest, study shows. 2011. Available from: https://www.theguardian.com/environment/2011/may/09/pet-food-asian-rainforest.

23 van der Goot AJ, Pelgrom PJM, Berghout JAM, et al. Concepts for further sustainable production of foods. *Journal of Food Engineering* 2016; 168: 42–51.

24 International Monetary Fund. Fossil fuel subsidies. 2019. Available from: https://www.imf.org/en/Topics/climate-change/energy-subsidies.

25 van der Goot et al, 2016.

26 National Food Strategy, 2021.

27 Rosane O. Humans and big ag livestock now account for 96 percent of mammal biomass. 2018. Available from: https://www.ecowatch.com/biomass-humans-animals-2571413930.html.

28 Bar-On YM, Phillips R, Milo R. The biomass distribution on Earth. *Proceedings of the National Academy of Sciences* 2018; 25: 6506–11.

29 Monteiro CA, Moubarac J-C, Bertazzi Levy R, et al. Household availability of ultra-processed foods and obesity in nineteen European countries. *Public Health Nutrition* 2018; 21: 18–26.

30 Lawrence, 2006.

31 Ritchie H, Roser M. Soy. 2021. Available from https://ourworldindata.org/soy.

32 National Food Strategy, 2021.

33 Lawrence, 2006.

34 Cliff C. Intensively farmed chicken: the effect on deforestation, environment and climate change. 2021. Available from: https://www.soilassociation.org/blogs/2021/august/4/intensively-farmed-chicken-and-its-affect-on-the-environment-and-climate-change/.

35 Worldwide Fund For Nature. Riskier business: the UK's overseas land footprint. 2020. Available from: https://www.wwf.org.uk/sites/default/files/2020–07/RiskierBusiness_July2020_V7_0.pdf.

36 Worldwide Fund for Nature. Appetite for Destruction. 2017._ Available from: https://www.wwf.org.uk/sites/default/files/2017–11/WWF_AppetiteForDestruction_Full_Report_Web_0.pdf.

37 Soil Association. Peak poultry – briefing for policy makers. 2022. Available from: https://www.soilassociation.org/media/22930/peak-poultry-briefing-for-policy-makers.pdf.

38 Worldwide Fund for Nature, 2017.

39 Soil Association, 2022.

40 Friends of the Earth Europe. Meat atlas: facts and figures about the animals we eat. Available from: https://friendsoftheearth.eu/wp-content/uploads/2014/01/foee_hbf_meatatlas_jan2014.pdf.

41 Leite-Filho AT, Costa MH, Fu R. The southern Amazon rainy season: the role of deforestation and its interactions with large-scale mechanisms. *International Journal of Climatology* 2020; 40: 2328–41.

42 Butt N, de Oliveira PA, Costa MH. Evidence that deforestation affects the onset of the rainy season in Rondonia, Brazil. *Journal of Geophysical Research* 2011; 116: D11120.

43 Gustavo Faleiros MA. Agro-suicide: Amazon deforestation hits Brazil's soy producers. 2020. Available from: https://dialogochino.net/en/agriculture/37887-agri-suicide-amazon-deforestation-hits-rain-brazils-soy-producers/.

44 Gatti LV, Basso LS, Miller JB, et al. Amazonia as a carbon source linked to deforestation and climate change. *Nature* 2021; 595: 388–93.

45 Carrington D. Amazon rainforest now emitting more CO2 than it absorbs. 2021. Available from: https://amp.theguardian.com/environment/2021/jul/14/amazon-rainforest-now-emitting-more-co2-than-it-absorbs.

46 Tilman D, Clark M. Global diets link environmental sustainability and human health. *Nature* 2014; 515: 518–22.

47 Soil Association, 2021.

48 International Assessment of Agricultural Knowledge, Science, Technology for Development. Agriculture at a crossroads – global report. 2009. Available from: https://wedocs.unep.org/handle/20.500.11822/8590.

49 Poux X, Aubert P-M. An agroecological Europe in 2050: multifunctional agriculture for healthy eating. Findings from the Ten Years

For Agroecology (TYFA) modelling exercise. 2018. Available from: https://www.soilassociation.org/media/18074/iddri-study-tyfa.pdf.

50 Aubert P-M, Schwoob M-H, Poux X. Agroecology and carbon neutrality: what are the issues? 2019. Available from: https://www.soilassociation.org/media/18564/iddri-agroecology-and-carbon-neutrality-what-are-the-issues.pdf.

51 Poux X, Schiavo M, Aubert P-M . Modelling an agroecological UK in 2050 – findings from TYFAREGIO. 2021. Available from: https://www.iddri.org/sites/default/files/PDF/Publications/Catalogue%20Iddri/Etude/202111-ST1021-TYFA%20UK_0.pdf.

52 Röös E, Mayer A, Muller A, et al. Agroecological practices in combination with healthy diets can help meet EU food system policy targets. *Science of the Total Environment* 2022; 847: 157612.

53 Muller A, Schader C, El-Hage Scialabba N, et al. Strategies for feeding the world more sustainably with organic agriculture. *Nature Communications* 2017; 8: 1290.

54 Fiolet et al, 2018.

55 Chen X, Zhang Z, Yang H, et al. Consumption of ultra-processed foods and health outcomes: a systematic review of epidemiological studies. *Nutrition Journal* 2020; 19: 86.

56 Dicken & Batterham, 2021.

57 Break Free From Plastic. Global brand audit report 2020. Available from: https://www.breakfreefromplastic.org/globalbrandauditreport2020/?utm_medium=email&utm_source=getresponse&utm_content=LIVE%3A+Plastic+Polluters+Brand+Audit+Report+%26+Invitation+to+Press+Briefing&utm_campaign=Breakfreefromplastic+Membership+Master+List.

58 Laville S. Report reveals 'massive plastic pollution footprint' of drinks firms. 2020. Available from: https://amp.theguardian.com/environment/2020/mar/31/report-reveals-massive-plastic-pollution-footprint-of-drinks-firms.

59 McVeigh K. Coca-Cola, Pepsi and Nestlé named top plastic polluters for third year in a row. 2020. Available from: https://amp.theguardian.com/environment/2020/dec/07/coca-cola-pepsi-and-nestle-named-top-plastic-polluters-for-third-year-in-a-row.

60 Laville S. Coca-Cola admits it produces 3m tonnes of plastic packaging a year. 2019. Available from: https://www.theguardian.com/business/2019/mar/14/coca-cola-admits-it-produces-3m-tonnes-of-plastic-packaging-a-year.

61 Geyer R, Jambeck JR, Law KL. Production, use, and fate of all plastics ever made. *Scientific Advances* 2017; 3: e1700782.

18. UPF is designed to be overconsumed

1 Yi J, Meemken E-M, Mazariegos-Anastassiou V, et al. Post-farmgate food value chains make up most of consumer food expenditures globally. *Nature Food* 2021; 2: 417–25.

2 Justia Patents. Patents by inventors Gary Norman Binley. 2022. Available from: https://patents.justia.com/inventor/gary-norman-binley.

3 Friedman M. A Friedman doctrine – the social responsibility of business is to increase its profits. 1970. Available from: https://www.nytimes.com/1970/09/13/archives/a-friedman-doctrine-the-social-responsibility-of-business-is-to.html.

4 Sorkin AR, Giang V, Gandel S, et al. The pushback on ESG investing. 2022. Available from: https://www.nytimes.com/2022/05/11/business/dealbook/esg-investing-pushback.html.

5 BlackRock. 2022 climate-related shareholder proposals more prescriptive than 2021. 2022. Available from: https://www.blackrock.com/corporate/literature/publication/commentary-bis-approach-shareholder-proposals.pdf.

6 MacAskill W. Does divestment work? 2015. Available from: https://www.newyorker.com/business/currency/does-divestment-work.

7 Nestlé. Nestlé enters weight management market – Jenny Craig acquisition enhances group's nutrition, health and wellness dimension. 2006. Available from: https://www.nestle.com/media/pressreleases/allpressreleases/weightmanagementmarketjennycraig-19jun06.

8 Jenny Craig. Jenny Craig Meals & Nutrition. 2022. Available from: https://www.jennycraig.com/nutrition-mission.

9 Reuters. Nestlé sells most of Jenny Craig to private equity firm. CNBC. 2013. Available from: https://www.cnbc.com/2013/11/07/nestle-sells-most-of-jenny-craig-to-private-equity-firm.html.

10 Nestlé. Acquisitions, partnerships & joint ventures. 2022. Available from: https://www.nestle.com/investors/overview/mergers-and-acqui sitions/nestle-health-science-acquisitions.

11 Kirchfeld A, David R, Nair D. Nestle eyed biggest-ever deal in aborted move for GSK unit. 2022. Available from: https://www.bloomberg.com/news/articles/2022–05-25/nestle-eyed-biggest-ever-deal-in-aborted-move-for-gsk-consumer.

12 Danone. Danone's subsidiaries and equity holdings as of December 31, 2020. Available from: https://www.danone.com/content/dam/danone-corp/danone-com/investors/danone-at-a-glance/List%20of%20subsidiairies%202020.pdf.

13 Ralph A. Philip Morris buys respiratory drugs company Vectura for £1bn. 2022. Available from: https://www.thetimes.co.uk/article/philip-morris-buys-respiratory-drugs-company-vectura-for-1bn-9mfts7jxq.

19. *What we could ask governments to do*

1 War on Want. The baby killer. 1974. Available from: http://archive.babymilkaction.org/pdfs/babykiller.pdf.

2 Quigley MA, Carson C. Breastfeeding in the 21st century. *Lancet* 2016; 387: 2087–88.

3 Stoltz T, Jones A, Rogers L, et al. 51 donor milk in the NICU: a community pediatrics perspective. *Paediatrics & Child Health* 2021; 26: e36–e36.

4 Lucas A, Cole TJ. Breast milk and neonatal necrotising enterocolitis. *Lancet* 1990; 336: 1519–23.

5 Johns Hopkins Medical Institutions. Formula-fed preemies at higher risk for dangerous GI condition than babies who get donor milk. 2011. Available from: https://www.sciencedaily.com/releases/2011/04/110430171122.htm.

6 Jelliffe DB. Commerciogenic malnutrition? *Nutrition Reviews* 1972; 30: 199–205.

7 Jelliffe, 1972.

8 War on Want, 1979.

9 Jelliffe, 1972.

10 *New Internationalist*. Action now on baby foods. 1973. Available from: https://newint.org/features/1973/08/01/baby-food-action-editorial.

11 Fitzpatrick I. Nestléd in controversy. *New Internationalist*. 2010. Available from: https://newint.org/columns/applause/2010/10/01/nestle-baby-milk-campaign.

12 UNICEF. Research on marketing and the code. 2022. Available from: https://www.unicef.org.uk/babyfriendly/news-and-research/baby-friendly-research/research-on-marketing-and-the-code/.

13 Save the Children. Don't push it: why the formula industry must clean up its act. 2018. Available from: https://resourcecentre.savethechildren.net/pdf/dont-push-it.pdf/.

14 Quigley & Carson, 2016.

15 Lamberti LM, Zakarija-Grković I, Fischer Walker CL, et al. Breast-feeding for reducing the risk of pneumonia morbidity and mortality in children under two: a systematic literature review and meta-analysis. *BMC Public Health* 2013; 13: S18.

16 Global Breastfeeding Collective. Nurturing the health and wealth of nations: the investment case for breastfeeding. Available from: https://www.globalbreastfeedingcollective.org/media/426/file/The%20invest ment%20case%20for%20breastfeeding.pdf.

17 Quigley & Carson, 2016.

18 Baker P, Smith J, Salmon L, et al. Global trends and patterns of commercial milk-based formula sales: is an unprecedented infant and young child feeding transition underway? *Public Health Nutrition* 2016; 19: 2540–50.

19 Forsyth BW, McCarthy PL, Leventhal JM. Problems of early infancy, formula changes, and mothers' beliefs about their infants. *Journal of Pediatrics* 1985; 106: 1012–17.

20 Polack FP, Khan N, Maisels MJ. Changing partners: the dance of infant formula changes. *Clinical Pediatrics* 1999; 38: 703–08.

21 Lakshman R, Ogilvie D, Ong KK. Mothers' experiences of bottle-feeding: a systematic review of qualitative and quantitative studies. *Archives of Disease in Childhood* 2009; 94: 596–601.

22 Lakshman R. Establishing a healthy growth trajectory from birth: the Baby Milk trial. Available from: https://heeoe.hee.nhs.uk/sites/default/files/docustore/baby_milk_trial_results18april17.pdf.

23 UK Food Standards Agency. Statement on the role of hydrolysed cows' milk formulae in influencing the development of atopic outcomes and autoimmune disease. Available at: https://cot.food.gov.uk/sites/default/files/finalstatement-hydrolysedformula.pdf.

24 Japanese guidelines for food allergy 2017. *Allergology* Int. 2017 Apr; 66(2): 248–64.

25 The Australasian Society of Clinical Immunology and Allergy infant feeding for allergy prevention guidelines. *Medical Journal of Australia* 2019, Feb; 210(2):89–93 doi: 10.5694/mja2.12102.

26 The Effects of Early Nutritional Interventions on the Development of Atopic Disease in Infants and Children: The Role of Maternal Dietary Restriction, Breastfeeding, Hydrolyzed Formulas, and Timing of Introduction of Allergenic Complementary Foods. *Pediatrics* 2019; 143: e20190281.

27 van Tulleken C. Overdiagnosis and industry influence: how cow's milk protein allergy is extending the reach of infant formula manufacturers. *British Medical Journal* 2018; 363: k5056.

28 Brown A. *Why Breastfeeding Grief and Trauma Matter.* London: Pinter & Martin, 2019.

29 Sankar MJ, Sinha B, Chowdhury R, et al. Optimal breastfeeding practices and infant and child mortality: a systematic review and meta-analysis. *Acta Paediatrica* 2015; 104: 3–13.

30 Horta BL, Loret de Mola C, Victora CG. Long-term consequences of breastfeeding on cholesterol, obesity, systolic blood pressure and type 2 diabetes: a systematic review and meta-analysis. *Acta Paediatrica* 2015; 104: 30–37.

31 Bowatte G, Tham R, Allen KJ, et al. Breastfeeding and childhood acute otitis media: a systematic review and meta-analysis. *Acta Paediatrica* 2015; 104: 85–95.

32 Victora CG, Bahl R, Barros AJD, et al. Breastfeeding in the 21st century: epidemiology, mechanisms, and lifelong effect. *Lancet* 2017; 387: 475–90.

33 Lodge CJ, Tan DJ, Lau MXZ, et al. Breastfeeding and asthma and allergies: a systematic review and meta-analysis. *Acta Paediatrica* 2015; 104: 38–53.

34 Thompson JMD, Tanabe K, Moon RY, et al. Duration of breastfeeding and risk of SIDS: an individual participant data meta-analysis. *Pediatrics* 2017; 140: e20171324.

35 Horta BL, Loret de Mola C, Victora CG. Breastfeeding and intelligence: a systematic review and meta-analysis. *Acta Paediatrica* 2015; 104: 14–29.

36 Baker et al, 2016.

37 British Nutrition Foundation. What we do. 2022. Available from: https://www.nutrition.org.uk/our-work/what-we-do/.

38 British Nutrition Foundation. Current members. 2022. Available from: https://www.nutrition.org.uk/our-work/support-what-we-do/corporate-partnerships/current-members/.

39 Carriedo A, Pinsky I, Crosbie E, et al. The corporate capture of the nutrition profession in the USA: the case of the Academy of Nutrition and Dietetics. *Public Health Nutrition* 2022; 25: 3568–82.

40 O'Connor A. Group shaping nutrition policy earned millions from junk food makers. 2022. Available from: https://www.washingtonpost.com/wellness/2022/10/24/nutrition-academy-processed-food-company-donations/.

41 Diabetes UK. Our current partners. 2022. Available from: https://www.diabetes.org.uk/get_involved/corporate/acknowledgements/partners.

42 Cancer Research UK. About our corporate partnership programme. 2022. Available from: https://www.cancerresearchuk.org/get-involved/become-a-partner/about-our-corporate-partnership-programme.

43 British Heart Foundation. Our current partners. 2022. Available from: https://www.bhf.org.uk/how-you-can-help/corporate-partnerships/our-corporate-partners.

44 The Association of UK Dietitians. BDA corporate members. 2022. Available from: https://www.bda.uk.com/news-campaigns/work-with-us/commercial-work/bda-corporate-members.html.

45 Greenpeace International. Top consumer companies' palm oil sustainability claims go up in flames. 2019. Available from: https://www.greenpeace.org/international/press-release/25675/burn ingthehouse/.

46 Taillie LS, Reyes M, Colchero MA, et al. An evaluation of Chile's law of food labeling and advertising on sugar-sweetened beverage purchases from 2015 to 2017: a before-and-after study. *PLoS Medicine* 2020; 17: e1003015.

47 Jacobs A. In sweeping war on obesity, Chile slays Tony the Tiger. 2018. Available from: https://www.nytimes.com/2018/02/07/health/obesity-chile-sugar-regulations.html.

48 Reyes M, Garmendia ML, Olivares S, et al. Development of the Chilean front-of-package food warning label. *BMC Public Health* 2019; 19: 906.

Afterword

1. Is ultra-processed food bad for you? Not always, scientists say. *The Times* [Internet]. [cited 2023 Dec 11]; Available from: https://www.the-times.co.uk/article/is-ultra-processed-food-bad-for-you-not-always-scientists-say-jd05qflg5.

2. Bawden T. 10 ultra-processed foods that are actually good for you. [Internet]. 2023 [cited 2023 Dec 11]. Available from: https://inews.co.uk/news/ultra-processed-foods-good-for-you-2646725.

3. Knapton S. Ultra-processed food can still be good for you, it depends on what is in it. *The Daily Telegraph* [Internet]. 2023 Sep 27 [cited 2023 Dec 11]; Available from: https://www.telegraph.co.uk/news/2023/09/27/ultra-processed-food-can-be-good-for-you-say-experts/.

4. Ultra-processed food isn't always unhealthy, say UK food officials. New Scientist [Internet]. [cited 2023 Dec 11]; Available from: https://www.newscientist.com/article/2394414-ultra-processed-food-isnt-always-unhealthy-say-uk-food-officials/.

5. Quinn I. Carbohydrates-probe scientists hit back at Dispatches industry bias claims. *The Grocer* [Internet]. 2014 [cited 2023 Dec 11]. Available from: https://www.thegrocer.co.uk/topics/carbohydrates-probe-scientists-hit-back-at-dispatches/353891.article.

6. Sugar's web of influence [Internet]. [cited 2023 Dec 11]. Available from: https://www.bmj.com/content/350/bmj.h231/infographic.

7. Sugar advisers have their cake and eat it. *The Times* [Internet]. [Cited 2023 Dec 11]; Available from: https://www.thetimes.co.uk/article/sugar-advisers-have-their-cake-and-eat-it-9cwrr3gb2sf.

8. Coombes R. Row over ultra-processed foods panel highlights conflicts of interest issue at heart of UK science reporting. BMJ [Internet]. 2023 Nov 1; 383: 2514. Available from: https://www.bmj.com/content/383/bmj.p2514.

9. Expert reaction to observational study of ultra processed food and risk of depression. [Internet]. [Cited 2023 Nov 30]. Available from: https://www.sciencemediacentre.org/expert-reaction-to-observational-study-of-ultra-processed-food-and-risk-of-depression-as-published-in-jama-network-open/.

10. Expert reaction to SACN (Scientific Advisory Committee on Nutrition) statement on processed foods and health. [Internet]. [Cited 2024 Jan 4]. Available from: https://www.sciencemediacentre.org/expert-reaction-to-sacn-scientific-advisory-committee-on-nutrition-statement-on-processed-and-health/.

11. Expert reaction to IARC press release and article in the Lancet Planetary Health looking at food processing and cancer risk in Europe. [Internet]. [Cited 2024 Jan 4]. Available from: https://www.sciencemediacentre.org/expert-reaction-to-iarc-press-release-and-article-in-the-lancet-planetary-health-looking-at-food-processing-and-cancer-risk-in-europe/.

12. Expert reaction to study looking at association of consumption of ultra-processed food and cognitive decline. [Internet]. [Cited 2024 Jan 4]. Available from: https://www.sciencemediacentre.org/expert-reaction-to-study-looking-at-association-of-consumption-of-ultra-processed-food-and-cognitive-decline/.

13. Schillinger D, Tran J, Mangurian C, Kearns C. Do Sugar-Sweetened Beverages Cause Obesity and Diabetes? Industry and the Manufacture of Scientific Controversy. *Annals of Internal Medicine*. 2016 Dec 20; 165(12): 895–97.

14. Tobacco Industry Research Committee [Internet]. TobaccoTactics. 2020 [cited 2023 Nov 30]. Available from: https://tobaccotactics.org/article/tobacco-industry-research-committee/.

15. Chang K, Gunter MJ, Rauber F, Levy RB, Huybrechts I, Kliemann N, et al. Ultra-processed food consumption, cancer risk and cancer mortality: a large-scale prospective analysis within the UK Biobank. EClinicalMedicine. 2023 Feb; 56: 101840.

16. Expert reaction to study looking at ultra-processed foods and risk of different cancers [Internet]. [Cited 2023 Nov 27]. Available from: https://www.sciencemediacentre.org/expert-reaction-to-study-looking-at-ultra-processed-foods-and-risk-of-different-cancers/.

17. Cordova R, Viallon V, Fontvieille E, Peruchet-Noray L, Jansana A, Wagner K-H, et al. Consumption of ultra-processed foods and risk of multimorbidity of cancer and cardiometabolic diseases: a multinational cohort study. The Lancet Regional Health – Europe [Internet]. 2023 Dec 1; 35. Available from: https://doi.org/10.1016/j.lanepe.2023.100771.

18. Fiolet T, Srour B, Sellem L, Kesse-Guyot E, Allès B, Méjean C, et al. Consumption of ultra-processed foods and cancer risk: results from NutriNet-Santé prospective cohort. BMJ. 2018 Feb 14; 360: k322.

19. Dicken SJ, Batterham RL. The Role of Diet Quality in Mediating the Association between Ultra-Processed Food Intake, Obesity and Health-Related Outcomes: A Review of Prospective Cohort Studies. Nutrients [Internet]. 2021 Dec 22; 14(1). Available from: http://dx.doi.org/10.3390/nu14010023.

20. Sellem L, Srour B, Javaux G, Chazelas E, Chassaing B, Viennois E, et al. Food additive emulsifiers and risk of cardiovascular disease in the Nutri-Net-Santé cohort: prospective cohort study. BMJ. 2023 Sep 6; 382: e076058.

21. Song Z, Song R, Liu Y, Wu Z, Zhang X. Effects of ultra-processed foods on the microbiota-gut-brain axis: The bread-and-butter issue. Food Res Int. 2023 May; 167: 112730.

22. Rios JM, Berg MK, Gearhardt AN. Evaluating Bidirectional Predictive Pathways between Dietary Restraint and Food Addiction in Adolescents. Nutrients [Internet]. 2023 Jun 30; 15(13); Available from: http://dx.doi.org/10.3390/nu15132977.

23. Gearhardt AN, Bueno NB, DiFeliceantonio AG, Roberto CA, Jiménez-Murcia S, Fernandez-Aranda F. Social, clinical, and policy implications of ultra-processed food addiction. BMJ. 2023 Oct 9; 383: e075354.

24. Ayton A, Ibrahim A, Dugan J, Galvin E, Wright OW. Ultra-processed foods and binge eating: A retrospective observational study. Nutrition. 2021 Apr; 84: 111023.

25. Martinez Steele E, Marrón Ponce JA, Cediel G, Louzada MLC, Khandpur N, Machado P, et al. Potential reductions in ultra-processed food consumption substantially improve population cardiometabolic-related dietary nutrient profiles in eight countries. Nutrition Metabolism Cardiovascular Diseases. 2022 Dec; 32(12): 2739–50.

26. Samuthpongtorn C, Nguyen LH, Okereke OI, Wang DD, Song M, Chan AT, et al. Consumption of Ultraprocessed Food and Risk of Depression. JAMA Network Open. 2023 Sep 5; 6(9): e2334770.

27. UNICEF. Engaging with the food and beverage industry: UNICEF programme guidance. 2023. Available from: https://www.unicef.org/media/142056/file/Programme%20Guidance%20on%20Engagement%20with%20the%20Food%20and%20Beverage%20Industry.pdf.

28. Counting the cost of UK poverty [Internet]. Joseph Rowntree Foundation. [Cited 2024 Jan 4]; Available from: https://www.jrf.org.uk/counting-the-cost-of-uk-poverty.

29. Ayton A, Ibrahim A. The Western diet: a blind spot of eating disorder research?-a narrative review and recommendations for treatment and research. *Nutrition Reviews.* 2020 Jul 1; 78(7): 579–96.

30. Expert reaction to study looking at consumption of ultra-processed foods and risk of multimorbidity of cancer and cardiometabolic diseases [Internet]. [Cited 2023 Nov 30]; Available from: https://www.sciencemediacentre.org/expert-reaction-to-study-looking-at-consumption-of-ultra-processed-foods-and-risk-of-multimorbidity-of-cancer-and-cardiometabolic-diseases/.

31. Zheng L, Sun J, Yu X, Zhang D. Ultra-Processed Food Is Positively Associated With Depressive Symptoms Among United States Adults. *Frontiers in Nutrition.* 2020 Dec 15; 7: 600449.

32. Adjibade M, Julia C, Allès B, Touvier M, Lemogne C, Srour B, et al. Prospective association between ultra-processed food consumption and incident depressive symptoms in the French NutriNet-Santé cohort. BMC Medicine. 2019 Apr 15; 17(1): 78.

33. Gómez-Donoso C, Sánchez-Villegas A, Martínez-González MA, Gea A, Mendonça R de D, Lahortiga-Ramos F, et al. Ultra-processed food consumption and the incidence of depression in a Mediterranean cohort: the SUN Project. *European Journal of Nutrition*. 2020 Apr; 59(3): 1093–103.

Index

Index

Index